PET Imaging

Editors

JONATHAN MCCONATHY
SAMUEL J. GALGANO

RADIOLOGIC CLINICS
OF NORTH AMERICA

www.radiologic.theclinics.com

Consulting Editor
FRANK H. MILLER

September 2021 • Volume 59 • Number 5

ELSEVIER

1600 John F. Kennedy Boulevard • Suite 1800 • Philadelphia, Pennsylvania, 19103-2899

http://www.theclinics.com

RADIOLOGIC CLINICS OF NORTH AMERICA Volume 59, Number 5
September 2021 ISSN 0033-8389, ISBN 13: 978-0-323-81070-8

Editor: John Vassallo (j.vassallo@elsevier.com)
Developmental Editor: Karen Solomon

Radiologic Clinics of North America (ISSN 0033-8389) is published bimonthly by Elsevier Inc., 360 Park Avenue South, New York, NY 10010-1710. Months of issue are January, March, May, July, September, and November. Periodicals postage paid at New York, NY and additional mailing offices. Subscription prices are USD 518 per year for US individuals, USD 1309 per year for US institutions, USD 100 per year for US students and residents, USD 611 per year for Canadian individuals, USD 1368 per year for Canadian institutions, USD 703 per year for international individuals, USD 1368 per year for international institutions, USD 100 per year for Canadian students/residents, and USD 315 per year for international students/residents. To receive student and resident rate, orders must be accompanied by name of affiliated institution, date of term and the signature of program/residency coordinatior on institution letterhead. Orders will be billed at individual rate until proof of status is received. Foreign air speed delivery is included in all *Clinics* subscription prices. All prices are subject to change without notice. **POSTMASTER:** Send address changes to *Radiologic Clinics of North America*, Elsevier Health Sciences Division, Subscription Customer Service, 3251 Riverport Lane, Maryland Heights, MO63043. **Customer Service: Telephone: 1-800-654-2452** (U.S. and Canada); **1-314-447-8871** (outside U.S. and Canada). **Fax: 1-314-447-8029.** E-mail: **journalscustomerservice-usa@elsevier.com (for print support); journalsonlinesupport-usa@elsevier.com (for online support)**.

Reprints. For copies of 100 or more of articles in this publication, please contact the Commercial Reprints Department, Elsevier Inc., 360 Park Avenue South, New York, New York 10010-1710. Tel.: +1-212-633-3874; Fax: +1-212-633-3820; E-mail: reprints@elsevier.com.

Radiologic Clinics of North America also published in Greek Paschalidis Medical Publications, Athens, Greece.

Radiologic Clinics of North America is covered in *MEDLINE/PubMed (Index Medicus), EMBASE/Excerpta Medica, Current Contents/Life Sciences, Current Contents/Clinical Medicine, RSNA Index to Imaging Literature, BIOSIS, Science Citation Index,* and *ISI/BIOMED*.

Printed in the United States of America.

Contributors

CONSULTING EDITOR

FRANK H. MILLER, MD, FACR
Lee F. Rogers MD Professor of Medical
Education, Chief, Body Imaging Section and
Fellowship Program, Medical Director, MRI,
Department of Radiology, Northwestern
Memorial Hospital, Northwestern University,
Feinberg School of Medicine, Chicago, Illinois,
USA

EDITORS

JONATHAN MCCONATHY, MD, PhD
Associate Professor, Department of Radiology,
Director, Division of Molecular Imaging and
Therapeutics, University of Alabama at
Birmingham, Birmingham, Alabama, USA

SAMUEL J. GALGANO, MD
Assistant Professor, Department of Radiology,
Director, Section of Abdominal Imaging,
O'Neal Comprehensive Cancer Center,
University of Alabama at Birmingham,
Birmingham, Alabama, USA

AUTHORS

EFSTATHIA ANDRIKOPOULOU, MD
Assistant Professor of Medicine and
Radiology, University of Alabama at
Birmingham, Birmingham, Alabama, USA

GREG AVEY, MD
Department of Radiology, University of
Wisconsin School of Medicine and Public
Health, Madison, Wisconsin, USA

NAVKARANBIR BAJAJ, MD
Asheville Cardiology Associates, Asheville,
North Carolina, USA

PRADEEP BHAMBHVANI, MD
Professor of Radiology, University of Alabama
at Birmingham, Birmingham, Alabama, USA

STEVE Y. CHO, MD
Professor, Nuclear Medicine and Molecular
Imaging Section, Department of Radiology,
University of Wisconsin School of Medicine
and Public Health, University of Wisconsin

Carbone Cancer Center, Madison, Wisconsin,
USA

CARLO CONTRERAS, MD
Assistant Professor, Division of Surgical
Oncology, Department of Surgery, The Ohio
State University Wexner Medical Center,
Columbus, Ohio, USA

FARROKH DEHDASHTI, MD
Division of Nuclear Medicine, Edward
Mallinckrodt Institute of Radiology, Alvin J.
Siteman Cancer Center, Washington University
School of Medicine, St Louis, Missouri, USA

MICHAEL D. FARWELL, MD
Department of Radiology, University of
Pennsylvania, Philadelphia, Pennsylvania, USA

AMY M. FOWLER, MD, PhD
Assistant Professor, Breast Imaging and
Intervention Section, Department of Radiology,
University of Wisconsin School of Medicine
and Public Health, Department of Medical

Physics, University of Wisconsin School of Medicine and Public Health, University of Wisconsin Carbone Cancer Center, Madison, Wisconsin, USA

SAUL N. FRIEDMAN, MD, PhD
Division of Nuclear Medicine, Edward Mallinckrodt Institute of Radiology, Washington University School of Medicine, St Louis, Missouri, USA

SAMUEL J. GALGANO, MD
Assistant Professor, Department of Radiology, Director, Section of Abdominal Imaging, O'Neal Comprehensive Cancer Center, University of Alabama at Birmingham, Birmingham, Alabama, USA

VICTOR H. GERBAUDO, PhD, MSHCA
Department of Radiology, Brigham and Women's Hospital and Harvard Medical School, Boston, Massachusetts, USA

GRAYSON R. GIMBLET, BS
MD-PhD Student, School of Medicine, University of Alabama at Birmingham, Birmingham, Alabama, USA

OLFAT KAMEL HASAN, MBChB, FRCR, FRCPC
Departments of Medicine and Radiology, McMaster University, Hamilton, Ontario, Canada

BRANDON A. HOWARD, MD, PhD
Assistant Professor, Department of Radiology, Division of Nuclear Medicine and Radiotheranostics, Duke University Medical Center, Durham, North Carolina, USA

NICOLA M. HUGHES, MBBChBAO, MRCSI, FFRRCSI
Fellow in Cancer Imaging Program, Department of Imaging and Radiology, Dana-Farber Cancer Institute, Brigham and Women's Hospital, Harvard Medical School, Boston, Massachusetts, USA

ANDREI IAGARU, MD
Professor, Department of Radiology, Stanford University, Stanford, California, USA

MALAK ITANI, MD
Section of Abdominal Imaging, Edward Mallinckrodt Institute of Radiology, Washington University School of Medicine, St Louis, Missouri, USA

OSIGBEMHE IYALOMHE, MD, PhD
Department of Radiology, University of Pennsylvania, Philadelphia, Pennsylvania, USA

HEATHER A. JACENE, MD
Associate Professor of Radiology, Department of Imaging and Radiology, Dana-Farber Cancer Institute, Brigham and Women's Hospital, Harvard Medical School, Boston, Massachusetts, USA

MICHAEL V. KNOPP, MD, PhD
Professor, Novartis Chair of Imaging Research, and Director of the Wright Center of Innovation in Biomedical Imaging, Department of Radiology, The Ohio State University Wexner Medical Center, Columbus, Ohio, USA

SUZANNE E. LAPI, PhD
Professor, Department of Radiology, Department of Chemistry, University of Alabama at Birmingham, Birmingham, Alabama, USA

JASON S. LEWIS, PhD
Professor, Department of Radiology, Memorial Sloan Kettering Cancer Center, Molecular Pharmacology Program, Memorial Sloan Kettering Cancer Center, Weill Cornell Medical College, New York, New York, USA

MATTHEW LUBANOVIC, MD, FRCPC
Department of Radiology, McMaster University, Hamilton, Ontario, Canada

PADMA PRIYA MANAPRAGADA, MD
Assistant Professor of Radiology, University of Alabama at Birmingham, Birmingham, Alabama, USA

CHARLES MARCUS, MD
Department of Nuclear Medicine and Molecular Imaging, Emory University Hospital, Atlanta, Georgia, USA

CHRISTIAN MASON, PhD
Postdoctoral Scholar, Department of Radiology, Memorial Sloan Kettering Cancer Center, New York, New York, USA

JONATHAN McCONATHY, MD, PhD
Associate Professor, Department of Radiology, Director, Division of Molecular Imaging and

Therapeutics, University of Alabama at Birmingham, Birmingham, Alabama, USA

ERIC D. MILLER, MD, PhD
Assistant Professor, Department of Radiation Oncology, James Cancer Center, The Ohio State University Wexner Medical Center, Columbus, Ohio, USA

FARSHAD MORADI, MD, PhD
Clinical Assistant Professor, Department of Radiology, Stanford University, Stanford, California, USA

J. BART ROSE, MD
Assistant Professor, O'Neal Comprehensive Cancer Center, Division of Surgical Oncology, Department of Surgery, University of Alabama at Birmingham, Birmingham, Alabama, USA

STEVEN P. ROWE, MD, PhD
Associate Professor, Division of Nuclear Medicine and Molecular Imaging, The Russell H. Morgan Department of Radiology and Radiological Science, Johns Hopkins University School of Medicine, Baltimore, Maryland, USA

BITAL SAVIR-BARUCH, MD
Associate Professor, Division of Nuclear Medicine, Department of Radiology, Loyola University Medical Center, Maywood, Illinois, USA

DAVID M. SCHUSTER, MD, FACR
Professor, Division of Nuclear Medicine and Molecular Imaging, Department of Radiology and Imaging Sciences, Emory University, Atlanta, Georgia, USA

SARA SHEIKHBAHAEI, MD
Department of Radiology, Johns Hopkins Medical Institutions, Baltimore, Maryland, USA

VEERESH KUMAR N. SHIVAMURTHY, MD
Epilepsy Center, St. Francis Hospital and Medical Center, Trinity Health of New England, Hartford, Connecticut, USA

RATHAN M. SUBRAMANIAM, MBBS, BMedSc, MClinEd, MPH, PhD, MBA, FRANZCR, FACNM, FSNMMI, FAUR
Dean's Office, Otago Medical School, University of Otago, Dunedin, New Zealand

BENJAMIN WEI, MD
Associate Professor, O'Neal Comprehensive Cancer Center, Division of Cardiothoracic Surgery, Department of Surgery, University of Alabama at Birmingham, Birmingham, Alabama, USA

RUDOLF A. WERNER, MD
Deputy Head, Department of Nuclear Medicine, University Hospital Würzburg, Würzburg, Germany

TERENCE Z. WONG, MD, PhD
Professor of Radiology and Chief, Division of Nuclear Medicine and Radiotheranostics; Professor in Medicine, Division of Medical Oncology, Duke University Medical Center, Durham, North Carolina, USA

CHADWICK L. WRIGHT, MD, PhD
Assistant Professor, Department of Radiology, Wright Center of Innovation in Biomedical Imaging, The Ohio State University Wexner Medical Center, Columbus, Ohio, USA

KATHERINE A. ZUKOTYNSKI, MD, PhD, FRCPC
Departments of Medicine and Radiology, McMaster University, Hamilton, Ontario, Canada

Contents

Precision medicine integrates molecular pathobiology, genetic make-up, and clinical manifestations of disease in order to classify patients into subgroups for the purposes of predicting treatment response and suggesting outcome. By identifying those patients who are most likely to benefit from a given therapy, interventions can be tailored to avoid the expense and toxicity of futile treatment. Ultimately, the goal is to offer the right treatment, to the right patient, at the right time. Lung cancer is a heterogeneous disease both functionally and morphologically. Further, over time, clonal proliferations of cells may evolve, becoming resistant to specific therapies. PET is a sensitive imaging technique with an important role in the precision medicine algorithm of lung cancer patients. It provides anatomo-functional insight during diagnosis, staging, and restaging of the disease. It is a prognostic biomarker in lung cancer patients that characterizes tumoral heterogeneity, helps predict early response to therapy, and may direct the selection of appropriate treatment.

Hematologic malignancies are a broad category of cancers arising from the lymphoid and myeloid cell lines. The 2016 World Health Organization classification system incorporated molecular markers as part of the diagnostic criteria and includes more than 100 subtypes. This article focuses on the subtypes for which imaging with positron emission tomography/computed tomography (PET/CT) has become an integral component of the patient's evaluation, that is, lymphoma and multiple myeloma. Leukemia and histiocytic and dendritic cell neoplasms are also discussed as these indications for PET/CT are less common, but increasingly seen in clinic.

Imaging plays an integral role in the clinical care of patients with breast cancer. This review article focuses on the use of PET imaging for breast cancer, highlighting the clinical indications and limitations of 2-deoxy-2-[^{18}F]fluoro-d-glucose (FDG) PET/CT, the potential use of PET/MRI, and 16α-[^{18}F]fluoroestradiol (FES), a newly approved radiopharmaceutical for estrogen receptor imaging.

Gastrointestinal malignancies encompass a variety of primary tumor sites, each with different staging criteria and treatment approaches. In this review we discuss technical aspects of 18F-FDG-PET/CT scanning to optimize information from both the

PET and computed tomography components. Specific applications for 18F-FDG-PET/CT are summarized for initial staging and follow-up of the major disease sites, including esophagus, stomach, hepatobiliary system, pancreas, colon, rectum, and anus.

Precision Nuclear Medicine: The Evolving Role of PET in Melanoma

Chadwick L. Wright, Eric D. Miller, Carlo Contreras, and Michael V. Knopp

The clinical management of melanoma patients has been rapidly evolving with the introduction of new targeted immuno-oncology (IO) therapeutics. The current diagnostic paradigms for melanoma patients begins with the histopathologic confirmation of melanoma, initial staging of disease burden with imaging and surgical approaches, treatment monitoring during systemic cytotoxic chemotherapy or IO therapeutics, restaging after completion of adjuvant systemic, surgical, and/or external radiation therapy, and the detection of recurrent malignancy/metastatic disease following therapy. New and evolving imaging approaches with positron-emission tomography (PET) imaging technologies, imaging methodologies, image reconstruction, and image analytics will likely continue to improve tumor detection, tumor characterization, and diagnostic confidence, enabling novel precision nuclear medicine practices for managing melanoma patients. This review will examine current concepts and challenges with existing PET imaging diagnostics for melanoma patients and introduce exciting new opportunities for PET in the current era of IO therapeutics.

PET Imaging for Head and Neck Cancers

Charles Marcus, Sara Sheikhbahaei, Veeresh Kumar N. Shivamurthy, Greg Avey, and Rathan M. Subramaniam

Head and neck cancers are commonly encountered cancers in clinical practice in the United States. Fluorine-18-fluorodeoxyglucose (^{18}F-FDG) PET/CT has been clinically applied in staging, occult primary tumor detection, treatment planning, response assessment, follow-up, recurrent disease detection, and prognosis prediction in these patients. Alternative PET tracers remain investigational and can provide additional valuable information such as radioresistant tumor hypoxia. The recent introduction of ^{18}F-FDG PET/MR imaging has provided the advantage of combining the superior soft tissue resolution of MR imaging with the functional information provided by ^{18}F-FDG PET. This article is a concise review of recent advances in PET imaging in head and neck cancer.

PET Imaging of Neuroendocrine Tumors

Samuel J. Galgano, Benjamin Wei, and J. Bart Rose

Neuroendocrine tumors (NETs) consist of a wide array of lesions arising from multiple organs throughout the body. Once diagnosed, accurate staging and tumor grading is needed to determine the optimal treatment algorithm for these patients, as they can range from slow-growing and indolent to highly aggressive. Molecular imaging has played a large role in the noninvasive diagnosis of NETs through the use of [111In]pentetreotide scintigraphy and now SSTR-PET radiotracers, which have become essential given the approval of [177Lu]DOTATATE therapy. The focus of this article is current and future applications of PET in several of the most common NETs, current PET radiotracers available for NET imaging, and pathologic considerations in molecular imaging of NETs.

The role of PET imaging with ^{11}C-choline and ^{18}F-fluciclovine in evaluating patients with prostate cancer (PCa) has become more important over the years and has been incorporated into the NCCN guidelines. A new generation of PET radiotracers targeting the prostate-specific membrane antigen (PSMA) is widely used outside the United States to evaluate patients with primary PCa and PCa recurrence. PET imaging influences treatment planning and demonstrates a significantly higher disease detection rate than conventional imaging such as computed tomography and MR imaging. Early data indicate that using PET radiotracers such as ^{18}F-fluciclovine and PSMA improves patient outcomes. 68-Ga-PSMA-11 and 18F-DCFPyL-PET/CT were recently approved by the US Food & Drug Administration (FDA) for clinical use. Other PSMA radiotracers, including fluorinated variants, will likely gain FDA approval in the not-too-distant future.

This review article summarizes the clinical applications of established and emerging PET tracers in the evaluation of the 5 most common gynecologic malignancies: endometrial, ovarian, cervical, vaginal, and vulvar cancers. Emphasis is given to 2-deoxy-2-[^{18}F]fluoro-d-glucose as the most widely used and studied tracer, with additional clinical tracers also explored. The common imaging protocols are discussed, including standard dose ranges and uptake times, established roles, as well as the challenges and future directions of these imaging techniques. The key points are emphasized with images from selected cases.

Cardiovascular disease is the leading cause of death worldwide. Given the increased availability of radiopharmaceuticals, improved positron emission tomography (PET) camera systems and proven higher diagnostic accuracy, PET is increasingly utilized in the management of various cardiovascular diseases. PET has high temporal and spatial resolution, when compared to Single Photon Emission Computed Tomography. In clinical practice, hybrid imaging with sequential PET and Computed Tomography acquisitions (PET/CT) or concurrent PET and Magnetic Resonance Imaging are standard. This article will review applications of cardiovascular PET/CT including myocardial perfusion, viability, cardiac sarcoidosis/inflammation, and infection.

PET/MR imaging is in routine clinical use and is at least as effective as PET/CT for oncologic and neurologic studies with advantages with certain PET radiopharmaceuticals and applications. In addition, whole body PET/MR imaging substantially reduces radiation dosages compared with PET/CT which is particularly relevant to pediatric and young adult population. For cancer imaging, assessment of hepatic, pelvic, and soft-tissue malignancies may benefit from PET/MR imaging. For neurologic imaging, volumetric brain MR imaging can detect regional volume loss relevant to cognitive impairment and epilepsy. In addition, the single-bed position acquisition enables dynamic brain PET imaging without extending the total study length which has the potential to enhance the diagnostic information from PET.

Immune PET Imaging

Osigbemhe Iyalomhe and Michael D. Farwell

18F-Fluorodeoxyglucose (FDG) PET/CT is sensitive to metabolic, immune-related, and structural changes that can occur in tumors in cancer immunotherapy. Unique mechanisms of immune checkpoint inhibitors (ICIs) occasionally make response evaluation challenging, because tumors and inflammatory changes are both FDG avid. These response patterns and sequelae of ICI immunotherapy, such as immune-related adverse events, are discussed. New immune-specific PET imaging probes in early clinical development are also reviewed, which may help guide the clinical management of cancer patients treated with immunotherapy and likely have applications outside of oncology for other diseases in which the immune system plays a role.

Novel Tracers and Radionuclides in PET Imaging

Christian Mason, Grayson R. Gimblet, Suzanne E. Lapi, and Jason S. Lewis

The use of PET imaging agents in oncology, cardiovascular disease, and neurodegenerative disease shows the power of this technique in evaluating the molecular and biological characteristics of numerous diseases. These agents provide crucial information for designing therapeutic strategies for individual patients. Novel PET tracers are in continual development and many have potential use in clinical and research settings. This article discusses the potential applications of tracers in diagnostics, the biological characteristics of diseases, the ability to provide prognostic indicators, and using this information to guide treatment strategies including monitoring treatment efficacy in real time to improve outcomes and survival.

PROGRAM OBJECTIVE

The objective of the *Radiologic Clinics of North America* is to keep practicing radiologists and radiology residents up to date with current clinical practice in radiology by providing timely articles reviewing the state of the art in patient care.

TARGET AUDIENCE

Practicing radiologists, radiology residents, and other healthcare professionals who provide patient care utilizing radiologic findings.

LEARNING OBJECTIVES

Upon completion of this activity, participants will be able to:
1. Describe common oncological indications for PET as well as the diagnostic benefits and limitations.
2. Discuss the current status of PET for clinical applications and perspectives on future developments.
3. Recognize newer technologies, such as PET/MRI, investigational PET agents, and immune system imaging, along with their clinical applications and future impact.

ACCREDITATION

The Elsevier Office of Continuing Medical Education (EOCME) is accredited by the Accreditation Council for Continuing Medical Education (ACCME) to provide continuing medical education for physicians.

The EOCME designates this journal-based CME activity for a maximum of 13 *AMA PRA Category 1 Credit*(s)™. Physicians should claim only the credit commensurate with the extent of their participation in the activity.

All other healthcare professionals requesting continuing education credit for this enduring material will be issued a certificate of participation.

DISCLOSURE OF CONFLICTS OF INTEREST

The EOCME assesses conflict of interest with its instructors, faculty, planners, and other individuals who are in a position to control the content of CME activities. All relevant conflicts of interest that are identified are thoroughly vetted by EOCME for fair balance, scientific objectivity, and patient care recommendations. EOCME is committed to providing its learners with CME activities that promote improvements or quality in healthcare and not a specific proprietary business or a commercial interest.

The planning committee, staff, authors, and editors listed below have identified no financial relationships or relationships to products or devices they or their spouse/life partner have with commercial interest related to the content of this CME activity:

Efstathia Andrikopoulou, MD; Greg Avey, MD; Navkaranbir Bajaj, MD; Pradeep Bhambhvani, MD; Regina Chavous-Gibson, MSN, RN; Steve Y. Cho, MD; Carlo Contreras, MD; Farrokh Dehdashti, MD; Michael D. Farwell, MD; Amy M. Fowler, MD, PhD; Saul N. Friedman, MD, PhD; Samuel J. Galgano, MD; Victor H. Gerbaudo, PhD, MSHCA; Grayson R. Gimblet, BS; Olfat Kamel Hasan, MBChB, FRCR, FRCPC; Brandon A. Howard, MD, PhD; Nicola M. Hughes, MBBChBAO, MRCSI, FFRRCSI; Malak Itani, MD; Osigbemhe Iyalomhe, MD, PhD; Michael V. Knopp, MD, PhD; Pradeep Kuttysankaran; Suzanne E. Lapi, PhD; Jason S. Lewis, PhD; Matthew Lubanovic, MD, FRCPC; Padma Priya Manapragada, MD; Charles Marcus, MD; Christian Mason, PhD; Eric D. Miller, MD, PhD; Farshad Moradi, MD, PhD; J. Bart Rose, MD; Sara Sheikhbahaei, MD; Veeresh Kumar N. Shivamurthy, MD; Rathan M. Subramaniam, MBBS, BMedSc, MClinEd, MPH, PhD, MBA, FRANZCR, FACNM, FSNMMI, FAUR; John Vassallo; Benjamin Wei, MD; Rudolf A. Werner, MD; Terence Z. Wong, MD, PhD; Chadwick L. Wright, MD, PhD; Katherine A. Zukotynski, MD, PhD, FRCPC.

The planning committee, staff, authors and editors listed below have identified financial relationships or relationships to products or devices they or their spouse/life partner have with commercial interest related to the content of this CME activity:

Andrei Iagaru, MD: Consultant/Advisor: GE Healthcare, ITM, Novartis AG, Progenics Pharmaceuticals, Inc.; Research Support: GE Healthcare, Novartis AG, Progenics Pharmaceuticals, Inc.

Heather A. Jacene, MD: Speakers Bureau: Janssen; Consultant/Advisor: Advanced Accelerator Applications

Jonathan McConathy, MD, PhD: Consultant/Advisor: Blue Earth Diagnostics, Lilly, GE Healthcare

Steven P. Rowe, MD, PhD: Consultant/Advisor: Progenics Pharmaceuticals, Inc., Precision Molecular, Inc., Plenary.ai, Inc.; Stock Ownership: Precision Molecular, Inc., Plenary.ai, Inc.; Research Support: Progenics Pharmaceuticals, Inc.; Co-founder: Precision Molecular, Inc., Plenary.ai, Inc.

Bital Savir-Baruch, MD: Consultant/Advisor and Speakers Bureau: Blue Earth Diagnostics

David M. Schuster, MD, FACR: Consultant/Advisor: AIM Specialty Health, Global Medical Solutions Taiwan, Ltd., Progenics Pharmaceuticals, Inc., Syncona

UNAPPROVED/OFF-LABEL USE DISCLOSURE

The EOCME requires CME faculty to disclose to the participants:

1. When products or procedures being discussed are off-label, unlabelled, experimental, and/or investigational (not US Food and Drug Administration [FDA] approved); and
2. Any limitations on the information presented, such as data that are preliminary or that represent ongoing research, interim analyses, and/or unsupported opinions. Faculty may discuss information about pharmaceutical agents that is outside of FDA-approved labelling. This information is intended solely for CME and is not intended to promote off-label use of these medications. If you have any questions, contact the medical affairs department of the manufacturer for the most recent prescribing information.

TO ENROLL

To enroll in the *Radiologic Clinics of North America* Continuing Medical Education program, call customer service at 1-800-654-2452 or sign up online at http://www.theclinics.com/home/cme. The CME program is available to subscribers for an additional annual fee of USD 356.00.

METHOD OF PARTICIPATION

In order to claim credit, participants must complete the following:
1. Complete enrolment as indicated above.
2. Read the activity.
3. Complete the CME Test and Evaluation. Participants must achieve a score of 70% on the test. All CME Tests and Evaluations must be completed online.

CME INQUIRIES/SPECIAL NEEDS

For all CME inquiries or special needs, please contact elsevierCME@elsevier.com.

RADIOLOGIC CLINICS OF NORTH AMERICA

Preface
Clinical Applications of PET

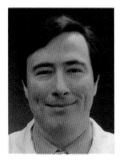   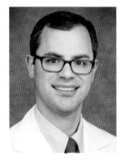

Jonathan McConathy, MD, PhD   Samuel J. Galgano, MD

Editors

The clinical roles of PET continue to grow with a number of exciting developments in recent years. In this issue of the *Radiologic Clinics of North America*, experts review the current status of PET for clinical applications and give their perspectives on future developments. Oncologic imaging with the glucose analogue [^{18}F]FDG remains the most frequent type of clinical PET study, but the number of Food and Drug Administration–approved PET tracers in the United States has grown substantially in the past decade, including ^{68}Ga- and ^{64}Cu-labeled somatostatin receptor ligands for neuroendocrine tumors, small molecule metabolic agents, and prostate-specific membrane antigen ligands for prostate cancer, [^{18}F]fluoroestradiol for estrogen receptor imaging in breast cancer, and amyloid and tau PET tracers for evaluation of cognitive impairment. Many of these recently approved PET agents are directly relevant to therapy, including targeted radionuclide therapies for neuroendocrine tumors and prostate cancer. Thus, PET is establishing a new paradigm in diagnostic imaging to characterize disease at the molecular level and directly inform selection of the most appropriate treatment.

Clinical PET imaging is expected to continue to increase as newer agents become established in clinical practice and investigational agents currently under development gain regulatory approval. The articles in this issue focus on relatively common clinical indications for PET and highlight the diagnostic benefits as well as limitations of PET for specific indications with a focus on oncology. We have also highlighted newer

technologies and applications, such as PET/MR imaging, investigational PET agents, and immune system imaging, which are expected to have increasing clinical impact in the near future. We could not cover every important topic in clinical PET, but we hope this issue will be a valuable resource for your current practice and will help you anticipate advances in the field.

We greatly appreciate the time and effort of all the authors who made this issue possible. We also thank Dr Frank Miller, the *Radiologic Clinics of North America* series editor, for the invitation and opportunity to lead this endeavor. We are also grateful to the Elsevier staff members, particularly Karen Solomon and John Vasallo, for their help, patience, and support throughout this process.

Jonathan McConathy, MD, PhD
University of Alabama at Birmingham
Molecular Imaging and Therapeutics
619 19th Street South, JT 773
Birmingham, AL 35249, USA

Samuel J. Galgano, MD
University of Alabama at Birmingham Radiology
Sections of Abdominal Imaging &
Molecular Imaging and Therapeutics
619 19th Street South, JT N325
Birmingham, AL 35249, USA

E-mail addresses:
jmcconathy@uabmc.edu (J. McConathy)
samuelgalgano@uabmc.edu (S.J. Galgano)

Radiol Clin N Am 59 (2021) xv
https://doi.org/10.1016/j.rcl.2021.06.002
0033-8389/21/© 2021 Published by Elsevier Inc.

Update on Molecular Imaging and Precision Medicine in Lung Cancer

Katherine A. Zukotynski, MD, PhD, FRCPC[a,b],
Olfat Kamel Hasan, MBChB, FRCR, FRCPC[a,b], Matthew Lubanovic, MD, FRCPC[b],
Victor H. Gerbaudo, PhD, MSHCA[c,*]

KEYWORDS

- Lung cancer • Positron emission tomography • Solitary pulmonary nodule • Cancer staging
- Targeted cancer therapy

KEY POINTS

- PET is helpful to stage patients with lung cancer.
- PET is a prognostic biomarker that is key in the initial treatment strategy of lung cancer patients by noninvasively assessing disease pathobiology so that appropriate therapy can be instituted.
- PET is helpful for the subsequent treatment strategy in lung cancer patients, including monitoring therapy response, detecting recurrence, and predicting outcomes.

LUNG CANCER AND PRECISION MEDICINE

Lung cancer is the second most commonly diagnosed malignancy in both men and women, accounting for approximately 235,760 new cases and 131,880 deaths in 2021 according to the American Cancer Society.[1] Although localized disease may be curable, metastatic lung cancer remains the leading cause of cancer-related death today, accounting for almost 25% of all cancer-related deaths and surpassing deaths from breast, prostate, and colorectal cancer combined.

Lung cancer is a spectrum of disease morphologically, both functionally and genetically.[2] Typically classified into two main subtypes, non-small cell lung cancer (NSCLC) accounts for approximately 85% of cases and includes adenocarcinoma and squamous cell carcinoma (among others), while small cell lung cancer (SCLC) accounts for approximately 15% of cases and is thought to be of neuroendocrine origin. While smoking tobacco is a risk factor for all lung cancer types, adenocarcinoma is more common in patients who have never smoked. Therapy may include surgery, radiation, chemotherapy, and immunotherapy, as well as an array of targeted drug therapies such as epidermal growth factor receptor (EGFR) inhibitors (eg, Erlotinib) and drugs targeting genetic mutations (eg, ALK, ROS1), among others. Localized NSCLC is often managed by surgery and adjuvant therapy; SCLC is rarely localized and tends to be treated nonsurgically.

Coupling the genetic underpinnings of malignancy with the use of molecular imaging to assess disease extent, its biologic behavior and metabolic response to therapy, contributes essential information to the personalized management of the lung cancer patient.[2,3] More specifically, it aids in the a priori identification of appropriate treatment for a specific patient at a given point in time, in order to maximize benefit while limiting toxicity. Positron emission tomography (PET) plays an important role in lung cancer patients both for initial staging and for planning the subsequent

[a] Department of Medicine, McMaster University, 1200 Main Street West, Hamilton, Ontario L9G 4X5, Canada;
[b] Department of Radiology, McMaster University, 1200 Main Street West, Hamilton, Ontario L9G 4X5, Canada;
[c] Department of Radiology, Brigham and Women's Hospital and Harvard Medical School, 75 Francis Street, Boston, MA 02492, USA
* Corresponding author.
E-mail address: gerbaudo@bwh.harvard.edu

Radiol Clin N Am 59 (2021) 693–703
https://doi.org/10.1016/j.rcl.2021.05.002

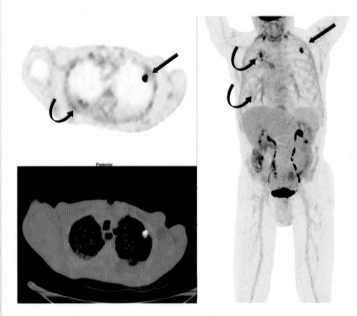

Fig. 1. Axial PET (*top*) and fused (*bottom*) images of the chest and a maximum intensity projection (MIP) image of the body (*right*) from an FDG-PET/CT, showing an intensely FDG-avid left upper lobe nodule biopsy-proven squamous cell carcinoma (*arrow*) and mildly FDG-avid inflammatory change in the right upper lobe (*curved arrows*).

treatment strategy (**Figs. 1–3**). PET contributes to precision medicine by characterizing tumor heterogeneity, by directing appropriate therapy at a metabolic-molecular level, and by providing predictive and prognostic insight into the therapy response. Further, PET can identify disease sites that are becoming resistant to treatment such that changes can be made at an earlier time point. The primary strength of PET has remained unchanged over the years, namely its ability to noninvasively evaluate in vivo tumor extent and heterogeneity over both time and space. Current scanners incorporate PET with computed tomography (CT) or magnetic resonance imaging (MRI). While PET/CT is more widely available than PET/MR, our experience with PET/MR will likely grow in the coming years. Further, technological advances are increasing our ability to image faster, with improved resolution and reduced patient radiation dose exposure. Ultimately, careful review of

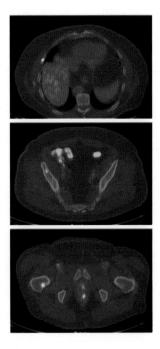

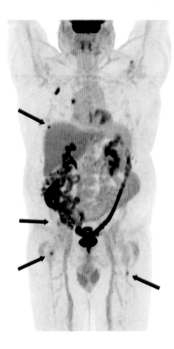

Fig. 2. Axial fused images of the ribs (*top*), pelvis (*middle*), and femurs (*bottom*), as well as an MIP image of the body (*right*) from an FDG-PET/CT, showing intensely FDG-avid sites of osseous metastatic disease in a right rib, the right iliac bone, and both femurs (*arrows*) in a patient with intensely FDG-avid right upper lobe non-small cell lung cancer and right hilar disease spread.

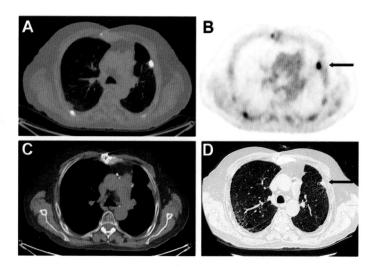

Fig. 3. Axial images of the chest from an FDG-PET/CT (*A*, *B*) and a diagnostic CT (*C*, *D*) showing intensely FDG-avid recurrent left upper lobe adenocarcinoma in the setting of anatomically stable postsurgical change.

all images and attention to artifacts (ie, respiratory motion or metal artifact) remains key. In our experience, nonattenuation corrected images are particularly helpful to detect small pulmonary nodules. Also, respiratory gating may be helpful to decrease artifacts,[4] although this is rarely done in routine clinical practice. Regardless of whether a PET/CT or PET/MR scanner is used, PET is important in evaluating lung cancer patients, with a significant impact on precision management including therapy intent (ie, cure vs palliation) and treatment selection (ie, surgery vs radiation).

There is ongoing investigation into radiopharmaceuticals that may be helpful for imaging lung cancer patients with PET. Neoplastic cells tend to have higher glucose metabolism than normal tissue and 2-deoxy-2-[^{18}F]fluoro-D-glucose (FDG), a radioactive glucose analogue, is preferentially taken up by neoplastic cells throughout the body and can be imaged with PET.[5,6] Also, changes in glucose metabolism may precede anatomic changes and both FDG-PET/CT and FDG-PET/MR are helpful to assess early therapy responses. Since the intensity of FDG uptake depends on factors such as cell density, aggressiveness, and technical parameters, among other things, using standardized parameters is important. Further, FDG uptake may be seen in lung cancer patients related to nonmalignant causes and evaluating imaging in the clinical context is critical (Figs. 4–6). There are several PET radiopharmaceuticals that may be helpful in imaging patient with lung cancer. For example, these include [^{18}F]fluoroazomycin arabinofuranoside (FAZA) and [^{18}F]fluoromisonidazole (1-(2-nitroimidazolyl)-2-hydroxy-3-fluoropropane) (FMISO) for hypoxia imaging, and more recently the quinoline-based ligands targeting cancer-associated fibroblasts (fibroblast-activating protein inhibitors or FAPI), among

others.[7,8] However, to date, FDG remains the only PET radiopharmaceutical used in routine clinical practice.

THE SOLITARY PULMONARY NODULE AND LUNG CANCER STAGING

FDG-PET/CT has proven to be helpful to: (1) characterize an indeterminate solitary solid pulmonary nodule that is greater than 8 mm on anatomic imaging; (2) guide biopsy to the site of most aggressive disease; and (3) evaluate disease extent including the primary disease, lymph node spread, and distant metastases. FDG-PET/CT should be interpreted in the clinical context since certain lung cancer subtypes such as carcinoid and rarely well-differentiated adenocarcinoma may have low metabolic activity, while benign processes such as infection or inflammation can be intensely FDG-avid. Further, intense FDG avidity can be associated with interventions such as talc pleurodesis and radiation, among others. In certain settings, such as talc pleurodesis, correlation with CT findings can be particularly helpful. In other cases, delaying imaging after an intervention may be key. For example, the general recommendation is to delay patient imaging for 3 to 4 months after radiation treatment to minimize false-positive FDG uptake due to inflammation, although there is some latitude on this. To wit, Hicks and colleagues showed inflammation after radical radiotherapy did not interfere with response assessment on PET if acquired at a median of 70 days after therapy completion.[9]

A *solitary pulmonary nodule* (SPN) is defined as less than 3 cm in size, may be solid or subsolid, and is often detected incidentally as a part of routine anatomic imaging.[10] Subsolid pulmonary

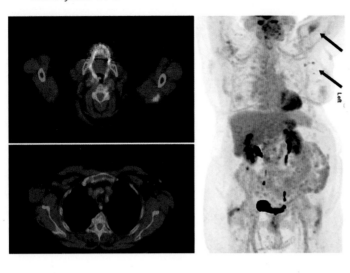

Fig. 4. Selected fused axial images focusing on the left deltoid muscle (*top*) and left axilla (*bottom*) and an MIP image of the body (*right*) from an FDG-PET/CT, showing uptake in the left deltoid muscle (*top arrow*) and in axillary lymph nodes (*bottom arrow*) associated with an influenza vaccination in a patient with biopsy-proven adenocarcinoma.

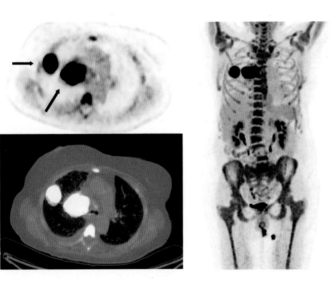

Fig. 5. Axial PET (*top*) and fused (*bottom*) images of the chest as well as an MIP image of the body from an FDG-PET/CT showing intensely FDG-avid biopsy-proven, poorly differentiated non-small cell lung cancer with spread to the right hilum (*arrows*) and diffuse uptake throughout the bone marrow related to anemia, possibly in conjunction with a paraneoplastic syndrome.

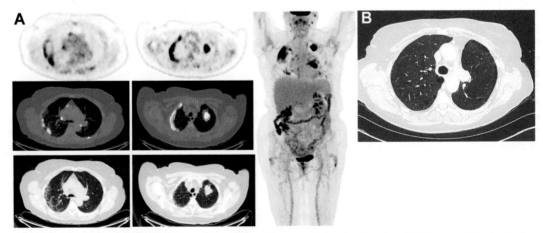

Fig. 6. Axial PET (*top*), fused (*middle*), and CT (*bottom*) images of the chest and an MIP image of the body from an FDG PET/CT (*A*) showing intensely FDG-avid peripheral ground-glass opacity consistent with COVID-19 infection in a patient with a left upper lobe adenocarcinoma. Selected axial CT image of the chest (*B*) post left upper lobe resection showing resolution of the incidentally detected COVID-19 pulmonary findings.

nodules are categorized as ground glass or mixed solid and ground glass. Typically, FDG-PET/CT is not included in the work-up of incidentally detected subsolid nodules, given the low metabolic activity and risk of false-negative results; in this case, the Fleishner Society guidelines recommend short-interval follow-up CT to establish stability, with continued CT surveillance for up to 5 years as needed.[11] FDG-PET/CT is helpful for the evaluation of solid nodules. FDG-PET/CT has high sensitivity and specificity to characterize an SPN as malignant, and high negative predictive value to exclude malignancy in nodules over 8 mm.[12–15] For example, in patients with an indeterminate SPN on CT and low probability of lung cancer, low FDG avidity suggests observation may be the most appropriate management. In patients with an indeterminate SPN on CT and intense FDG avidity, histopathology is suggested with surgical resection if this is the only site of malignant disease. The Society of Nuclear Medicine and Molecular Imaging (SNMMI) recommends FDG-PET/CT to: (1) detect a potentially malignant SPN early in the course of disease and potentially enable curative surgery in high-risk patients; (2) to exclude malignancy in low-risk patients with an indeterminate lesion; and (3) to improve healthcare outcomes by avoiding futile surgery in these patients.[16]

PET/CT is helpful for *lung cancer staging* and impacts management, since treatment strategy is related to staging, as well as tumor biology and genetic mutations. Locoregional and oligometastatic disease may be amenable to surgical resection, adjuvant chemotherapy, and/or targeted radiation. Chemotherapy, molecular targeted treatment, and immunotherapy are typically preferred for patients with distant metastases. The 5-year overall survival for patients with lung cancer localized to a small pulmonary nodule post surgery is 90% or higher;[17,18] survival remains poor (<10%) for patients with distant metastases.[1] While contrast-enhanced CT is preferred to evaluate size, location, and invasion of adjacent structures by lung cancer, PET provides complementary metabolic information.[19] In terms of the *primary disease* (T status), FDG-PET/CT helps distinguish metabolically active tissue from an adjacent benign process such as atelectasis.[20] For disease that has spread to *lymph nodes* (N status), an irregular margin or measurement of more than 1 cm in lymph node short axis on diagnostic CT is suggestive of disease spread. FDG-PET/CT is more accurate than CT for evaluating mediastinal disease.[21] However, false-negative results may be seen in the setting of micrometastases or when the primary disease avidity is low and false-positive results may occur in the setting of inflammation or

infection. Ultimately, tissue sampling is recommended for the purpose of confirmation.[22] A major strength of FDG-PET/CT is its ability to detect *distant metastases* (M status). It is estimated that over 50% of patients with lung cancer have metastases at presentation, with common sites including the adrenal glands, liver, brain, and bones.[23] Also, the incidence of occult disease using anatomic imaging is relatively high; in clinical stage I disease it exceeds 10%.[24,25] Metabolic imaging can be very helpful in this setting; the sensitivity, specificity, and accuracy of PET for detecting systemic metastases are higher than 90%[26] to identify occult systemic disease on anatomic imaging.[27] To date, PET/CT and PET/MR have shown similar results for lung cancer staging.[28–30]

PET/CT-BASED MOLECULAR IMAGING AND PRECISION MEDICINE IN SUBSEQUENT LUNG CANCER TREATMENT STRATEGY

Precision medicine integrates the molecular pathobiology and genetic make-up of a disease to suggest targeted therapy, and predict treatment response and outcomes. In this way, "preventive or therapeutic interventions" can be tailored to provide benefit while avoiding the expense and toxicity of futile treatment given to those who will not respond. The goal is to offer the right treatment, to the right patient, at the right time. Tissue biopsy or circulating free-cell DNA is becoming increasingly important to genotype the disease and help select optimal therapy. For oncogene-driven lung cancer that includes any of EGFR, ALK, ROS1, BRAF, TRK, RET, and MET, among others, specific targeted drug therapies may be suggested. For patients that lack an actionable tumor oncogenic driver, immune-checkpoint therapy may be preferred.[31] Discussion is ongoing regarding the best first-line therapy, the potential need for combination therapy and the role of neo-adjuvant therapy prior to resection. Further, there remains a risk of recurrence in patients with NSCLC following initial treatment.

PET-based molecular imaging of lung cancer is a *predictive biomarker* of response to cytotoxic and cytostatic therapy, radiotherapy, and image-guided interventions as well as a *biomarker of prognosis*. This contributes to precision medicine by influencing the decision to treat and the type of treatment to give.[32] Accurate timely treatment response assessment is critical for adjusting treatment to achieve maximal impact on outcome, although adopting a standardized definition of treatment "success" remains enigmatic. PET is also helpful to detect residual disease following therapy. He and colleagues[33] performed a meta-analysis including 1035 patients and 13 articles. The authors concluded that the pooled sensitivity (95% confidence interval [CI]) for the detection of lung cancer recurrence by PET/CT versus conventional imaging techniques (CITs) was: 0.90 (0.84–0.95) versus 0.78 (0.71–0.84), respectively. The pooled specificity (95% CI) was 0.90 (0.87–0.93) versus 0.80 (0.75–0.84), respectively.[33] According to the Society for Nuclear Medicine and Molecular Imaging, FDG-PET/CT is appropriate for: (1) restaging patients with lung cancer after treatment; (2) detection of recurrence; and (3) treatment response evaluation.[34]

PET AS A BIOMARKER OF RESPONSE TO LUNG CANCER THERAPY

The criteria for response assessment have evolved over the years. The first criteria to be widely adopted were based on anatomic findings (ie, WHO, RECIST); however, these had shortcomings for assessing therapy response in lung cancer patients. While cytolytic therapy may cause tumor mass reduction, cytostatic therapy tends to slow or stop tumor cell proliferation without a reduction in tumor mass. More recently, Wahl and colleagues[35] proposed criteria (ie, PERCIST) that included an assessment of metabolic response (PET) to monitor treatment effect. The clinical superiority of FDG-PET/CT as a predictive biomarker of lung cancer response to cytotoxic and cytostatic therapies is largely attributable to the fact that metabolic and pathophysiological changes can precede alterations in lesion morphology. Thus, PET-based molecular imaging may predict treatment response earlier than anatomic imaging modalities (ie, CT and MRI). Further, in general, the earlier the response, the better the progression-free and overall survival of the cancer patient.

The advent of immunotherapy, however, has made response assessment more challenging. Efficacy rests on proliferation of immune cells with tumor infiltration that may lead to a response within days and can include an early, transient, increase in tumor burden and metabolic activity including the development of new lesions, despite apparent clinical benefit. Typically, these imaging findings stabilize or improve after 3 to 4 months. This phenomenon, termed *pseudo-progression*, may be seen in approximately 10% of patients and has suggested the need for new response assessment criteria in patients treated with immunotherapy. Response assessment criteria such as iRECIST, PECRIT, and PERCIMIT have been proposed.[36–39] Validation of these criteria and their use in the lung cancer treatment arena remains a topic of current research. Ultimately, correlation of imaging findings with the clinical condition of the patient is key. For example, in patients with lung cancer treated with immunotherapy, imaging progression in the context of an improving or stable clinical condition suggests pseudoprogression. In this case treatment might be continued with response confirmed by follow-up imaging. On the other hand, patients with imaging progression and clinical deterioration are most likely progressing and discontinuing therapy may be warranted. Rarely, patients may experience rapid disease progression or *hyperprogression* in the setting of clinical deterioration. Also, immune-related adverse events such as thyroiditis, pneumonitis, myalgias, and reactive lymph node enlargement, among others, may be detected with FDG-PET/CT, sometimes weeks before these complications become clinically apparent.[40]

Response Assessment to Chemotherapy and Radiotherapy

Several years ago, PET was shown to be a reliable way to assess response to chemotherapy and radiation treatment. In addition, response on PET, both early in the course of treatment and at the end of therapy, was shown to portend improved survival. There are several supporting studies. Among them, for example, Eschmann and colleagues[41] reported on a study of 70 patients with stage III NSCLC who had FDG-PET before and at the conclusion of neoadjuvant radiochemotherapy. The authors found that a negative PET or a reduction in the standardized uptake value (SUV) by more than 80% at the end of therapy suggested a better outcome. Also, FDG-PET detected residual viable primary tumor with a sensitivity, specificity, and overall accuracy of 94.5%, 80%, and 91%, respectively. MacManus and colleagues[42] showed in their study of 88 patients with NSCLC treated with either concurrent platinum-based radical chemoradiotherapy (73 patients) or radical radiotherapy alone (15 patients), that complete metabolic responders had a 1-year survival rate of 93% compared to 47% for nonresponders, and a 2-year survival rate of 62% versus 30%, respectively. Dooms and colleagues in their study of 30 patients with stage IIIA-N2 NSCLC, found that a decrease of 60% in primary tumor uptake and mild residual FDG avidity in mediastinal nodes after induction chemotherapy were associated with significantly longer 5-year overall survival and benefit.[43] In Hoekstra and colleagues' study of 47 patients with stage IIIA-N2 NSCLC, a 35% reduction in tumor FDG uptake after one cycle of induction therapy correlated with improved overall survival.[44]

Assessment of Response to Targeted Drug Therapy and Immunotherapy

Studies of targeted drug therapy in lung cancer started to appear in the literature several years ago. In 2004, Paez and colleagues, and Lynch and colleagues showed that the tyrosine kinase inhibitor (TKI) gefitinib stopped the growth of lung tumors expressing somatic mutations of the epidermal growth factor receptor gene (EGFR).[45,46] Today, oncogene-targeted drug therapies are often used to treat lung cancer, thus the subclassification of malignancy as a result of identifying genetic mutations (genomic profiling) at the time of diagnosis is critical to determining optimal therapy.[31,32,47]

With the advent of cytostatic drug-targeted therapy, a change in tumor size was not always consistent with efficacy and the use of RECIST or WHO criteria could underestimate the efficacy. PET-based molecular imaging was thought to be more appropriate to monitor the effect of these therapies. However, the ideal timing of PET during and after targeted therapy, as well as what should be considered a significant reduction in radiopharmaceutical uptake to be consistent with successful response to therapy, remains a topic of debate to this day. Several studies suggest that FDG and FLT uptake at the site of the primary lung lesion tends to increase in nonresponding patients, while earlier and larger reductions in radiotracer uptake with TKI therapy suggest longer survival and better quality of life.[48–58] Other studies have shown that response to targeted therapy such as erlotinib and gefitinib on FDG-PET can be predicted early in the course of treatment, sometimes as early as 2 days after the start of therapy.[48,49] Additional reports have suggested an accurate prediction of response on FDG and FLT-PET was possible within 3 weeks of treatment initiation, as confirmed by conventional imaging and clinical evaluation 4 to 6 weeks later.[50–58]

More recently, immune-checkpoint inhibitor (ICI) therapy targeting programmed cell death-1 (PD-1) and programmed cell death-ligand 1 (PD-L1) is becoming a prevalent therapy for patients with advanced NSCLC.[59] In 2019, Yu and colleagues studied the association of survival and immune-related biomarkers with immunotherapy in patients with NSCLC through a meta-analysis including 14,395 patients. The authors concluded that immunotherapy was promising in terms of clinical outcome for patients with NSCLC and that the combined predictive utility of PD-L1 expression and tumor mutation burden was associated with prognosis.[60] Several recent studies have assessed the role of PET response to immunotherapy and the potential value of radiomic features for predicting benefit.[61–63] Currently, the choice of optimal therapy and response assessment (in the case of immunotherapy) remain topics of research.

PET IMAGE PHENOTYPE AS A BIOMARKER OF PROGNOSIS IN LUNG CANCER

The PET image phenotype may facilitate identification of patients at high risk of disease progression regardless of their clinical stage at diagnosis. This information can then be used to personalize therapy. Examples of PET image phenotypes include the: intensity and patterns of tumor metabolic activity (SUV), the metabolically active tumor mass [total tumor glycolysis (TLG)], and tumoral metabolic heterogeneity assessed with texture analysis.

Tumor FDG Avidity

Intensity FDG uptake is associated with lung cancer aggressiveness and has prognostic value. Evidence suggests that high tumor uptake correlates with poor prognosis across different stages and histologic types of lung cancer.[64] Since Ahuja and colleagues[65] suggested primary lung tumor FDG uptake was an independent predictor of overall survival back in 1998, many studies have confirmed a good correlation between outcome and intensity of tumor uptake in patients with early as well as advanced stage NSCLC.[66–68] For example, Ohtsuka and colleagues[66] found that increased FDG avidity in the primary lung tumor correlated with shorter progression-free survival and a higher rate of recurrence. Based on their results, the authors recommended that in early-stage disease, the intensity of tumor uptake could be used to identify those patients who might benefit from adjuvant chemotherapy. Cerfolio and colleagues[67] analyzed progression-free survival within different lung cancer stages as a function of FDG avidity and concluded that a higher primary tumor uptake within the same stage predicted progression of disease and a shorter overall survival. A National Cancer Institute-funded American College of Radiology Imaging Network/Radiation Therapy Oncology Group study (ACRIN 6668/RTOG 0235) found that in 253 patients with stage III NSCLC and FDG-PET obtained before and at 14 weeks of concurrent platinum-based chemoradiotherapy, a higher posttreatment SUV_{peak} and SUV_{max} were associated with poor survival.[68] Studies have also been conducted to understand associations of FDG avidity with underlying protein expression in lung cancer patients. For example, Nair and colleagues correlated FDG avidity with NK-κBp65 expression and prognosis in 355 lung cancer patients, where NK-κBp65 controls DNA transcription, cytokine production, and tumor cell survival. The investigators found that a high tumor SUV coupled with high NF-κBp65 expression was seen in patients with more extensive disease, tumor invasion, and worse prognosis.[69]

Metabolically Active Tumor Volumes

Tumor bulk is also a prognostic indicator in lung cancer patients. Three-dimensional volumetric indices of metabolic tumor activity can be derived using PET, namely the: (1) metabolic tumor volume (MTV) estimated using semiautomatic tumor-contouring software with a predefined SUV threshold to segment metabolic tumor boundaries and (2) total lesion glycolysis (TLG) estimated by multiplying the tumor's mean SUV by the MTV. Whole-body MTV and TLG are obtained by summing the values for each lesion in the body.[70] Studies of metabolically active lung cancer volumes suggest this may be a predictor of survival.[64,71-76]

Metabolic Heterogeneity of Lung Cancer

Tumor heterogeneity has been shown to correlate with aggressiveness, therapeutic resistance, and therefore, poor survival.[77] Various texture parameters can be used to noninvasively characterize tumor metabolic heterogeneity.[78,79] There are emerging data suggesting that measures of tumoral metabolic heterogeneity have a prognostic role in lung cancer patients. For example, Cook and colleagues[80] reported on the role of FDG-PET-derived tumor textural features as biomarkers of response and outcomes in 47 NSCLC patients treated with TKIs. The investigators found that reduced metabolic heterogeneity at week 6 during treatment was consistent with a good response to erlotinib confirmed by CT at week 12. In addition, PET image-derived texture parameters were independent predictors of survival. These metabolic signatures of tumor heterogeneity have prognostic potential, although prospective, randomized trials are needed for further evaluation.

SUMMARY

PET imaging has become an integral decision-making tool in the precision medicine algorithm of lung cancer patients. It provides anatomo-molecular insight during the course of care of the cancer patient. This PET-derived information is now used to make treatment decisions, to predict metabolic response during and after therapy, and as a clinical biomarker of survival in lung cancer patients.

CLINICS CARE POINTS

- PET and PET/CT imaging are very accurate imaging modalities for the non-invasive metabolic characterization of lung lesions as benign or malignant.
- However, FDG uptake in lung lesions is not always specific for malignancy, and therefore, evaluating imaging findings in the patient's clinical context is critical.
- PET and PET/CT are very accurate imaging techniques to stage and restage lung cancer.
- PET and PET/CT imaging patterns serve as biomarkers of response to treatment and prognosis.

DISCLOSURE

Dr K.A. Zukotynski, Dr O. Kamel Hasan, Dr M. Lubanovic, and Dr V.H. Gerbaudo have no disclosures to make.

REFERENCES

1. American Cancer Society. Key statistics for lung cancer. 2020. Available at: http://www.cancer.org/cancer/lungcancer-non-smallcell/detailedguide/non-small-cell-lung-cancer-key-statistics. Accessed June 11, 2021.
2. Herbst RS, Morgensztern D, Boshoff C. The biology and management of non-small cell lung cancer. Nature 2018;553:446–54.
3. Mena E, Yanamadala A, Cheng G, et al. The current and evolving role of PET in personalized management of lung cancer. PET Clin 2016;11(3):243–59.
4. Crivellaro C, Guerra L. Respiratory gating and the performance of PET/CT in pulmonary lesions. Curr Radiopharm 2020;13:218–27.
5. Warburg O, Wind F, Negelein E. The metabolism of tumours in the body. J Gen Physiol 1927;8(6):519–30.
6. Warburg O. On respiratory impairment in cancer cells. Science 1956;124(3215):269–70.
7. Kinoshita T, Fujii H, Hayashi Y, et al. Prognostic significance of hypoxic PET using (18)F-FAZA and (62) Cu-ATSM in non-small-cell lung cancer. Lung Cancer 2016;91:56–66.
8. Giesel FL, Adeberg S, Syed M, et al. FAPI-74 PET/CT using either 18F-AlF or cold-kit 68Ga-labeling: biodistribution, radiation dosimetry and tumor

delineation in lung cancer patients. J Nucl Med 2021;62(2):201–7.

9. Hicks RJ, Mac Manus MP, Matthews JP, et al. Early FDG-PET imaging after radical radiotherapy for non-small-cell lung cancer: inflammatory changes in normal tissues correlate with tumor response and do not confound therapeutic response evaluation. Int J Radiat Oncol Biol Phys 2004;60(2):412–8.

10. Gould MK, Tang T, Liu IL, et al. Recent trends in the identification of incidental pulmonary nodules. Am J Respir Crit Care Med 2015;192(10):1208–14.

11. MacMahon H, Naidich DP, Goo JM, et al. Guidelines for management of incidental pulmonary nodules detected on CT images: from the Fleischner Society 2017. Radiology 2017;284(1):228–43.

12. Gould MK, Maclean CC, Kuschner WG, et al. Accuracy of positron emission tomography for diagnosis of pulmonary nodules and mass lesions: a meta-analysis. JAMA 2001;287:914–24.

13. Gambhir SS, Czernin J, Schwimmer J, et al. A tabulated summary of the FDG PET literature. J Nucl Med 2001;42:1S–93S.

14. Cronin P, Dwamena B, Kelly AM, et al. Solitary pulmonary nodules: meta-analytic comparison of cross-sectional imaging modalities for diagnosis of malignancy. Radiology 2008;246:772–82.

15. Garcia-Velloso MJ, Bastarrika G, de-Torres JP, et al. Assessment of indeterminate pulmonary nodules detected in lung cancer screening: diagnostic accuracy of FDG PET/CT. Lung Cancer 2016;97:81–6.

16. Fletcher JW, Djulbegovic B, Soares HP, et al. Recommendations on the use of ^{18}F-FDG PET in oncology. J Nucl Med 2008;49(3):480–508.

17. Kodama K, Higashiyama M, Okami J, et al. Oncologic outcomes of segmentectomy versus lobectomy for clinical T1a N0 M0 non-small cell lung cancer. Ann Thorac Surg 2016;101(2):504–11.

18. Carr SR, Schuchert MJ, Pennathur A, et al. Impact of tumor size on outcomes after anatomic lung resection for stage 1A non-small cell lung cancer based on the current staging system. J Thorac Cardiovasc Surg 2012;143(2):390–7.

19. Lardinois D, Weder W, Hany TF, et al. Staging of non–small-cell lung cancer with integrated positron emission tomography and computed tomography. N Engl J Med 2003;348:2500–7.

20. Gerbaudo VH, Julius B. Anatomo-metabolic characteristics of atelectasis in F-18 FDG-PET/CT imaging. Eur J Radiol 2007;64(3):401–5.

21. Gould MK, Kuschner WG, Rydzak CE, et al. Test performance of positron emission tomography and computed tomography for mediastinal staging in patients with non-small-cell lung cancer: a meta-analysis. Ann Intern Med 2003;139:879–92.

22. Fischer BM, Mortensen J, Hansen H, et al. Multimodality approach to mediastinal staging in non-small

cell lung cancer. Faults and benefits of PET-CT: a randomised trial. Thorax 2011;66(4):294–300.

23. National cancer institute. Cancer state facts: lung and bronchus cancer. Available at: https://seer.cancer.gov/statfacts/html/lungb.html. Accessed January 23, 2020.

24. Robinson EM, Ilonen IK, Tan KS, et al. Prevalence of occult peribronchial N1 nodal metastasis in peripheral clinical N0<2cm NSCLC. Ann Thorac Surg 2020;109(1):270–6.

25. Sider L, Horejs D. Frequency of extrathoracic metastases from bronchogenic carcinoma in patients with normal-sized hilar and mediastinal lymph nodes on CT. AJR Am J Roentgenol 1988;151(5):893–5.

26. Hellwig D, Ukena D, Paulsen F, et al, Onko-PET der Deutschen Gesellschaft fur Nuklearmedizin. Meta-analysis of the efficacy of positron emission tomography with F-18-fluorodeoxyglucose in lung tumors. Basis for discussion of the German Consensus Conference on PET in Oncology 2000. Pneumologie 2001;55(8):367–77.

27. MacManus MP, Hicks RJ, Matthews JP, et al. High rate of detection of unsuspected distant metastases by PET in apparent stage III non-small-cell lung cancer: implications for radical radiation therapy. Int J Radiat Oncol Biol Phys 2001;50(2):287–93.

28. Lee SM, Goo JM, Park CM, et al. Preoperative staging of non-small cell lung cancer: prospective somparison of PET/MR and PET/CT. Eur Radiol 2016; 26(11):3850–7.

29. Huellner MW, Barbosa FdG, Husmann L, et al. TNM staging of non-small cell lung cancer: comparison of PET/MR and PET/CT. J Nucl Med 2016;57(1):21–6.

30. Schaarschmidt B, Grueneisen J, Metzenmacher M, et al. Thoracic staging with 18F-FDG PET/MR in non-small cell lung cancer – does it change therapeutic decisions in comparison to 18F-FDG PET/CT? Eur Radiol 2017;27(2):681–8.

31. Yang SR, Schultheis AM, Yu H, et al. Precision medicine in non-small cell lung cancer: current applications and future directions. Semin Cancer Biol 2020. S1044-579X(20)30164-4.

32. Park H, Sholl LM, Hatabu H, et al. Imaging of precision therapy for lung cancer: current state of the art. Radiology 2019;293:15–29.

33. He Y, Gong H, Deng Y, et al. Diagnostic efficacy of PET and PET/CT for recurrent lung câncer: a meta-analysis. Acta Radiol 2014;55(3):309–17.

34. Jadvar H, Colletti PM, Delgado-Bolton R, et al. Appropriate use criteria for 18F-FDG PET/CT in restaging and treatment response assessment of malignant disease. J Nucl Med 2017;58(12):2026–37.

35. Wahl RL, Jacene H, Kasamon Y, et al. From RECIST to PERCIST: evolving considerations for PET response criteria in solid tumors. J Nucl Med 2009; 50(Suppl 1):122S–50S.

36. Cho SY, Lipson EJ, Im HJ, et al. Prediction of response to immune checkpoint inhibitor therapy using early-time-point ^{18}F-FDG PET/CT imaging in patients with advanced melanoma. J Nucl Med 2017; 58:1421–8.

37. Anwar H, Sachpekidis C, Winkler J, et al. Absolute number of new lesions on ^{18}F-FDG PET/CT is more predictive of clinical response than SUV changes in metastatic melanoma patients receiving ipilimumab. Eur J Nucl Med Mol Imaging 2018;45:376–83.

38. Sachpekidis C, Anwar H, Winkler J, et al. The role of interim ^{18}F-FDG PET/CT in prediction of response to ipilimumab treatment in metastatic melanoma. Eur J Nucl Med Mol Imaging 2018;45:1289–96.

39. Seymour L, Bogaerts J, Perrone A, et al. iRECIST: guidelines for response criteria for use in trials testing immunotherapeutics. Lancet Oncol 2017; 18(3):e143–52.

40. Kwak JJ, Tirumani SH, Van den Abbeele AD, et al. Cancer immunotherapy: imaging assessment of novel treatment response patterns and immune-related adverse events. Radiographics 2015;35: 424–37.

41. Eschmann SM, Friedel G, Paulsen F, et al. 18F-FDG PET for assessment of therapy response and preoperative re-evaluation after neoadjuvant radiochemotherapy in stage III non-small cell lung cancer. Eur J Nucl Med Mol Imaging 2007;34(4):463–71.

42. Mac Manus MP, Hicks RJ, Matthews JP, et al. Metabolic (FDG-PET) response after radical radiotherapy/chemoradiotherapy for non-small cell lung cancer correlates with patterns of failure. Lung Cancer 2005;49(1):95–108.

43. Dooms C, Verbeken E, Stroobants S, et al. Prognostic stratification of stage IIIA-N2 non-small-cell lung cancer after induction chemotherapy: a model based on the combination of morphometric-pathologic response in mediastinal nodes and primary tumor response on serial 18-fluoro-2-deoxy-glucose positron emission tomography. J Clin Oncol 2008;26(7):1128–34.

44. Hoekstra CJ, Stroobants SG, Smit EF, et al. Prognostic relevance of response evaluation using [18F]-2-fluoro-2-deoxy-D-glucose positron emission tomography in patients with locally advanced non-small-cell lung cancer. J Clin Oncol 2005;23(33): 8362–70.

45. Paez JG, Jänne PA, Lee JC, et al. EGFR mutations in lung cancer: correlation with clinical response to gefitinib therapy. Science 2004;304(5676):1497–500.

46. Lynch TJ, Bell DW, Sordella R, et al. Activating mutations in the epidermal growth factor receptor underlying responsiveness of non-small-cell lung cancer to gefitinib. N Engl J Med 2004;350(21): 2129–39.

47. Osmani L, Askin F, Gabielson E, et al. Current WHO guidelines and the critical role of immunohistochemical markers in the subclassification of non-small cell lun carcinoma (NSCLC): moving from targeted therapy to immunotherapy. Semin Cancer Biol 2018; 52(Pt 1):103–9.

48. Sunaga N, Oriuchi N, Kaira K, et al. Usefulness of FDG-PET for early prediction of the response to gefitinib in non-small cell lung cancer. Lung Cancer 2008;59(2):203–10.

49. Takahashi R, Hirata H, Tachibana I, et al. Early [18F] fluorodeoxyglucose positron emission tomography at two days of gefitinib treatment predicts clinical outcome in patients with adenocarcinoma of the lung. Clin Cancer Res 2012;18(1):220–8.

50. van Gool MH, Aukema TS, Schaake EE, et al, NEL Study Group. Timing of metabolic response monitoring during erlotinib treatment in non-small cell lung cancer. J Nucl Med 2014;55(7):1081–6.

51. Benz MR, Herrmann K, Walter F, et al. (18)F-FDG PET/CT for monitoring treatment responses to the epidermal growth factor receptor inhibitor erlotinib. J Nucl Med 2011;52(11):1684–9.

52. Hachemi M, Couturier O, Vervueren L, et al. [18F] FDG positron emission tomography within two weeks of starting erlotinib therapy can predict response in non-small cell lung cancer patients. PLoS One 2014;9(2):e87629.

53. van Gool MH, Aukema TS, Schaake EE, et al. (18)F-fluorodeoxyglucose positron emission tomography versus computed tomography in predicting histopathological response to epidermal growth factor receptor-tyrosine kinase inhibitor treatment in resectable non-small cell lung cancer. Ann Surg Oncol 2014;21(9):2831–7.

54. Ullrich RT, Zander T, Neumaier B, et al. Early detection of erlotinib treatment response in NSCLC by 3'-deoxy-3'-[F]-fluoro-L-thymidine ([F]FLT) positron emission tomography (PET). PLoS One 2008;3(12): e3908.

55. Sohn HJ, Yang YJ, Ryu JS, et al. [18F]Fluorothymidine positron emission tomography before and 7 days after gefitinib treatment predicts response in patients with advanced adenocarcinoma of the lung. Clin Cancer Res 2008;14(22):7423–9.

56. Kahraman D, Scheffler M, Zander T, et al. Quantitative analysis of response to treatment with erlotinib in advanced non-small cell lung cancer using 18F-FDG and 3'-deoxy-3'-18F-fluorothymidine PET. J Nucl Med 2011;52(12):1871–7.

57. Zander T, Scheffler M, Nogova L, et al. Early prediction of nonprogression in advanced non-small-cell lung cancer treated with erlotinib by using [(18)F]fluorodeoxyglucose and [(18)F]fluorothymidine positron emission tomography. J Clin Oncol 2011; 29(13):1701–8.

58. Bhoil A, Singh B, Singh N, et al. Can 3'-deoxy-3'-(18)F-fluorothymidine or 2'-deoxy-2'-(18)F-fluoro-d-glucose PET/CTbetter assess response after 3-weeks treatment by epidermal growth factor receptor kinase

inhibitor, in non-small lung cancer patients? Preliminary results. Hell J Nucl Med 2014;17(2):90–6.

59. Proto C, Ferrara R, Signorelli D, et al. Choosing wisely first line immunotherapy in non-small cell lung cancer (NSCLC): what to add and what to leave out. Caner Treat Rev 2019;75:39–51.

60. Yu Y, Zeng D, Ou Q, et al. Association of survival and immune-related biomarkers with immunotherapy in patients with non-small cell lung cancer: a meta-analysis and individual patient-level analysis. JAMA Netw Open 2019;2(7):e196879.

61. Mu W, Tunali I, Gray JE, et al. Radiomics of 18F-FDG PET/CT images predicts clinical benefit of advanced NSCLC patients to checkpoint blockade immunotherapy. Eur J Nucl Med Mol Imaging 2020;47(5):1168–82.

62. Rossi G, Bauckneht M, Genova C, et al. Comparison between 18F-FDG PET-based and CT-based criteria in non-small cell lung cancer patients treated with nivolumab. J Nucl Med 2020;61(7):990–8.

63. Evangelista L, Cuppari L, Menis J, et al. 18F-FDG PET/CT in non-small-cell lung cancer patients: a potential predictive biomarker of response to immunotherapy. Nucl Med Commun 2019;40(8):802–7.

64. Paesmans M, Berghmans T, Dusart M, et al. Primary tumor standardized uptake value measured on fluorodeoxyglucose positron emission tomography is of prognostic value for survival in non-small cell lung cancer: update of a systematic review and meta-analysis by the European Lung Cancer Working Party for the International Association for the Study of Lung Cancer Staging Project. J Thorac Oncol 2010;5(5):612–9.

65. Ahuja V, Coleman RE, Herndon J, et al. The prognostic significance of fluorodeoxyglucose positron emission tomography imaging for patients with non-small cell lung carcinoma. Cancer 1998;83(5):918–24.

66. Ohtsuka T, Nomori H, Watanabe K, et al. Prognostic significance of [(18)F]fluorodeoxyglucose uptake on positron emission tomography in patients with pathologic stage I lung adenocarcinoma. Cancer 2006;107(10):2468–73.

67. Cerfolio RJ, Bryant AS, Ohja B, et al. The maximum standardized uptake values on positron emission tomography of a non-small cell lung cancer predict stage, recurrence, and survival. J Thorac Cardiovasc Surg 2005;130(1):151–9.

68. Machtay M, Duan F, Siegel BA, et al. Prediction of survival by [18F]fluorodeoxyglucose positron emission tomography in patients with locally advanced non-small-cell lung cancer undergoing definitive chemoradiation therapy: results of the ACRIN 6668/RTOG 0235 trial. J Clin Oncol 2013;31(30):3823–30.

69. Nair VS, Gevaert O, Davidzon G, et al. NF-κB protein expression associates with (18)F-FDG PET tumor uptake in non-small cell lung cancer: a radiogenomics validation study to understand tumor metabolism. Lung Cancer 2014;83(2):189–96.

70. Larson SM, Erdi Y, Akhurst T, et al. Tumor treatment response based on visual and quantitative changes in global tumor glycolysis using PET-FDG imaging. The visual response score and the change in total lesion glycolysis. Clin Positron Imaging 1999;2(3):159–71.

71. Lee P, Weerasuriya DK, Lavori PW, et al. Metabolic tumor burden predicts for disease progression and death in lung cancer. Int J Radiat Oncol Biol Phys 2007;69(2):328–33.

72. Dehing-Oberije C, De Ruysscher D, van der Weide H, et al. Tumor volume combined with number of positive lymph node stations is a more important prognostic factor than TNM stage for survival of non-small-cell lung cancer patients treated with (chemo)radiotherapy. Int J Radiat Oncol Biol Phys 2008;70(4):1039–44.

73. Liao S, Penney BC, Zhang H, et al. Prognostic value of the quantitative metabolic volumetric measurement on 18F-FDG PET/CT in stage IV nonsurgical small-cell lung cancer. Acad Radiol 2012;19(1):69–77.

74. Zhang H, Wroblewski K, Liao S, et al. Prognostic value of metabolic tumor burden from (18)F-FDG PET in surgical patients with non-small-cell lung cancer. Acad Radiol 2013;20(1):32–40.

75. Park SY, Cho A, Yu WS, et al. Prognostic value of total lesion glycolysis by 18F-FDG PET/CT in surgically resected stage IA non-small cell lung cancer. J Nucl Med 2015;56(1):45–9.

76. Ohri N, Duan F, Machtay M, et al. Pretreatment FDG-PET metrics in stage III non-small cell lung cancer: ACRIN 6668/RTOG 0235. J Natl Cancer Inst 2015;107(4):djv004.

77. Jamal-Hanjani M, Hackshaw A, Ngai Y, et al. Tracking genomic cancer evolution for precision medicine: the lung TRACERx study. PLoS Biol 2014;12(7):e1001906.

78. Davnall F, Yip CS, Ljungqvist G, et al. Assessment of tumor heterogeneity: an emerging imaging tool for clinical practice? Insights Imaging 2012;3(6):573–89.

79. van Gómez López O, García Vicente AM, Honguero Martínez AF, et al. Heterogeneity in [18F]fluorodeoxyglucose positron emission tomography/computed tomography of non-small cell lung carcinoma and its relationship to metabolic parameters and pathologic staging. Mol Imaging 2014;13:1–12.

80. Cook GJ, O'Brien ME, Siddique M, et al. Non-small cell lung cancer treated with erlotinib: heterogeneity of (18)F-FDG uptake at PET-association with treatment response and prognosis. Radiology 2015;276(3):883–93.

PET Imaging for Hematologic Malignancies

Nicola M. Hughes, MBBChBAO, MRCSI, FFRRCSI, Heather A. Jacene, MD*

KEYWORDS

- Hematologic malignancies • PET/CT • Lymphoma • Myeloma • Leukemia • Histiocytosis • Staging
- Response assessment

KEY POINTS

- FDG-PET/CT is the imaging modality of choice for staging and assessing end of treatment response for FDG-avid lymphomas. Interim FDG-PET/CT has prognostic value, which has led to risk-adapted treatment strategies with many clinical trials evaluating escalation and de-escalation strategies.
- FDG-PET/CT can be used as an alternative to whole-body CT or whole-body MRI for evaluation of many plasma cell disorders and is the recommended modality of choice for assessing response to treatment in multiple myeloma.
- FDG-PET/CT can detect extramedullary disease in patients with leukemia although the prognostic relevance and applications for assessing response are unclear.
- FDG-PET/CT can detect sites of disease in patients with histiocytosis but the definitive role of FDG-PET/CT has yet to be defined.
- Many patients with hematologic malignancies use medications that lead to false-positive and false-negative results on FDG-PET/CT such as immunomodulatory drugs, steroids, and G-CSF, so it is important that the interpreter be aware of these potential pitfalls.

INTRODUCTION

Hematologic malignancies are a broad category of cancers arising from the lymphoid and myeloid cell lines. The 2016 World Health Organization classification system incorporated molecular markers as part of the diagnostic criteria and includes more than 100 subtypes.[1,2] This article focuses on the subtypes for which imaging with positron emission tomography/computed tomography (PET/CT) has become an integral component of the patient's evaluation, that is, lymphoma and multiple myeloma (MM). Leukemia and histiocytic and dendritic cell neoplasms are also discussed because FDG-PET/CT for these indications, although less common, are increasingly being seen in clinic.

NORMAL ANATOMY AND PHYSIOLOGY

The lymphatic system comprises lymph nodes, lymphatic ducts, thymus, spleen, tonsils, and Peyer's patches in the small bowel. The bone marrow is also considered part of the lymphatic system, but does not have any lymphatic drainage. Lymph nodes are bean-shaped structures of lymphatic tissue contained in a fibrous capsule that filter interstitial fluid from afferent vessels and return it to the circulation via efferent vessels. The major structural components of lymph nodes are as follows: (1) inner medulla layer; (2) outer cortex containing multiple germinal centers; and (3) inner cortical layer (paracortex) containing deep cortical units. B-lymphocytes (B-cells) are found in the cortex and medulla, whereas T-lymphocytes (T-cells) are in the paracortex. On imaging, normal lymph nodes have a smooth, well-defined borders, are less than 1 cm, and have a fatty hilum. The spleen is composed of many lobules, each containing peripheral red pulp and core white pulp, within a connective tissue sheath. The upper limit of

Department of Imaging and Radiology, Dana-Farber Cancer Institute, Brigham and Women's Hospital, Harvard Medical School, 450 Brookline Avenue, Boston, MA 02215, USA
* Corresponding author.
E-mail address: hjacene@bwh.harvard.edu

Radiol Clin N Am 59 (2021) 705–723
https://doi.org/10.1016/j.rcl.2021.05.003

normal for spleen size is 12 cm in maximum longitudinal dimension; however, emerging evidence suggests normal splenic size should be adjusted for sex and height.[3]

The thymus is a bilobed, triangular-shaped primary lymphatic organ located in the anterior mediastinum and its major function is to mature and educate T-lymphocytes. The thymus is large in childhood, grows to peak size during puberty, and then begins involuting in early adulthood with progressive fatty infiltration, often with no residual thymic tissue visible on imaging in adults older than 40 years. The bone marrow consists of richly vascularized red marrow where hematopoiesis occurs and fatty yellow marrow containing inactive hematopoietic tissue. Red marrow predominates at birth occupying most of the skeleton. The normal adult distribution of marrow is reached at about 25 years of age with active red marrow persisting in the axial and proximal appendicular skeleton.

PROTOCOL AND IMAGING TECHNIQUE

The most commonly used radiotracer for PET/CT to evaluate hematologic malignancies is fluorine-2-deoxy-2-[^{18}F]fluoro-D-glucose (^{18}F-FDG). Detailed imaging protocols are found in the European Association of Nuclear Medicine and American College of Radiology procedure guidelines[4,5] Briefly, ^{18}F-FDG is injected intravenously followed by an uptake phase (goal 60 minutes, acceptable range 50–75 minutes), then sequential PET and CT images. ^{18}F-FDG activity administered ranges from 5 to 20 mCi (185–740 MBq) depending on the PET scanner, local acquisition and reconstruction protocols, and patient weight. CT protocols also vary from low dose for attenuation correction to fully diagnostic with intravenous contrast administration. In preparation for the scan, patients should fast 4 to 6 hours, avoid strenuous activity for 24 hours before the examination, and be well hydrated. It is generally recommended that blood glucose levels are less than 200 mg/dL immediately before injection of ^{18}F-FDG; however, some circumstances, like a research trial, might require stricter cut-offs.

Most patients with lymphoma have a standard PET/CT from the base of the skull through the mid-thigh, with exceptions including known sites of disease outside that range whereby the field of view can be tailored accordingly. A total body PET/CT is performed for patients with myeloma and for patients with leukemia requiring assessment for extramedullary disease.

LYMPHOMA
Classification

Lymphoma is classified into two major categories: non-Hodgkin lymphoma (NHL) and Hodgkin lymphoma (HL). NHL is the most common with more than 30 subtypes described based on the abnormal cell lineage of origin—B-cell, T-cell, or rarely natural killer cell (NK-cell).[1] The most common subtypes of NHL in the USA are diffuse large B-cell lymphoma (DLBCL) and follicular lymphoma (FL). HL represents approximately 10% of all lymphoma diagnoses and is subcategorized as classical Hodgkin lymphoma (cHL) and lymphocyte-predominant Hodgkin lymphoma (lpHL, 5% of all HL).

Clinical Presentation and Natural History

NHL usually presents as painless lymphadenopathy with approximately 40% of patients reporting "B-symptoms" of fever, night sweats, and/or weight loss at diagnosis.[6] The natural history of NHL is variable between and within each histologic subtype. DLBCL typically has a more aggressive course, whereas FL is usually considered indolent but can behave indolently or aggressively depending on the histologic grade.[7]

NHL mostly involves lymph nodes, but extranodal sites of disease are more frequent in NHL compared with HL. The spleen is considered an extranodal site in NHL, but nodal in HL. The most common sites of extranodal disease include the stomach, spleen, Waldeyer's ring, the central nervous system (CNS), lung, bone, and skin.[8] The pattern of spread in NHL is less predictable than HL; however, there are some patterns that favor one entity over the other. For example, mediastinal disease is less common in NHL (~20% of patients), whereas mesenteric or epitrochlear lymphadenopathy or involvement of Waldeyer's ring is more common in NHL compared with HL.[9]

HL also usually presents as painless supradiaphragmatic lymphadenopathy and about 30% of patients experience "B-symptoms." Classical HL is considered as a more aggressive disease, whereas lpHL behaves more like a low-grade NHL. Roth and colleagues evaluated patterns of lymph node spread in 297 patients with HL who underwent pathologic staging by assuming either right or left cervical nodes as the primary site of origin as 70% of patients with stage I disease had involvement of cervical nodes.[10] They found two distinct patterns of disease determined by laterality. In patients with right cervical nodes, the disease spreads first to the upper mediastinum, then pulmonary hilar nodes, upper abdominal nodes, and then to the spleen. In patients with left cervical nodes, the spread was directly to the upper abdomen bypassing the mediastinum, then back up to pulmonary hilar nodes, upper mediastinum, the contralateral cervical chain, and then on to axillary and finally inguinal nodes.[10]

Clinical Applications of Imaging and Diagnostic Criteria: Diagnosis and Histologic Grading

Most lymphomas are FDG-avid.[11,12] In general, aggressive NHL is intensely FDG-avid, whereas the more indolent subtypes such as small lymphocytic lymphoma (SLL), enteropathy-type T-cell lymphoma, extranodal marginal zone lymphoma (MZL), mucosa-associated lymphoid tissue (MALT) MZL, lymphoid papulosis, and primary cutaneous anaplastic large T-cell lymphoma have lower levels of FDG uptake.[12–14]

There is no set value defining high versus low levels of FDG uptake in NHL; however, Schoder and colleagues found that an SUV less than 10 identified 81% of indolent NHL and an SUV $\geq$13 indicated aggressive disease.[13] FDG-PET/CT is not a replacement for histologic grading but may guide tissue sampling to areas of higher FDG uptake that may harbor more aggressive disease. This is especially important for identifying high-grade transformation in the setting of existing low-grade disease.

Transformation to a high-grade lymphoma may be seen in a variety of indolent NHL subtypes, including chronic lymphocytic leukemia (CLL)/SLL (ie, Richters transformation), FL, mantle cell lymphoma (MCL), and MALT, and is associated with poor outcomes. Several studies evaluated the use of FDG-PET/CT for identifying high-grade transformation. In patients with CLL, which typically has low-level homogeneous FDG uptake, the strength of FDG-PET/CT is its high negative predictive value of 97% using a cut-off point of SUVmax 5 to exclude Richter's transformation.[15] In a more heterogeneous group of patients with NHL including FL, CLL, Waldenstrom's macroglobulinemia, and MZL and clinical concern for transformation, FDG-PET/CT was prospectively used to guide biopsy at the site of highest SUVmax; an SUVmax less than 11.7 was always associated with indolent lymphoma and SUVmax greater than 17 was always associated with high-grade transformation.[16] The larger the gradient between the indolent lymphoma and potential site of transformation, the more specific FDG-PET/CT is for identifying high-grade transformation (**Fig. 1**).

Both forms of HL are FDG-avid. A limited number of studies have suggested that lpHL may be less FDG-avid than cHL.[17,18] Results regarding

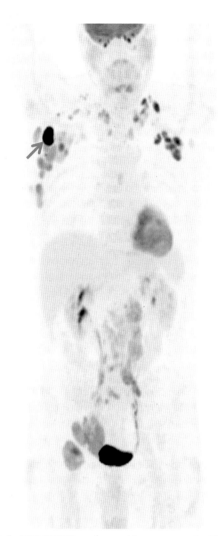

Fig. 1. FDG-PET/CT performed for assessment of transformation in the setting of known low-grade follicular lymphoma. FDG-PET/CT maximum-intensity projection (MIP) image showed an enlarged intensely FDG-avid right axillary lymph node (*arrow*), which showed much more intense uptake than the other sites of known follicular lymphoma. Biopsy of this right axillary node confirmed the transformation of follicular lymphoma to diffuse large B-cell lymphoma.

differences in levels of uptake between cHL subtypes were mixed.

Clinical Applications and Diagnostic Criteria: Initial Staging and Treatment Response

FDG-PET/CT is the imaging modality of choice for the initial staging of FDG-avid lymphoma. FDG-PET/CT changes initial staging in 10% to 30% of patients compared to CT, although this does not necessarily result in a management change for all cases.[19] The 2014 Lugano classification is the current system for staging and response assessment for lymphoma,[20] and includes criteria for FDG-PET/CT as well as CT for non–FDG-avid lymphoma subtypes or when PET/CT is not available. The Lugano classification includes a modified Ann Arbor staging system, but current management strategies rely more on prognostic and risk factors than stage alone.[19]

One major change in the Lugano classification is more judicious recommendations for using bone marrow biopsy as an initial staging procedure based on studies demonstrating that FDG-PET/CT is more accurate than standard iliac crest biopsy, particularly in HL and aggressive NHL subtypes.[21–24] In the current Lugano classification, FDG-PET/CT obviates the need for bone marrow biopsy in HL, and bone marrow biopsy in DLBCL is only recommended in the setting of a negative FDG-PET/CT and the need to identify a discordant lymphoma subtype in the bone marrow where management would be altered by a positive result.[19]

FDG-PET/CT is also now the modality of choice to assess response to treatment for FDG-avid lymphoma. This is based on the ability of PET to differentiate residual active tumor from post-treatment changes in residual mass on CT during and after treatment.[25] End of therapy (EOT) FDG-PET/CT is routinely performed approximately 6 to 8 weeks after completion of first-line systemic therapy or 2 to 3 months or more after completion of radiotherapy to determine remission status.[26] A positive EOT FDG-PET/CT portends a poor prognosis across most lymphoma subtypes and for DLBCL and HL, treatment is typically escalated in the setting of a positive EOT FDG-PET/CT scan,[27,28] although management changes are specific for different stages and risk factors and a complete review is beyond the scope of this paper. Interim FDG-PET/CT (iPET) is performed midway through treatment to determine chemosensitivity and early treatment response and provides prognostic information. Integration of how this information affects management has been more variable than EOT FDG-PET/CT and across lymphoma subtypes and is discussed further below.

For both EOT and interim FDG-PET/CT, the 5-point Deauville score (DS) is used to assess metabolic activity in tumor compared to internal references of mediastinal blood pool and normal liver uptake by visual assessment[19,29] (Figs. 2–4, Table 1). A DS of 1 or 2 is considered a complete metabolic response. A DS of 3 is interpreted depending on the timing of the PET/CT, the clinical context, type of treatment, and whether the patient is on a clinical trial. A DS of 4 or 5 on iPET is considered a partial treatment response if the FDG uptake has decreased from the baseline study or treatment failure if unchanged or increased from baseline. On EOT PET/CT, a DS of 4 or 5 is considered a treatment failure.

The prognostic value of the DS on iPET has been validated in both HL and NHL with patients receiving a DS score of 1 to 3 (interpreted as a negative PET) having a better outcome than those with a DS of 4 or 5 (interpreted as a positive PET).[30–32] This has led to risk-adapted therapy approaches based on iPET results and clinical trials have explored both escalation and de-escalation strategies and consider both efficacy and toxicity in regards to survival outcomes depending on disease stage and clinical prognostic factors.

In the RAPID trial, patients with early-stage HL and negative iPET after 3 cycles of adriamycin, vinblastine, bleomycin, and dacarbazine (ABVD) chemotherapy were randomly assigned to receive involved-field radiotherapy (IFRT) or no further treatment. A lower rate of progression and longer 3-year progression-free survival (PFS) was seen in the IFRT group, and the de-escalation strategy was not deemed noninferior to IFRT.[33] Another important finding in the RAPID trial was that the IFRT group had a higher rate of death because of nonprogression raising the question regarding late toxicity from radiation therapy. A more recent meta-analysis showed decreased PFS in patients with early HL by omitting radiotherapy based on negative iPET; however, overall survival (OS) was not changed.[34] The EORTC H10 trial investigated both escalation and de-escalation strategies in early-stage I/II HL depending on iPET results. Patients with a negative iPET after 2 cycles of ABVD were randomized to receive additional chemotherapy ± radiation therapy. The chemotherapy alone arm was closed early because of higher recurrence rates. In the iPET positive arm after 2 cycles of ABVD, patients randomized to the escalated to bleomycin, etoposide, adriamycin, cyclophosphamide, vincristine, procarbazine, and prednisone (BEACOPP) and IFRT arm had improved 5-year PFS compared with those randomized to ABVD + IFRT.[35] The role of iPET response assessment was evaluated in advanced HL on the RATHL trial, which found that the omission of bleomycin for those with negative iPET resulted in less pulmonary toxicity but not significantly lower efficacy.[36] Although the 2020 NCCN guidelines for HL recognize the potential value of iPET for some specific clinical scenarios and regimens in HL, caution is also advised that its role is not established for all clinical scenarios.[28]

Baseline FDG-PET/CT   Follow up FDG-PET/CT

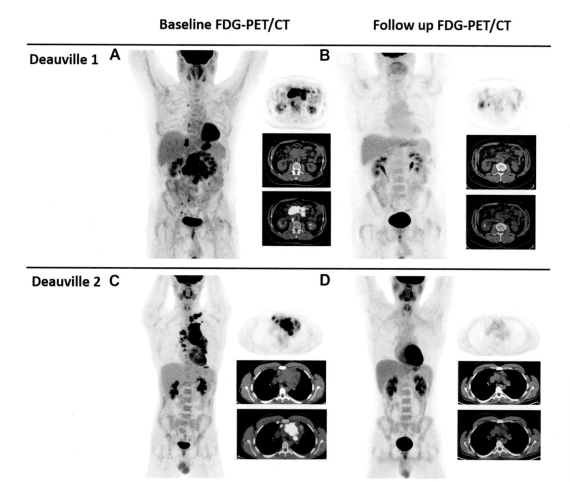

Fig. 2. (A) and (B) FDG-PET/CT performed for staging and response assessment of diffuse large B-cell lymphoma. (A) FDG-PET/CT MIP image performed at diagnosis before treatment showed an FDG-avid pancreatic mass, multiple FDG-avid nodules in the paravertebral fat, and FDG-avid mesenteric, right common iliac and right external iliac lymph nodes at sites of lymphoma. (B) End of treatment FDG-PET/CT MIP image performed 6 weeks after completing R-CHOP with interval resolution of FDG uptake at all sites of disease. Deauville 1. (C) and (D) FDG-PET/CT performed for staging and response assessment of classical Hodgkin lymphoma. (C) FDG-PET/CT MIP image performed at diagnosis before treatment showed an FDG-avid large mediastinal mass, with FDG-avid left supraclavicular, left epiphrenic, prevascular, and right internal mammary lymph nodes. (D) End of treatment FDG-PET/CT MIP image after completion of 4 cycles of ABVD and IFRT showed interval decrease in size and intensity of FDG uptake at all sites of disease, with small volume mediastinal soft tissue remaining with the intensity of uptake similar to that of mediastinal blood pool. Deauville 2.

Similar trials investigating iPET in patients with NHL have also been performed; however, the predictive value of the iPET for residual disease and outcome in DLBCL has been more mixed because of high false-positive rates.[37] The NCCN guidelines for DLBCL recommend against iPET for guiding therapy as well as confirmatory biopsies or follow-up imaging in the setting of a positive iPET and consideration of therapy change.[27]

Semiquantitative measures on iPET using SUV have also been proposed as an alternative to the qualitative DS. Several studies have found that a decrease in SUVmax of 66% between baseline and iPET is an optimal cut-off to determine whether patients with DLBCL were good responders or poor responders and using this has also proved to be predictive of response.[31,38,39] In these studies, iPET was performed after two cycles of chemotherapy and other studies have shown that when iPET is performed later, after 3 or 4 cycles, the predictive value is not superior to DS.[40,41] More recently, Schöder and colleagues reported that the change in SUVmax was predictive of OS in patients with DLBCL.[42] Other studies have reported methods of using SUVmax of residual tumor expressed as a ratio to SUVmax of the

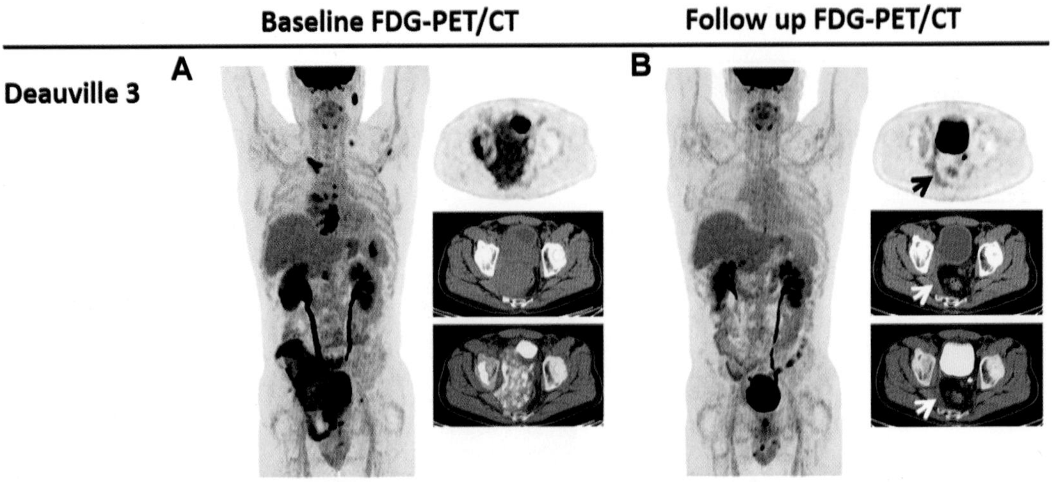

Baseline FDG-PET/CT   **Follow up FDG-PET/CT**

Deauville 3   A   B

Fig. 3. FDG-PET/CT performed for staging and response assessment of recurrent follicular lymphoma. (*A*) FDG-PET/CT performed at diagnosis before treatment showed a large FDG-avid mass centered in the right bony pelvis with extensive soft tissue extension into the pelvis, FDG-avid soft tissue in the right paracolic gutter, lateral to left temporalis muscle, at the splenic hilum, in the right anterior and mid chest wall, as well as left supraclavicular and right inguinal lymph nodes, and in the sternum, left scapula, right clavicle, T12, and left acetabulum at sites of lymphoma. (*B*) End of treatment FDG-PET/CT after 6 cycles of bendamustine and rituximab showed interval decrease in size and intensity of FDG uptake with the most avid uptake remaining in residual soft tissue in the right hemipelvis (*arrows*), with the intensity of uptake similar to normal liver parenchyma. Deauville 3.

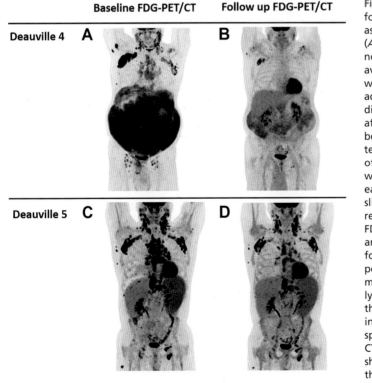

Baseline FDG-PET/CT   **Follow up FDG-PET/CT**

Deauville 4   A   B

Deauville 5   C   D

Fig. 4. (*A*) and (*B*) FDG-PET/CT performed for staging and response assessment of mantle cell lymphoma. (*A*) FDG-PET/CT performed at diagnosis before treatment showed FDG-avid peritoneal disease and ascites as well as multistation FDG-avid lymphadenopathy above and below the diaphragm. (*B*) Interim FDG-PET/CT after 3 cycles of rituximab-bendamustine showed significant interval decrease in size and intensity of FDG-avid tumor burden; however, with residual metabolically active disease demonstrating FDG uptake slightly greater than normal liver parenchyma. Deauville 4. (*C*) and (*D*) FDG-PET/CT performed for staging and response assessment of recurrent follicular lymphoma. (*C*) FDG-PET/CT performed at diagnosis before treatment showed multistation FDG-avid lymphadenopathy above and below the diaphragm, with mild diffusely increased FDG uptake in the enlarged spleen. (*D*) End of treatment FDG-PET/CT after treatment on a clinical trial showed slight interval decrease of the burden of metabolically active disease; however, the intensity of uptake still remained markedly greater than the uptake in the normal liver parenchyma. Deauville 5.

Table 1
Deauville score based on visual assessment of metabolic activity on FDG-PET

Deauville Score	Visual Assessment of Metabolic Activity on FDG-PET/CT
1	No uptake
2	Uptake less than or equal to mediastinal blood pool
3	Uptake greater than mediastinal blood pool and less than or equal to liver
4	Uptake moderately increased compared to liver
5	Uptake markedly increased compared to liver or any new site of uptake
X	Uptake not attributed to lymphoma

normal liver parenchyma which also showed predictive value.[43,44] Hasenclever and colleagues created a semiautomatic quantification measure qPET, which functions as an extension of the DS using SUVpeak of residual tumor, SUVmean of liver and mediastinal blood pool in a pediatric population with HL,[45] which has since been reproduced in adults.[46] These semiquantitative and quantitative measures are being evaluated with the aim of reducing interobserver variability for interpretation, although for now, the DS is still the official recommendation for response assessment.

The use of FDG-PET/CT in lymphomas other than DLBCL and HL and for follow-up after primary response assessment was recently reviewed by Karls and colleagues, which serves to provide more details for these indications.[47]

MULTIPLE MYELOMA
Classification

Multiple myeloma represents ~10% of hematologic malignancies and results from abnormal proliferation of malignant monoclonal plasma cells. Monoclonal gammopathy of undetermined significance (MGUS) and smoldering multiple myeloma (SMM) are asymptomatic premalignant precursors to MM.[48–50] The rate of progression to MM is ~1% per year for patients with MGUS and ~10% per year for those with SMM.[50,51] The diagnostic criteria for MGUS and SMM are shown in **Table 2**

and both require the absence of a myeloma-defining event. Myeloma-defining events indicate end-organ damage caused by the malignancy and include hypercalcemia, renal failure, anemia, and osteolytic bone lesions. Updated diagnostic criteria now include the presence of at least one of the biomarkers of malignancy as a myeloma-defining event, including findings on advanced imaging (see **Table 2**).[52] Solitary plasmacytoma is an early-stage malignancy in the plasma cell neoplasm spectrum and can occur in bone or be extramedullary and progress to MM. The risk of a solitary plasmacytoma progressing to MM is higher in the presence of minimal bone marrow involvement (20%–60% at 3 years) than no marrow involvement (~10%).[52] Throughout the spectrum of the plasma cell neoplasms, whole-body imaging is of the utmost importance as the presence or absence of lesions directly influences diagnosis.

Clinical Applications of Imaging and Diagnostic Criteria

Skeletal surveys have been replaced by whole-body CT, whole-body MRI, or FDG-PET/CT in the routine work-up for identifying MM-defining lesions. Both MRI and FDG-PET/CT have the benefit of assessing marrow replacing lesions before osseous destruction is visible on CT alone. Choosing the appropriate whole-body imaging modality can be difficult and the International Myeloma Working Group (IMWG) has devised recommendations for initial work-up, follow-up, and treatment response assessment for each subtype of plasma cell neoplasm (**Table 3**).[53] A detailed discussion of each modality is beyond the scope of this article and we have focused on the indications for FDG-PET/CT.

FDG-PET/CT is recommended for high-risk MGUS if initial whole-body CT is positive, as the first-line whole-body imaging study for patients with extramedullary solitary plasmacytoma, and in SMM if CT or MRI is unavailable.[53] Whole-body CT or FDG-PET/CT is recommended as first-line imaging for patients with MM, and again for these patients, FDG-PET/CT can also be considered in place of MRI.[53]

Bone lesions that fulfill criteria for initiating treatment for MM include the presence of more than one focal lesion on MRI and one or more osteolytic lesion on CT or FDG-PET/CT. Bone marrow lesions can also be detected on FDG-PET/CT in the absence of corresponding morphologic changes in the bone on CT. Three patterns of marrow disease are described: focal with one or more lesion (**Fig. 5**), diffuse infiltration (**Fig. 6**), or

Table 2
Diagnostic criteria for plasma cell neoplasms

	Monoclonal Gammopathy of Unknown Significance	Smoldering Multiple Myeloma	Multiple Myeloma
Serum monoclonal protein	<3 g/dL	≥3 g/dL	—
Urinary monoclonal protein	-	≥500 mg/24 h	—
Clonal bone marrow plasma cells	<10%	10%–60%	≥10% or biopsy proven plasmacytoma
Myeloma-defining events	Absent	Absent	Hypercalcemia Renal insufficiency Anemia Lytic bone lesion on XR, CT, PET/CT[a] >5 mm or >1 focal marrow signal abnormality on MRI Clonal bone marrow plasma cells 20%–60% Serum FLC ratio ≥100 (if involved FLC ≥100 mg/L)

[a] Presence of focal FDG uptake in the absence of a lytic lesion is not sufficient to fulfill the criteria for a bone lesion.

Table 3
International Myeloma Working Group imaging recommendations for initial work-up of myeloma

	1st Line Imaging Modality	2nd Line Imaging Modality
Monoclonal gammopathy of unknown significance	WB CT[a] [a]If unavailable, X-ray skeletal survey or WB MRI[b]	Negative WB CT: annual clinical surveillance Indeterminate WB CT: WB MRI[b] Positive WB CT: FDG-PET/CT
Smoldering multiple myeloma	WB CT or FDG-PET/CT	Negative: WB MRI[b] Indeterminate: WB MRI[b]
Solitary plasmacytoma	Bone: WB MRI[b] Extramedullary: FDG-PET/CT	
Multiple myeloma	WB CT or FDG-PET/CT	Negative: WB MRI[b] Indeterminate: WB MRI[b] If one unequivocal lesion on MRI, alternate imaging with WB CT and WB MRI every 6 mo and treat when increase in size or number of lesions

Abbreviation: WB, whole-body.
[a] If WB CT unavailable, X-ray skeletal survey or WB MRI[b].
[b] If WB MRI unavailable, MRI spine/pelvis or alternatively FDG-PET/CT can be performed.

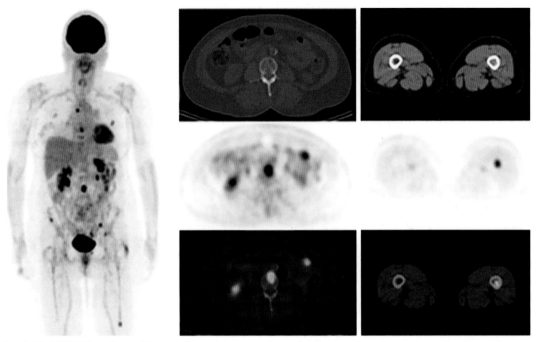

Fig. 5. FDG-PET/CT performed in a patient with new pain and a history of previously treated solitary plasmacytoma in the sacrum. FDG-PET/CT showed multiple focal sites of FDG-avid myeloma.

variegated (typically described on MRI). A combination of more than one pattern may also be seen. MRI is superior to FDG-PET/CT for evaluating diffuse marrow involvement,[54–56] but FDG-PET/CT detects lesions outside the MRI field of view and better assesses for extramedullary disease.[57]

FDG-PET/CT is the recommended imaging modality for assessing response to treatment in MM[58] because of its ability to distinguish metabolically active versus inactive (or treated) sites of disease (**Figs. 7** and **8**). FDG-PET/CT detects response to treatment earlier than MRI[59] and demonstrates superior prognostic value compared with MRI.[60] Negative FDG-PET/CT before autologous stem cell transplant (ASCT) is predictive of favorable post-transplant outcomes[61,62] and a decrease in FDG-avid disease or a negative FDG-PET/CT after transplant correlates with longer PFS.[63,64] FDG-PET/CT has also been shown to detect minimal residual disease (MRD) with clinical complete response after ASCT, which confers a poorer prognosis.[65]

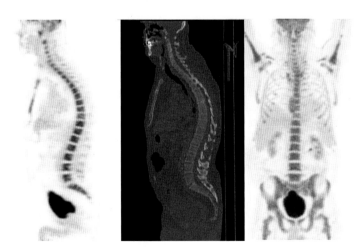

Fig. 6. FDG-PET/CT performed for assessment for multiple myeloma with bone marrow aspirate showing 80% marrow involvement with plasma cells. PET showed moderately increased diffuse FDG uptake throughout the marrow with no correlation on the CT component.

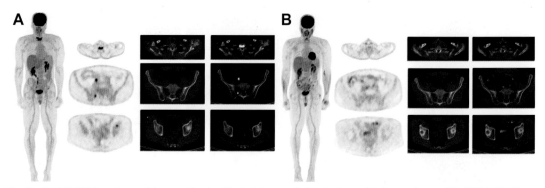

Fig. 7. FDG-PET/CT performed in a patient with IgG kappa light chain multiple myeloma. (*A*) FDG-PET/CT performed at initial diagnosis showed FDG-avid lytic lesions in T1 and in the pelvis. (*B*) FDG-PET/CT performed after 3 cycles of systemic therapy before autologous stem cell transplant showed interval resolution of the FDG uptake in all lytic lesions.

The IMWG defines categories of response, which include stringent complete response (sCR), complete response (CR), very good partial response (VGPR), partial response (PR), minimal response (MR), stable disease (SD), progressive disease (PD), and MRD.[66] Lesion size is part of the response assessment criteria and the presence of residual FDG uptake is considered in the MRD category,[66] but other potential useful predictors of outcome on FDG-PET/CT are not. To date, there are no standardized interpretation criteria for evaluating FDG-PET/CT in MM. An Italian group proposed diagnostic criteria in 2016 called Italian Myeloma criteria for PET Use (IMPeTUs) that combined a descriptive assessment with visual assessment,[67] modeled on the DS for lymphoma. IMPeTUs included a description of bone marrow uptake using the DS, the number and location of FDG-avid osseous lesions using DS with or without an associated osteolytic component on CT, the presence and location of extramedullary and paramedullary disease using DS, and the presence of fractures.[67] Initial assessments of this criteria suggested that it is easy to apply, reproducible,[67] and prospective clinical validation is currently awaited.[68]

LEUKEMIA
Classification and Diagnosis

Leukemia is subcategorized based on the malignant cell lineage of origin and whether the disease is acute affecting immature cells or chronic affecting mature cells. Initial diagnosis is based on complete blood count and peripheral blood smear, and then confirmed with bone marrow biopsy. Bone marrow biopsy is also used to assess the disease extent and to follow treatment response. The role of imaging in leukemia is limited and this article will specifically focus on extramedullary acute myeloid leukemia (AML).

Clinical Presentation and Natural History

Extramedullary AML, also known as myeloid sarcoma (MS), chloroma or granulocytic sarcoma, can present at initial diagnosis or relapse, with or without bone marrow involvement. Extramedullary AML is associated with a poor prognosis[69,70] and patients often require treatment intensification and allogeneic hematopoietic stem cell transplant.[71]

The detection of extramedullary AML on conventional anatomic imaging is challenging because of the wide spectrum of potential sites and manifestations. When extramedullary AML occurs without bone marrow involvement, the most common sites of disease are connective/soft tissue, breast/cutaneous tissue, and the gastrointestinal tract.[72]

Clinical Applications of Imaging and Diagnostic Criteria

Although there is a paucity of literature, several studies have suggested a role of FDG-PET/CT in the evaluation of extramedullary AML (**Fig. 9**). Reported sensitivities for detecting extramedullary AML with FDG-PET/CT range from 77% to 93%, with specificities of 70% to 97%.[71,73] A few studies reported that FDG-PET/CT finds additional disease not detected on clinical examination and SUVmax in sites of extramedullary disease ranged from 2 to 10 in 2 studies,[73,74] but a larger range of uptake was found in a third study.[75] Stölzel and colleagues found discordance with FDG-PET/CT response and bone marrow response in 6 of 10 patients[75]; 4 of these 6 had persistent metabolically active extramedullary disease post-treatment but remission on bone marrow biopsy and 3 of the 4 patients had subsequent relapses despite consolidative therapy.[75] Although it seems clear that extramedullary AML is detectable on

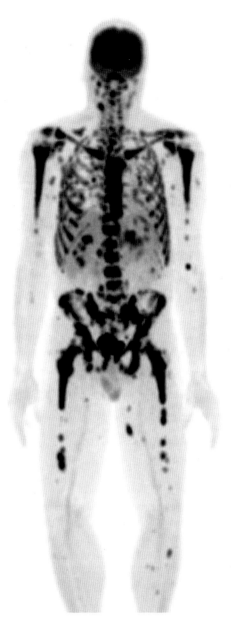

Fig. 8. FDG-PET/CT performed in a patient with IgG kappa multiple myeloma after 4 cycles of RVD, 2 cycles of DCEP, and prior peripheral blood stem cell transplant with widespread FDG-avid disease and no response to treatment.

FDG-PET/CT, the prognostic relevance and applications for assessing response still need to be defined.

HISTIOCYTOSIS
Classification

Histiocytoses are rare disorders characterized by abnormal proliferation of macrophages, monocytes, or dendritic cells. With more than 100

disease subtypes, the most recent classification was published in 2016 by the Histiocyte Society and defines 5 different categories of disease including Langerhans-related disorders (L group), cutaneous and myocutaneous disorders (C group), malignant histiocytoses (M group), Rosai-Dorfman disease (R group), and hemophagocytic lymphohistiocytosis and macrophage activation syndrome (H group).[76] Langerhans cell histiocytosis (LCH) is the most common subtype and is the focus of this section.

Clinical Presentation and Natural History

LCH can involve any organ resulting in a wide range of clinical manifestations in adults and children with significant variability of disease outcomes ranging from self-limiting to widespread disease with significant morbidity and mortality. The most common sites of disease in children include the bones (80% of cases), skin (33%), pituitary gland (25%), liver (15%), spleen (15%), marrow (15%), lungs (15%), lymph nodes (5%–10%), or the CNS (2%–4%), and pulmonary disease is more common in adults.[76] Single system involvement of LCH, either single-site or multisite, is considered as a low-risk disease and has a higher rate of spontaneous remission and more favorable outcomes,[77] whereas multisystem disease is frequently associated with a poor prognosis, especially when risk organs (lungs, liver, spleen, and marrow) are involved.[78,79]

Clinical Applications of Imaging and Diagnostic Criteria

Several small studies have evaluated the role of FDG-PET/CT for initial staging and assessing response to treatment for histiocytosis (**Fig. 10**). A common finding among the studies is the detection of occult sites of disease on conventional imaging leading to upstaging.[80,81] In a small number of these cases, upstaging led to a change in management.[82] Limitations of FDG-PET/CT for initial staging of LCH seem to be detection of pulmonary disease compared to CT[82] and detection of pituitary involvement compared to MRI.[81] FDG-PET/CT may detect partial or complete metabolic response to treatment earlier than conventional imaging,[82] which is important for these patients as rapid response to initial therapy is a prognostic factor.[83] Interestingly, one study reported higher SUVmax in lesions of multisite single organ and multisystem organ involvement compared with single organ, single-site involvement.[80] Although the role of FDG-PET/CT in patients with LCH still needs to be defined, a tailored approach depending on individual pattern of disease could be

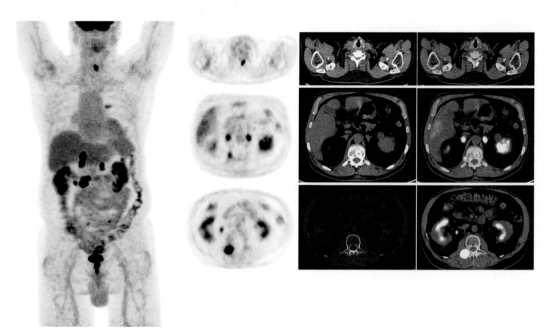

Fig. 9. FDG-PET/CT performed to assess for extramedullary disease in a patient with recurrent acute myeloid leukemia confirmed multifocal FDG-avid paravertebral disease, FDG-avid adrenal disease, and FDG-avid osseous disease.

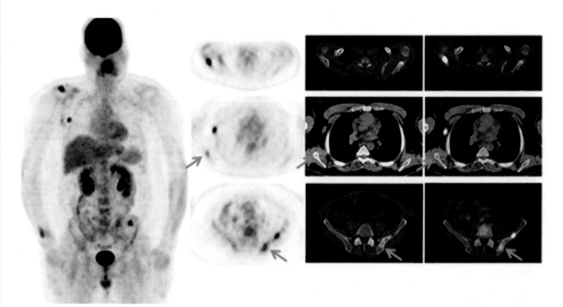

Fig. 10. FDG-PET/CT performed in a patient with known single system multisite Langerhans cell histiocytosis involving the right inferior scapula and right iliac bone previously treated with 6 cycles of vinblastine. FDG-PET/CT upstaged the disease, now with multisystem involvement with new FDG-avid lytic lesions in the right scapula and left iliac bone as well as an FDG-avid right axillary lymph node. Persistent low-level FDG uptake was also seen in the right inferior scapula and left iliac bone (arrows) at sites of partially treated disease.

considered and larger prospective studies are needed to further investigate.

DIAGNOSTIC CHALLENGES

A major diagnostic challenge that has emerged for interpreting FDG-PET/CT in hematologic malignancies is the approval of new immunotherapy agents. New patterns of response were first reported in solid tumors, but similar findings were subsequently seen in lymphoma.[84–86] Consequently, the Lugano classification was adapted for considerations of immunotherapy in the Lymphoma Response to Immunomodulatory Therapy Criteria (LYRIC).[87] Efforts have also been made to align the Lugano classification with the traditional Response Evaluation Criteria in Solid Tumors (RECIST),[88,89] called the Response Evaluation Criteria In Lymphoma (RECIL).[90] RECIL is mostly CT-based and some of the major differences from the Lugano classification are use of unidimensional measurements, maximum of 3 target lesions, and the addition of a Minor Response category for those with decreased tumor burden, but not meeting criteria for Partial Response.[90]

In LYRIC, the new response category "Indeterminate Response" was introduced to account for the different response patterns to immunotherapy that were seen in solid tumors,[87] specifically the pattern of pseudoprogression, which can be difficult to discern from true disease progression in the early phase of treatment. Applying LYRIC allows those with an overall increase in tumor burden without clinical deterioration, those with a new lesion or growth of more than 50% of one or more pre-existing lesions without overall progression, and those with an increase of FDG uptake in one or more lesions without an increase in size or number of lesions to be assigned Indeterminate Response[87] and continue on treatment for reassessment (in about 12 weeks) to make the determination of delayed response and pseudoprogression or true disease progression.[87] The authors of LYRIC anticipate that this indeterminate response category is temporary until there is a better understanding of how to distinguish true progression from delayed response and pseudoprogression.

Immune-related adverse events (irAEs) are often detectable on imaging before the development of symptoms,[85] and as a result allow for early intervention improving patient outcome. This is especially relevant for the interpretation of FDG-PET/CT as it is a highly sensitive imaging modality for detecting inflammatory change. In the setting of lymphoma, the diagnosis of a sarcoid-like postimmunotherapy granulomatosis can be difficult to discern from progressive disease (**Fig. 11**). Sarcoid-like postimmunotherapy granulomatosis typically presents with FDG-avid mediastinal and hilar lymphadenopathy and pulmonary nodules.[91,92] Pulmonary parenchymal findings can

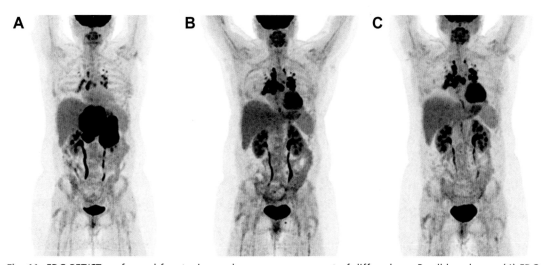

Fig. 11. FDG-PET/CT performed for staging and response assessment of diffuse large B-cell lymphoma. (*A*) FDG-PET/CT performed at baseline showed intense FDG uptake in hepatic and gastric masses; the biopsy-proven sites of lymphoma. There were also mildly FDG-avid mediastinal and bilateral hilar lymph nodes, with much less intense uptake than at the sites of lymphoma considered to represent sarcoid (*arrows*). (*B*) Interim FDG-PET/CT performed after 3 cycles of R-CHOP showed resolution of the FDG-avid hepatic and gastric masses. In contrast, the FDG-avid hilar and mediastinal lymph nodes increased in size and intensity; likely sarcoid or sarcoid-like reaction. (*C*) End of treatment FDG-PET/CT showed continued resolution of lymphoma (Deauville 1), but persistent FDG-avid intrathoracic lymph nodes consistent with sarcoid (Deauville X).

also be found in the absence of intrathoracic lymphadenopathy.[93] Other lymph node chain involvement has also been reported,[94] as well as other organ systems including skin,[95] spleen,[94,96] liver,[94] kidney,[94,97,98] and the CNS,[99] although much of the literature to date is generated from studies in patients with melanoma on ipilimumab. It is thought that sarcoid-like granulomatosis is less common with anti–PD-1 and anti–PD-L1 antibodies[100] nevertheless it is important when interpreting FDG-PET/CT for these patients to be aware of the wide spectrum of imaging findings associated with irAEs.[85]

As always when interpreting FDG-PET/CT, physiologic FDG uptake can be difficult to discern from pathologic uptake. This can be particularly challenging in the setting physiologic joint surface uptake in patients with myeloma mimicking a site of active disease, with metabolically active brown adipose tissue in patients with lymphoma limiting assessment for metabolically active lymph nodes or with physiologic uptake in the thymus or with rebound thymic hyperplasia in patients with lymphoma. Thymic FDG uptake can be challenging in patients with HL and lymphoblastic NHL who often have mediastinal disease.

False negatives can occur in the setting of transient metabolic suppression as a result of high-dose steroid use[58] that are used as part of the treatment regimen in many patients with hematologic malignancies. Other medications commonly used in patients with hematologic malignancies that can lead to false negatives as well as false positives include recombinant human granulocyte colony-stimulating factors (G-CSF) such as filgrastim and pegfilgrastim. These hematopoietic agents result in transient intense FDG uptake throughout the marrow[101–103] and also the spleen,[103,104] which can mimic diffuse malignant marrow involvement resulting in false-positive interpretation or masking of residual disease. The intense marrow uptake also accumulates FDG leading to altered biodistribution and less FDG available for tumor cell uptake leading to false-negative interpretation at sites of active disease. For patients with MM, calvarial lytic lesions can be falsely negative if they are obscured by the intense physiologic FDG uptake in the adjacent brain.[105] False negatives have been reported in certain sites of extramedullary AML including the meninges, the oral cavity, and skin, most likely as a result of the spatial resolution of FDG-PET/CT.[71]

SUMMARY

FDG-PET/CT has become an integral part in staging and evaluating response to treatment in many hematologic malignancies, particularly in lymphoma and MM. There is also a role for FDG-PET/CT in evaluating for less common manifestations of other hematologic malignancies such as detecting extramedullary acute leukemia as well as evaluating response to treatment. Histiocytoses are a rare group of disorders for which the role of FDG-PET/CT is much less defined; however, in time as more studies evaluate its use, FDG-PET/CT may also prove useful for the staging and response assessment for these disorders as well.

CLINICS CARE POINTS

- FDG-PET/CT is the imaging modality of choice for staging and assessing response to treatment for most lymphomas.
- FDG-PET/CT is useful for detecting high grade transformation of more indolent lymphomas and can be used to guide biopsy to areas of more intense uptake that may harbour more aggressive disease.
- Interim PET has prognostic value in patients with lymphoma and this had led to risk-adapted therapy approaches.
- In patients with multiple myeloma FDG-PET/CT can detect sites of marrow involvement before a lytic lesion is visible on CT, but the presence of FDG uptake alone without a lytic lesion does not meet the criteria for a myeloma-defining event.
- FDG-PET/CT has prognostic value in patients with multiple myeloma and detects response to treatment earlier than MRI.
- Extramedullary AML and histiocytosis are detectable on FDG-PET/CT although the prognostic relevance and clinical applications for assessing treatment response are yet to be defined.
- New immunotherapy agents have been approved for treating lymphoma. These drugs have different response patterns to conventional chemotherapy and patients can develop immune-related adverse events as a result of treatment that are detectable on PET/CT before the patient is symptomatic, both of which can mimic worsening lymphoma.

DISCLOSURE

N.M. Hughes has nothing to disclose. H.A. Jacene discloses the following: Advanced

Accelerator Applications, consulting; American Roentgen Ray Society, stipend; Australian and New Zealand Urogenital and Prostate Cancer Clinical Trial Group, honoraria; Cambridge University Press, royalties; Janssen, honoraria; and Siemens Healthcare and GTx, Inc: research support to the institution.

REFERENCES

1. Swerdlow SH, Campo E, Pileri SA, et al. The 2016 revision of the World Health Organization classification of lymphoid neoplasms. Blood 2016. https://doi.org/10.1182/blood-2016-01-643569.

2. Arber DA, Orazi A, Hasserjian R, et al. The 2016 revision to the World Health Organization classification of myeloid neoplasms and acute leukemia. Blood 2016. https://doi.org/10.1182/blood-2016-03-643544.

3. Chow KU, Luxembourg B, Seifried E, et al. Spleen size is significantly influenced by body height and sex: Establishment of normal values for spleen size at US with a cohort of 1200 healthy individuals. Radiology 2016. https://doi.org/10.1148/radiol.2015150887.

4. Boellaard R, Delgado-Bolton R, Oyen WJG, et al. FDG PET/CT: EANM procedure guidelines for tumour imaging: version 2.0. Eur J Nucl Med Mol Imaging 2015. https://doi.org/10.1007/s00259-014-2961-x.

5. Kevin P, Banks MD, Chair Helen R, et al. ACR–SPR practice parameter for performing FDG-PET/CT in oncology. Am Coll Radiol 2014. Available at: https://www.acr.org/-/media/ACR/Files/Practice-Parameters/fdg-pet-ct.pdf.

6. Anderson T, Chabner BA, Young RC, et al. Malignant lymphoma I. The histology and staging of 473 patients at the national cancer institute. Cancer 1982. https://doi.org/10.1002/1097-0142(19821215)50:12<2699::AID-CNCR2820501202>3.0.CO;2-A.

7. Wahlin BE, Yri OE, Kimby E, et al. Clinical significance of the WHO grades of follicular lymphoma in a population-based cohort of 505 patients with long follow-up times. Br J Haematol 2012. https://doi.org/10.1111/j.1365-2141.2011.08942.x.

8. Paes FM, Kalkanis DG, Sideras PA, et al. FDG PET/CT of extranodal involvement in non-Hodgkin lymphoma and Hodgkin disease. Radiographics 2010. https://doi.org/10.1148/rg.301095088.

9. Freedman ASNL. In: Kufe DW, Pollock RE, Weichselbaum RR, et al, editors. Holland-Frei Cancer Medicine. 6th editio. Hamilton (ON): BC Decker; 2003.

10. Roth SL, Sack H, Havemann K, et al. Contiguous pattern spreading in patients with Hodgkin's disease. Radiother Oncol 1998;47(1):7–16. https://doi.org/10.1016/S0167-8140(97)00208-9.

11. Newman JS, Francis IR, Kaminski MS, et al. Imaging of lymphoma with PET with 2-[F-18]-fluoro-2-deoxy-D-glucose: Correlation with CT. Radiology 1994. https://doi.org/10.1148/radiology.190.1.8259386.

12. Weiler-Sagie M, Bushelev O, Epelbaum R, et al. 18F-FDG avidity in lymphoma readdressed: A study of 766 patients. J Nucl Med 2010. https://doi.org/10.2967/jnumed.109.067892.

13. Schöder H, Noy A, Gönen M, et al. Intensity of 18fluorodeoxyglucose uptake in positron emission tomography distinguishes between indolent and aggressive non-Hodgkin's lymphoma. J Clin Oncol 2005. https://doi.org/10.1200/JCO.2005.12.072.

14. Rodriguez M, Rehn S, Ahlstrom H, et al. Predicting malignancy grade with PET in non-Hodgkin's lymphoma. J Nucl Med 1995;36(10):1790–6.

15. Bruzzi JF, Macapinlac H, Tsimberidou AM, et al. Detection of Richter's transformation of chronic lymphocytic leukemia by PET/CT. J Nucl Med 2006;47(8):1267–73.

16. Bodet-Milin C, Kraeber-Bodéré F, Moreau P, et al. Investigation of FDG-PET/CT imaging to guide biopsies in the detection of histological transformation of indolent lymphoma. Haematologica 2008. https://doi.org/10.3324/haematol.12013.

17. Holalkere N, Hochberg EP, Takvorian R, et al. Intensity of FDG Uptake on PET Scan Varies by Histologic Subtype of Hodgkin Lymphoma. Blood 2007. https://doi.org/10.1182/blood.v110.11.4393.4393.

18. Hutchings M, Loft A, Hansen M, et al. Different histopathological subtypes of Hodgkin lymphoma show significantly different levels of FDG uptake. Hematol Oncol 2006. https://doi.org/10.1002/hon.782.

19. Cheson BD, Fisher RI, Barrington SF, et al. Recommendations for initial evaluation, staging, and response assessment of hodgkin and non-hodgkin lymphoma: The lugano classification. J Clin Oncol 2014. https://doi.org/10.1200/JCO.2013.54.8800.

20. Cheson BD, Pfistner B, Juweid ME, et al. Revised response criteria for malignant lymphoma. J Clin Oncol 2007. https://doi.org/10.1200/JCO.2006.09.2403.

21. Pakos EE, Fotopoulos AD, Ioannidis JPA. 18F-FDG PET for evaluation of bone marrow infiltration in staging of lymphoma: A meta-analysis. J Nucl Med 2005;46(6):958–63.

22. Adams HJA, Kwee TC, de Keizer B, et al. Systematic review and meta-analysis on the diagnostic performance of FDG-PET/CT in detecting bone marrow involvement in newly diagnosed Hodgkin lymphoma: is bone marrow biopsy still necessary? Ann Oncol 2014. https://doi.org/10.1093/annonc/mdt533.

23. Adams HJA, Kwee TC, De Keizer B, et al. FDG PET/CT for the detection of bone marrow

involvement in diffuse large B-cell lymphoma: systematic review and meta-analysis. Eur J Nucl Med Mol Imaging 2014. https://doi.org/10.1007/s00259-013-2623-4.

24. Chen YK, Yeh CL, Tsui CC, et al. F-18 FDG PET for evaluation of bone marrow involvement in non-hodgkin lymphoma: A meta-analysis. Clin Nucl Med 2011. https://doi.org/10.1097/RLU.0b013e318217aeff.

25. Kim EE, Chung SK, Haynie TP, et al. Differentiation of residual or recurrent tumors from post-treatment changes with F-18 FDG PET. Radiographics 1992. https://doi.org/10.1148/radiographics.12.2.1561416.

26. Barrington SF, Mikhaeel NG, Kostakoglu L, et al. Role of imaging in the staging and response assessment of lymphoma: Consensus of the international conference on malignant lymphomas imaging working group. J Clin Oncol 2014. https://doi.org/10.1200/JCO.2013.53.5229.

27. Zelenetz AD, Gordon LI, Abramson JS, et al. NCCN Guidelines Insights: B-Cell Lymphomas, Version 3.2019. J Natl Compr Cancer Netw 2019. https://doi.org/10.6004/jnccn.2019.0029.

28. Hoppe RT, Advani RH, Ai WZ, et al. Hodgkin Lymphoma, Version 2.2020, NCCN Clinical Practice Guidelines in Oncology. J Natl Compr Cancer Netw 2020. https://doi.org/10.6004/jnccn.2020.0026.

29. Meignan M, Gallamini A, Haioun C. Report on the First International Workshop on interim-PET scan in lymphoma. Leuk Lymphoma 2009. https://doi.org/10.1080/10428190903040048.

30. Gallamini A, Barrington SF, Biggi A, et al. The predictive role of interim positron emission tomography for Hodgkin lymphoma treatment outcome is confirmed using the interpretation criteria of the Deauville five-point scale. Haematologica 2014. https://doi.org/10.3324/haematol.2013.103218.

31. Itti E, Meignan M, Berriolo-Riedinger A, et al. An international confirmatory study of the prognostic value of early PET/CT in diffuse large B-cell lymphoma: comparison between Deauville criteria and ΔsUVmax. Eur J Nucl Med Mol Imaging 2013. https://doi.org/10.1007/s00259-013-2435-6.

32. Qian L, Yan M, Zhang W, et al. Prognostic value of interim 18F-FDG PET/CT in T-cell lymphomas. Leuk Lymphoma 2020. https://doi.org/10.1080/10428194.2019.1697815.

33. Radford J, Illidge T, Counsell N, et al. Results of a trial of PET-directed therapy for early-stage Hodgkin's lymphoma. N Engl J Med 2015. https://doi.org/10.1056/NEJMoa1408648.

34. Shaikh PM, Alite F, Pugliese N, et al. Consolidation radiotherapy following positron emission tomography complete response in early-stage Hodgkin lymphoma: a meta-analysis. Leuk Lymphoma 2020. https://doi.org/10.1080/10428194.2020.1725506.

35. André MPE, Girinsky T, Federico M, et al. Early positron emission tomography response-adapted treatment in stage I and II hodgkin lymphoma: final results of the randomized EORTC/LYSA/FIL H10 trial. J Clin Oncol 2017. https://doi.org/10.1200/JCO.2016.68.6394.

36. Johnson P, Federico M, Kirkwood A, et al. Adapted treatment guided by interim PET-CT scan in advanced Hodgkin's lymphoma. N Engl J Med 2016. https://doi.org/10.1056/NEJMoa1510093.

37. Coughlan M, Elstrom R. The use of FDG-PET in diffuse large B cell lymphoma (DLBCL): predicting outcome following first line therapy. Cancer Imaging 2014. https://doi.org/10.1186/s40644-014-0034-9.

38. Casasnovas RO, Meignan M, Berriolo-Riedinger A, et al. SUVmax reduction improves early prognosis value of interim positron emission tomography scans in diffuse large B-cell lymphoma. Blood 2011. https://doi.org/10.1182/blood-2010-12-327767.

39. Lin C, Itti E, Haioun C, et al. Early 18F-FDG PET for prediction of prognosis in patients with diffuse large B-cell lymphoma: SUV-based assessment versus visual analysis. J Nucl Med 2007. https://doi.org/10.2967/jnumed.107.042093.

40. Fuertes S, Setoain X, Lopez-Guillermo A, et al. Interim FDG PET/CT as a prognostic factor in diffuse large B-cell lymphoma. Eur J Nucl Med Mol Imaging 2013. https://doi.org/10.1007/s00259-012-2320-8.

41. Yang DH, Ahn JS, Byun BH, et al. Interim PET/CT-based prognostic model for the treatment of diffuse large B cell lymphoma in the post-rituximab era. Ann Hematol 2013. https://doi.org/10.1007/s00277-012-1640-x.

42. Schöder H, Polley MYC, Knopp MV, et al. Prognostic value of interim FDG-PET in diffuse large cell lymphoma: results from the CALGB 50303 Clinical Trial. Blood 2020. https://doi.org/10.1182/blood.2019003277.

43. Annunziata S, Cuccaro A, Calcagni ML, et al. Interim FDG-PET/CT in Hodgkin lymphoma: the prognostic role of the ratio between target lesion and liver SUVmax (rPET). Ann Nucl Med 2016. https://doi.org/10.1007/s12149-016-1092-9.

44. Fan Y, Zhang Y, Yang Z, et al. Evaluating early interim fluorine-18 fluorodeoxyglucose positron emission tomography/computed tomography with the SUVmax-liver-based interpretation for predicting the outcome in diffuse large B-cell lymphoma. Leuk Lymphoma 2017. https://doi.org/10.1080/10428194.2016.1277384.

45. Hasenclever D, Kurch L, Mauz-Körholz C, et al. qPET - A quantitative extension of the Deauville

scale to assess response in interim FDG-PET scans in lymphoma. Eur J Nucl Med Mol Imaging 2014. https://doi.org/10.1007/s00259-014-2715-9.

46. Georgi TW, Kurch L, Hasenclever D, et al. Quantitative assessment of interim PET in Hodgkin lymphoma: an evaluation of the qPET method in adult patients in the RAPID trial. PLoS One 2020. https://doi.org/10.1371/journal.pone.0231027.

47. Karls S, Shah H, Jacene H. PET/CT for lymphoma post-therapy response assessment in other lymphomas, response assessment for autologous stem cell transplant, and lymphoma follow-up. Semin Nucl Med 2018. https://doi.org/10.1053/j.semnuclmed.2017.09.004.

48. Landgren O, Kyle RA, Pfeiffer RM, et al. Monoclonal gammopathy of undetermined significance (MGUS) consistently precedes multiple myeloma: a prospective study. Blood 2009. https://doi.org/10.1182/blood-2008-12-194241.

49. Weiss BM, Abadie J, Verma P, et al. A monoclonal gammopathy precedes multiple myeloma in most patients. Blood 2009. https://doi.org/10.1182/blood-2008-12-195008.

50. Kyle RA, Remstein ED, Therneau TM, et al. Clinical course and prognosis of smoldering (asymptomatic) multiple myeloma. N Engl J Med 2007. https://doi.org/10.1056/nejmoa070389.

51. Kyle RA, Therneau TM, Rajkumar SV, et al. A long-term study of prognosis in monoclonal gammopathy of undetermined significance. N Engl J Med 2002. https://doi.org/10.1056/nejmoa01133202.

52. Rajkumar SV. Updated diagnostic criteria and staging system for multiple myeloma. Am Soc Clin Oncol Educ B 2016. https://doi.org/10.1200/edbk_159009.

53. Hillengass J, Usmani S, Rajkumar SV, et al. International myeloma working group consensus recommendations on imaging in monoclonal plasma cell disorders. Lancet Oncol 2019. https://doi.org/10.1016/S1470-2045(19)30309-2.

54. Zamagni E, Nanni C, Patriarca F, et al. A prospective comparison of 18F-fluorodeoxyglucose positron emission tomography-computed tomography, magnetic resonance imaging and whole-body planar radiographs in the assessment of bone disease in newly diagnosed multiple myeloma. Haematologica 2007. https://doi.org/10.3324/haematol.10554.

55. Fonti R, Salvatore B, Quarantelli M, et al. 18F-FDG PET/CT, 99mTc-MIBI, and MRI in evaluation of patients with multiple myeloma. J Nucl Med 2008. https://doi.org/10.2967/jnumed.107.045641.

56. Pawlyn C, Fowkes L, Otero S, et al. Whole-body diffusion-weighted MRI: A new gold standard for assessing disease burden in patients with multiple myeloma? Leukemia 2016. https://doi.org/10.1038/leu.2015.338.

57. Salaun PY, Gastinne T, Frampas E, et al. FDG-positron-emission tomography for staging and therapeutic assessment in patients with plasmacytoma. Haematologica 2008. https://doi.org/10.3324/haematol.12654.

58. Cavo M, Terpos E, Nanni C, et al. Role of 18F-FDG PET/CT in the diagnosis and management of multiple myeloma and other plasma cell disorders: a consensus statement by the International Myeloma Working Group. Lancet Oncol 2017; 18(4):e206–17. https://doi.org/10.1016/S1470-2045(17)30189-4.

59. Spinnato P, Bazzocchi A, Brioli A, et al. Contrast enhanced MRI and 18F-FDG PET-CT in the assessment of multiple myeloma: A comparison of results in different phases of the disease. Eur J Radiol 2012. https://doi.org/10.1016/j.ejrad.2012.06.028.

60. Moreau P, Attal M, Caillot D, et al. Prospective evaluation of magnetic resonance imaging and [18F]fluorodeoxyglucose positron emission tomography-computed tomography at diagnosis and before maintenance therapy in symptomatic patients with multiple myeloma included in the IFM/DFCI 2009 trial. J Clin Oncol 2017. https://doi.org/10.1200/JCO.2017.72.2975.

61. Bartel TB, Haessler J, Brown TLY, et al. F18-fluorodeoxyglucose positron emission tomography in the context of other imaging techniques and prognostic factors in multiple myeloma. Blood 2009. https://doi.org/10.1182/blood-2009-03-213280.

62. Usmani SZ, Mitchell A, Waheed S, et al. Prognostic implications of serial 18-fluoro-deoxyglucose emission tomography in multiple myeloma treated with total therapy 3. Blood 2013. https://doi.org/10.1182/blood-2012-08-451690.

63. Beksac M, Gunduz M, Ozen M, et al. Impact of PET-CT response on survival parameters following autologous stem cell transplantation among patients with multiple myeloma: comparison of two cut-off values. Blood 2014. https://doi.org/10.1182/blood.v124.21.3983.3983.

64. Patriarca F, Carobolante F, Zamagni E, et al. The role of positron emission tomography with 18F-fluorodeoxyglucose integrated with computed tomography in the evaluation of patients with multiple myeloma undergoing allogeneic stem cell transplantation. Biol Blood Marrow Transpl 2015. https://doi.org/10.1016/j.bbmt.2015.03.001.

65. Zamagni E, Patriarca F, Nanni C, et al. Prognostic relevance of 18-F FDG PET/CT in newly diagnosed multiple myeloma patients treated with up-front autologous transplantation. Blood 2011. https://doi.org/10.1182/blood-2011-06-361386.

66. Kumar S, Paiva B, Anderson KC, et al. International Myeloma Working Group consensus criteria for response and minimal residual disease

assessment in multiple myeloma. Lancet Oncol 2016. https://doi.org/10.1016/S1470-2045(16)30206-6.

67. Nanni C, Zamagni E, Versari A, et al. Image interpretation criteria for FDG PET/CT in multiple myeloma: a new proposal from an Italian expert panel. IMPeTUs (Italian Myeloma criteria for PET USe). Eur J Nucl Med Mol Imaging 2016. https://doi.org/10.1007/s00259-015-3200-9.

68. Nanni C, Versari A, Chauvie S, et al. Interpretation criteria for FDG PET/CT in multiple myeloma (IMPeTUs): final results. IMPeTUs (Italian myeloma criteria for PET USe). Eur J Nucl Med Mol Imaging 2018. https://doi.org/10.1007/s00259-017-3909-8.

69. Schmid C, Schleuning M, Schwerdtfeger R, et al. Long-term survival in refractory acute myeloid leukemia after sequential treatment with chemotherapy and reduced-intensity conditioning for allogeneic stem cell transplantation. Blood 2006. https://doi.org/10.1182/blood-2005-10-4165.

70. Schaich M, Schlenk RF, Al-Ali HK, et al. Prognosis of acute myeloid leukemia patients up to 60 years of age exhibiting trisomy 8 within a non-complex karyotype: individual patient data-based meta-analysis of the German Acute Myeloid Leukemia Intergroup. Haematologica 2007. https://doi.org/10.3324/haematol.11100.

71. Zhou WL, Wu HB, Wang LJ, et al. Usefulness and pitfalls of F-18-FDG PET/CT for diagnosing extramedullary acute leukemia. Eur J Radiol 2016. https://doi.org/10.1016/j.ejrad.2015.11.019.

72. Goyal G, Bartley AC, Patnaik MM, et al. Clinical features and outcomes of extramedullary myeloid sarcoma in the United States: Analysis using a national data set. Blood Cancer J 2017. https://doi.org/10.1038/bcj.2017.79.

73. Stölzel F, Röllig C, Radke J, et al. 18F-FDG-PET/CT for detection of extramedullary acute myeloid leukemia. Haematologica 2011. https://doi.org/10.3324/haematol.2011.045047.

74. Cribe ASWI, Steenhof M, Marcher CW, et al. Extramedullary disease in patients with acute myeloid leukemia assessed by (18)F-FDG PET. Eur J Haematol 2013. https://doi.org/10.1111/ejh.12085.

75. Stölzel F, Lüer T, Löck S, et al. The prevalence of extramedullary acute myeloid leukemia detected by 18FDG-PET/CT: Final results from the prospective PETAML trial. Haematologica 2020. https://doi.org/10.3324/haematol.2019.223032.

76. Emile JF, Abla O, Fraitag S, et al. Revised classification of histiocytoses and neoplasms of the macrophage-dendritic cell lineages. Blood 2016. https://doi.org/10.1182/blood-2016-01-690636.

77. Titgemeyer C, Grois N, Minkov M, et al. Pattern and course of single-system disease in langerhans cell histiocytosis data from the DAL-HX 83- and 90-study. Med Pediatr Oncol 2001. https://doi.org/10.1002/mpo.1178.

78. Lahey ME. Prognostic factors in histiocytosis X. Am J Pediatr Hematol Oncol 1981.

79. Gadner H, Grois N, Arico M, et al. A randomized trial of treatment for multisystem Langerhans' cell histiocytosis. J Pediatr 2001. https://doi.org/10.1067/mpd.2001.111331.

80. Lee HJ, Ahn BC, Lee SW, et al. The usefulness of F-18 fluorodeoxyglucose positron emission tomography/computed tomography in patients with Langerhans cell histiocytosis. Ann Nucl Med 2012. https://doi.org/10.1007/s12149-012-0635-y.

81. Obert J, Vercellino L, Van Der Gucht A, et al. 18F-fluorodeoxyglucose positron emission tomography-computed tomography in the management of adult multisystem Langerhans cell histiocytosis. Eur J Nucl Med Mol Imaging 2017. https://doi.org/10.1007/s00259-016-3521-3.

82. Albano D, Bosio G, Giubbini R, et al. Role of 18F-FDG PET/CT in patients affected by Langerhans cell histiocytosis. Jpn J Radiol 2017. https://doi.org/10.1007/s11604-017-0668-1.

83. Gadner H, Grois N, Pötschger U, et al. Improved outcome in multisystem Langerhans cell histiocytosis is associated with therapy intensification. Blood 2008. https://doi.org/10.1182/blood-2007-08-106211.

84. Wolchok JD, Hoos A, O'Day S, et al. Guidelines for the evaluation of immune therapy activity in solid tumors: Immune-related response criteria. Clin Cancer Res 2009. https://doi.org/10.1158/1078-0432.CCR-09-1624.

85. Kwak JJ, Tirumani SH, Van den Abbeele AD, et al. Cancer immunotherapy: Imaging assessment of novel treatment response patterns and immune-related adverse events. Radiographics 2015. https://doi.org/10.1148/rg.352140121.

86. Pianko MJ, Moskowitz AJ, Lesokhin AM. Immunotherapy of lymphoma and myeloma: Facts and hopes. Clin Cancer Res 2018. https://doi.org/10.1158/1078-0432.CCR-17-0539.

87. Cheson BD, Ansell S, Schwartz L, et al. Refinement of the Lugano Classification lymphoma response criteria in the era of immunomodulatory therapy. Blood 2016. https://doi.org/10.1182/blood-2016-05-718528.

88. Eisenhauer EA, Therasse P, Bogaerts J, et al. New response evaluation criteria in solid tumours: Revised RECIST guideline (version 1.1). Eur J Cancer 2009. https://doi.org/10.1016/j.ejca.2008.10.026.

89. Schwartz LH, Litière S, De Vries E, et al. RECIST 1.1 - Update and clarification: From the RECIST committee. Eur J Cancer 2016. https://doi.org/10.1016/j.ejca.2016.03.081.

90. Younes A, Hilden P, Coiffier B, et al. International Working Group consensus response evaluation criteria in lymphoma (RECIL 2017). Ann Oncol 2017. https://doi.org/10.1093/annonc/mdx097.

91. Wilgenhof S, Morlion V, Seghers AC, et al. Sarcoidosis in a patient with metastatic melanoma sequentially treated with anti-CTLA-4 monoclonal antibody and selective BRAF inhibitor. Anticancer Res 2012.

92. Eckert A, Schoeffler A, Dalle S, et al. Anti-CTLA4 monoclonal antibody induced sarcoidosis in a metastatic melanoma patient. Dermatology 2008. https://doi.org/10.1159/000161122.

93. Nishino M, Sholl LM, Awad MM, et al. Sarcoid-like granulomatosis of the lung related to immune-checkpoint inhibitors: Distinct clinical and imaging features of a unique immune-related adverse event. Cancer Immunol Res 2018. https://doi.org/10.1158/2326-6066.CIR-17-0715.

94. Chowdhury FU, Sheerin F, Bradley KM, et al. Sarcoid-like reaction to malignancy on whole-body integrated 18F-FDG PET/CT: prevalence and disease pattern. Clin Radiol 2009. https://doi.org/10.1016/j.crad.2009.03.005.

95. Dimitriou F, Frauchiger AL, Urosevic-Maiwald M, et al. Sarcoid-like reactions in patients receiving modern melanoma treatment. Melanoma Res 2018. https://doi.org/10.1097/CMR.0000000000000437.

96. Andersen R, Nørgaard P, Al-Jailawi MKM, et al. Late development of splenic sarcoidosis-like lesions in a patient with metastatic melanoma and long-lasting clinical response to ipilimumab. Oncoimmunology 2014. https://doi.org/10.4161/21624011.2014.954506.

97. Izzedine H, Gueutin V, Gharbi C, et al. Kidney injuries related to ipilimumab. Invest New Drugs 2014. https://doi.org/10.1007/s10637-014-0092-7.

98. Thajudeen B, Madhrira M, Bracamonte E, et al. Ipilimumab granulomatous interstitial nephritis. Am J Ther 2015. https://doi.org/10.1097/MJT.0b013e3182a32ddc.

99. Murphy KP, Kennedy MP, Barry JE, et al. New-onset mediastinal and central nervous system sarcoidosis in a patient with metastatic melanoma undergoing CTLA4 monoclonal antibody treatment. Oncol Res Treat 2014. https://doi.org/10.1159/000362614.

100. Gkiozos I, Kopitopoulou A, Kalkanis A, et al. Sarcoidosis-like reactions induced by checkpoint inhibitors. J Thorac Oncol 2018. https://doi.org/10.1016/j.jtho.2018.04.031.

101. Sugawara Y, Fisher SJ, Zasadny KR, et al. Preclinical and clinical studies of bone marrow uptake of fluorine-18- fluorodeoxyglucose with or without granulocyte colony-stimulating factor during chemotherapy. J Clin Oncol 1998. https://doi.org/10.1200/JCO.1998.16.1.173.

102. Hollinger EF, Alibazoglu H, Ali A, et al. Hematopoietic cytokine-mediated FDG uptake simulates the appearance of diffuse metastatic disease on whole-body PET imaging. Clin Nucl Med 1998. https://doi.org/10.1097/00003072-199802000-00007.

103. Jacene HA, Ishimori T, Engles JM, et al. Effects of pegfilgrastim on normal biodistribution of 18F-FDG: Preclinical and clinical studies. J Nucl Med 2006.

104. Sugawara Y, Zasadny KR, Kison PV, et al. Splenic fluorodeoxyglucose uptake increased by granulocyte colony- stimulating factor therapy: PET imaging results. J Nucl Med 1999;40(9):1456–62.

105. Van Lammeren-Venema D, Regelink JC, Riphagen II, et al. 18F-fluoro-deoxyglucose positron emission tomography in assessment of myeloma-related bone disease: A systematic review. Cancer 2012. https://doi.org/10.1002/cncr.26467.

PET Imaging for Breast Cancer

Amy M. Fowler, MD, PhD[a,b,c,]*, Steve Y. Cho, MD[c,d]

KEYWORDS

- Breast cancer • Positron emission tomography • Computed tomography
- Magnetic resonance imaging • ^{18}F-FDG • ^{18}F-FES

KEY POINTS

- Clinical indications of FDG PET/CT for breast cancer include initial systemic staging, suspected recurrence, and treatment response assessment.
- FDG PET/CT is not recommended for primary breast cancer detection, distinguishing benign from malignant breast lesions, or local tumor staging for newly diagnosed breast cancer.
- FDG PET/MRI has less radiation dose and may have superior performance for detecting hepatic and osseous metastases than FDG PET/CT.
- FES has recently obtained FDA approval for clinical use with PET imaging to detect ER-positive lesions in patients with recurrent or metastatic breast cancer.

INTRODUCTION

Breast cancer is the most common malignancy diagnosed in women and is the leading cause of cancer-related deaths for women worldwide.[1] In 2020, approximately 276,480 women will be diagnosed with invasive breast cancer and 42,170 women will die from breast cancer in the United States.[2] Breast cancer can also occur in men, although much less often than in women.[2]

Breast cancer is a heterogeneous disease with several histologic and molecular subtypes associated with distinct prognoses and therapeutic options. The most common invasive histologic subtypes are invasive ductal carcinoma and invasive lobular carcinoma.[3] Molecular subtypes of invasive breast cancer are classified by the expression of tumor biomarkers including estrogen receptor (ER), progesterone receptor (PR), and human epidermal growth factor receptor-2 (HER2). Hormone receptor positive (ER and/or PR positive), HER2-negative breast cancer is the most common molecular subtype (73%).[4]

Imaging with mammography, ultrasound, magnetic resonance imaging (MRI), computed tomography (CT), and bone scintigraphy plays an integral part in the detection, staging, and monitoring of breast cancer. Positron emission tomography (PET) has also demonstrated clinical utility for breast cancer. This article reviews the use of PET imaging for patients with breast cancer, highlighting the clinical indications and limitations of 2-deoxy-2-[^{18}F]fluoro-D-glucose (FDG) PET/CT, the potential use of PET/MRI, and 16α-[^{18}F]fluoroestradiol (FES), a newly approved radiopharmaceutical for estrogen receptor imaging.

CLINICAL INDICATIONS FOR FDG PET/CT

The Society of Nuclear Medicine and Molecular Imaging (SNMMI) and the European Association of Nuclear Medicine (EANM) have published

[a] Breast Imaging and Intervention Section, Department of Radiology, University of Wisconsin School of Medicine and Public Health, 600 Highland Avenue, Madison, WI 53792-3252, USA; [b] Department of Medical Physics, University of Wisconsin School of Medicine and Public Health, 1111 Highland Avenue, Madison, WI 53705, USA; [c] University of Wisconsin Carbone Cancer Center, 600 Highland Avenue, Madison, WI 53792, USA; [d] Nuclear Medicine and Molecular Imaging Section, Department of Radiology, University of Wisconsin School of Medicine and Public Health, 600 Highland Avenue, Madison, WI 53792-3252, USA
* Corresponding author. Breast Imaging and Intervention Section, Department of Radiology, University of Wisconsin School of Medicine and Public Health, 600 Highland Avenue, Madison, WI 53792-3252.
E-mail address: afowler@uwhealth.org

Radiol Clin N Am 59 (2021) 725–735
https://doi.org/10.1016/j.rcl.2021.05.004
0033-8389/21/© 2021 Elsevier Inc. All rights reserved.

procedure guidelines for oncologic imaging with FDG PET/CT.[5,6] These guidelines detail the clinical indications, performance, interpretation, and reporting of FDG PET/CT examinations. FDG PET/CT can be used for systemic staging of breast cancer, evaluation of suspected disease recurrence, and assessment of treatment response.

Initial Staging

Staging provides prognostic information regarding survival outcomes and is used to guide local, regional, and systemic therapy decisions. Breast cancer staging follows the American Joint Committee on Cancer (AJCC) TNM classification system.[7] The anatomic stage includes the primary tumor size (T stage), regional lymph node status (N stage), and distant metastasis (M stage). Physical examination and conventional breast imaging (mammography, ultrasound, and MRI, if performed) are used to determine T and N clinical anatomic staging. Pathologic anatomic staging is based on surgical specimens from lumpectomy or mastectomy for T staging and sentinel lymph node biopsy or full axillary dissection for axillary N staging.

Approximately, 6% of all patients with newly diagnosed breast cancer have distant metastatic disease (M1; stage IV) at presentation.[8] The most common sites are bone, lung, brain, liver, and distant lymph nodes. The use of imaging for the evaluation of distant sites of disease depends on the clinical stage and the presence of symptoms or laboratory abnormalities. For asymptomatic patients with early-stage disease (clinical stage 0-IIB), systemic imaging is not recommended by the National Comprehensive Cancer Network (NCCN) and the American College of Radiology (ACR).[9,10] Systemic imaging is indicated for patients with suspicious symptoms or laboratory abnormalities and for those with stage III, locally advanced and inflammatory breast cancers.[9] Imaging options include CT, MRI, bone scintigraphy, and FDG PET/CT (**Figs. 1** and **2**). Discovery of unsuspected distant metastases during initial staging is significant because clinical management then shifts from curative to palliative intent.

The relative utilization of conventional imaging with CT and bone scintigraphy versus FDG PET/CT for systemic staging is variable in clinical practice.[11] NCCN guidelines consider FDG PET/CT use optional when conventional imaging is equivocal or suspicious. However, recent studies of patients with stages II–III breast cancer planning neoadjuvant chemotherapy have demonstrated that FDG PET/CT has less false-positive findings, comparable cost, and lower radiation exposure

compared with conventional imaging.[11,12] Furthermore, FDG PET/CT has been shown to have higher sensitivity compared with conventional imaging for diagnosing distant metastases in patients with breast cancer.[13,14] Thus, FDG PET/CT could be considered an alternative, rather than adjunct, to CT and bone scintigraphy for systemic staging.

Consideration of additional prognostic factors beyond clinical stage may further refine the most appropriate patient population for FDG PET/CT imaging for systemic staging. These factors include histologic subtype, molecular subtype, and patient age. Hogan and colleagues demonstrated that FDG PET/CT more frequently identified unsuspected distant metastatic disease in patients with stage III invasive ductal carcinoma compared with stage III invasive lobular carcinoma.[15] In a retrospective study of 232 patients with triple-negative breast cancer, FDG PET/CT discovered distant metastases in 15% with stage IIB disease.[16] In a retrospective study of 144 women younger than 40 years, Riedl and colleagues demonstrated that FDG PET/CT identified unsuspected distant metastases in 17% with stage IIB disease.[17] These data are slightly higher than the previously reported 11% yield of detecting distant metastases overall for stage IIB disease in a prospective study of 254 consecutive patients.[18] Thus, systemic staging with FDG PET/CT may be justified starting as early as stage IIB, particularly for patients who are younger than 40 years with triple-negative invasive ductal carcinoma.

A major change in the AJCC staging system for breast cancer occurred with the 8th edition reflecting the new era of precision medicine. Biologic factors with established prognostic significance (histologic grade, ER, PR, and HER2 status, multigene panel recurrence scores) have been incorporated with the traditional anatomic stage to yield a prognostic stage for more accurate estimation of individual outcomes.[7] Although not currently used as a biomarker in the AJCC prognostic stage, FDG PET/CT may provide additional prognostic information because breast cancers with high FDG avidity have been shown to correlate with poorer outcomes.[19]

Suspected Disease Recurrence

More than 3.8 million women are living in the United States with a personal history of breast cancer.[20] Approximately, 30% to 40% of breast cancer recur as metastatic disease and the risk of recurrence continues for decades after initial treatment, particularly for patients with hormone

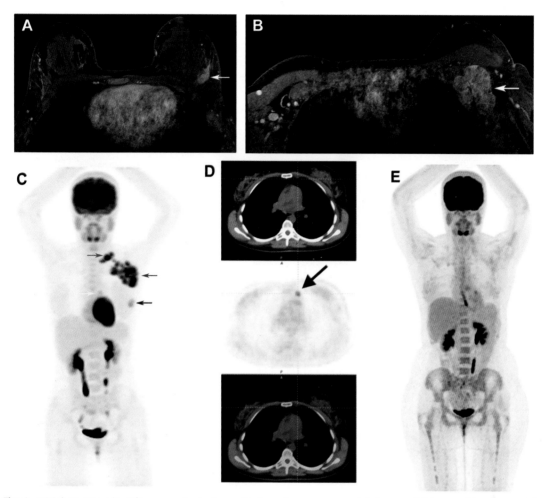

Fig. 1. Initial staging identifies supraclavicular and internal mammary nodal disease. A 27-year-old woman with newly diagnosed 4.2 cm left breast cancer (ER-/PR-/HER2- invasive ductal carcinoma) (*A*) and biopsy-proven axillary nodal metastasis (*B*) as demonstrated on axial postcontrast T1-weighted images from breast MRI. (*C*) Whole-body PET maximal intensity projection (MIP) image from FDG PET/CT shows abnormal FDG uptake in the left breast at the site of primary malignancy (*black arrow*; SUV_{max} 5.1), multiple left level I-III axillary lymph nodes (*blue arrow*; SUV_{max} 12.7), left supraclavicular lymph nodes (*red arrow*; SUV_{max} 13.5), and a left internal mammary lymph node (*yellow arrow*; SUV_{max} 4.1) seen on transaxial CT, PET, and fused PET/CT images (crosshairs and *arrow* on PET in (*D*). There was no evidence of distant metastases. The patient underwent neoadjuvant chemotherapy, mastectomy and axillary nodal dissection, post-mastectomy radiation therapy including the supraclavicular fossa and internal mammary chain, and adjuvant chemotherapy. (*E*) Whole-body PET MIP image from FDG PET/CT after completion of adjuvant therapy shows interval resolution of the hypermetabolic left supraclavicular and internal mammary lymph nodes. Moderate diffuse osseous FDG uptake is compatible with reactive bone marrow secondary to recent chemotherapy.

receptor-positive breast cancer.[21] The American Cancer Society (ACS), American Society of Clinical Oncologists (ASCO), and NCCN recommend regular clinical assessment (history and physical examination) and annual mammography for breast cancer survivors.[9,22] Breast MRI is also recommended in addition to mammography by the ACR for women with a personal history of treated breast cancer who are diagnosed before the age of 50 years or have mammographically dense breasts.[23] Laboratory tests and systemic imaging

are not recommended for asymptomatic breast cancer survivors.[22] For patients presenting with symptoms, physical examination findings, or laboratory abnormalities suspicious for disease recurrence, systemic imaging is indicated. Imaging options include CT, MRI, bone scintigraphy, and FDG PET/CT (**Fig. 3**).

FDG PET/CT can be performed for the detection of distant metastases as well as locoregional recurrences (chest wall, axillary and internal mammary lymph nodes) in patients previously treated

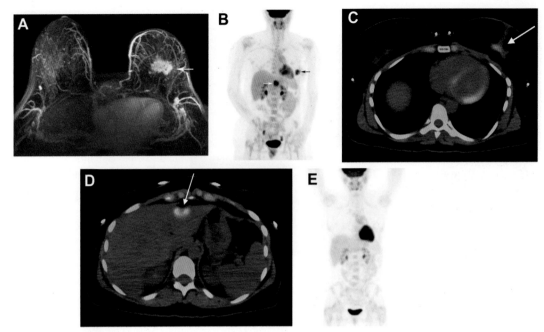

Fig. 2. Initial staging identifies solitary liver metastasis. 39-year-old woman with newly diagnosed 4.3 cm left breast cancer (ER+/PR+/HER2- invasive mammary carcinoma; *white arrow*) as demonstrated on dynamic contrast enhanced breast MRI MIP image (*A*). Whole-body PET MIP image (*B*) and axial fused images from FDG PET/CT show an FDG-avid left breast mass corresponding to the primary malignancy (*black arrow* in *B* and *white arrow* in *C*; SUV$_{max}$ 7.3) (*C*) and a hypermetabolic mass in the left hepatic lobe (*white arrow* in *B* and *D*; SUV$_{max}$ 7.7) (*D*), which was confirmed via biopsy as metastatic breast carcinoma. No other sites of metastatic disease were identified, with note of physiologic bilateral ovarian activity on the PET MIP image. The patient was treated with chemotherapy followed by endocrine therapy. (*E*) Whole-body PET MIP image from FDG PET/CT during treatment showed complete metabolic response.

for breast cancer.[24–27] In a meta-analysis of 26 studies of FDG PET or PET/CT with 1752 patients, summary sensitivity and specificity for detecting recurrent breast cancer was 0.90 [0.88–0.92 95% CI] and 0.81 [0.78–0.84 95% CI], respectively.[24] FDG PET/CT has been shown to have increased sensitivity compared with CT for the diagnosis of breast cancer recurrence.[25] FDG PET/CT may also be more accurate than contrast-enhanced CT alone or contrast-enhanced CT combined with bone scintigraphy for diagnosing breast cancer recurrences.[28]

Treatment Response—Primary Setting

Neoadjuvant chemotherapy can be used to treat patients with breast cancer before surgery to reduce tumor size, allowing for lumpectomy instead of mastectomy, and to minimize the extent of axillary surgery. Importantly, long-term survival outcomes for patients who received neoadjuvant chemotherapy are comparable to those with adjuvant chemotherapy.[29] As a complement to physical examination, imaging provides important information for evaluating response to

neoadjuvant therapy.[30,31] Imaging before neoadjuvant chemotherapy may be helpful for predicting which patients are most likely to respond.[32] Imaging can also be performed during therapy to confirm clinical suspicion of disease progression and to identify early nonresponders to therapy to allow for a change in treatment or to expedite surgery.[32] Imaging performed after completion of neoadjuvant therapy can be used for planning the extent of surgery.[32] Current standard of care is to perform surgery even if no residual imaging abnormality remains after neoadjuvant therapy because microscopic residual disease on final surgical pathology is possible.[9]

Several meta-analyses have investigated FDG PET/CT for assessing response to neoadjuvant chemotherapy.[33–40] FDG PET and PET/CT have a pooled sensitivity of 71% to 87% and specificity of 66% to 85% for determining pathologic response.[33–40] For studies in which patients underwent both FDG PET/CT and breast MRI, there was comparable accuracy for predicting therapy response.[37–39] Some studies found that FDG PET/CT had higher sensitivity and MRI had higher specificity for determining pathologic response.[37,40,41]

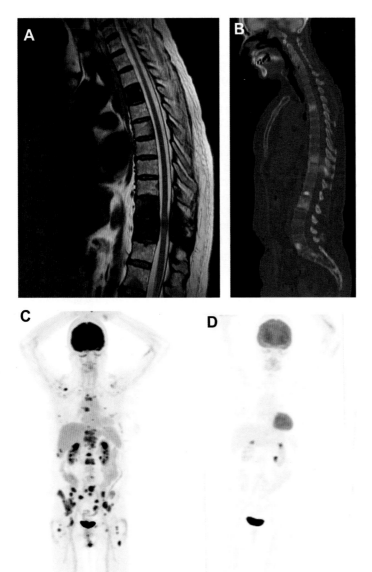

Fig. 3. Breast cancer recurrence and treatment response. A 71-year-old woman with a personal history of treated invasive lobular breast cancer presents with back pain and multiple suspicious vertebral body lesions identified on thoracolumbar spine MRI (A; T2-weighted sagittal). Fused FDG PET/CT sagittal (B) and whole-body PET MIP images (C) show numerous FDG-avid lesions involving the axial and appendicular skeleton and no sites of lymphadenopathy or visceral disease. CT-guided right iliac bone biopsy confirmed ER+/PR+/HER2- metastatic breast carcinoma. (D) Whole-body PET MIP image from FDG PET/CT after starting therapy with an aromatase inhibitor combined with a cyclin-dependent kinase 4/6 inhibitor shows complete metabolic response.

Although MRI may be better at assessing residual disease burden post-therapy, FDG-PET/CT may be better at assessing early response, between 1 and 3 cycles of chemotherapy.[39,40] Response to neoadjuvant chemotherapy on FDG PET/CT also has prognostic significance as it has been shown to predict disease recurrence and survival.[42]

Treatment Response—Metastatic Setting

Imaging is used, together with symptom assessment, physical examination, and blood tests, to monitor for disease progression in patients undergoing treatment for metastatic breast cancer. Conventional imaging to assess treatment efficacy includes CT and/or bone scintigraphy with a suggested interval of every 2–6 months.[9] To assess interval changes in tumor burden, standardized criteria have been established for defining complete response, partial response, stable disease, and disease progression as an objective measurement of response to therapy.[43] Determination of disease progression is clinically significant as it triggers a change to a subsequent line of therapy.

FDG PET/CT can be used to assess response to therapy for patients with metastatic breast cancer by measuring therapy-induced changes in tumor metabolism and glycolytic activity (see **Figs. 2** and **3**). Metabolic changes typically occur earlier than changes in tumor size measurements.

Reduced FDG uptake after the first cycle of chemotherapy has been shown to predict clinical response defined by conventional imaging.[44,45] Furthermore, the metabolic response after 3 cycles of chemotherapy has been shown to predict both the clinical response at the completion of 6 cycles of chemotherapy and overall survival.[46] For bone-dominant metastatic breast cancer, changes in tumor metabolic activity may more closely reflect treatment response than CT or bone scintigraphy.[47–49] Guidelines for reproducible imaging acquisition methods[50] and standardized criteria for metabolic response assessment[51,52] are important for accurately evaluating therapy response with FDG PET/CT.

Relatively, few studies directly compare FDG PET/CT with conventional imaging for predicting survival outcomes.[53,54] In a study of 65 patients with metastatic breast cancer undergoing first- or second-line therapy, Riedl and colleagues demonstrated that metabolic response on PET/CT was a better predictor of progression-free survival and disease-specific survival than anatomic response on contrast-enhanced CT.[55] Thus, additional prospective data are needed.

For patients with hormone receptor-positive metastatic breast cancer, FDG PET/CT has also been studied for assessing response to endocrine therapy. The metabolic response based on the difference in SUV_{max} between FDG PET/CT performed at baseline and during endocrine therapy has been shown in small pilot studies to predict progression-free survival.[56,57] The timing of imaging is important because a transient paradoxic increase in FDG uptake ("metabolic flare") can be observed if performed during the first 2 weeks of therapy with tamoxifen that correlates with clinical benefit.[58]

Limitations of FDG PET/CT

FDG PET/CT is not indicated for primary breast cancer detection, for distinguishing benign from malignant breast lesions, or for local tumor staging in patients with newly diagnosed breast cancer. The spatial resolution of whole-body PET/CT scanners limits the sensitivity for detecting cancers smaller than 1 cm.[59] Also, an inherent biologic limitation of FDG PET/CT is that breast cancers have a wide spectrum of glycolytic activity. For example, low-grade invasive carcinoma and ductal carcinoma in situ can have low FDG avidity resulting in reduced sensitivity of FDG PET/CT for detection.[59,60] Lower FDG uptake and reduced PET/CT sensitivity have also been observed for invasive lobular carcinoma compared with invasive ductal carcinoma.[59,60] Furthermore, certain benign etiologies may be FDG avid resulting in

false-positive findings, such as silicone granuloma, fat necrosis, fibroadenoma, postsurgical changes, inflammation/abscess, granulomatous mastitis, gynecomastia, and lactational change.[61]

Although FDG PET/CT has limitations for evaluating breast lesions, it is important to identify and appropriately evaluate abnormal FDG uptake in the breast. There is a 55% to 60% likelihood of malignancy (primary breast cancer, lymphoma, non-breast metastases) for incidentally detected FDG-avid breast lesions.[62,63] Thus, further evaluation is warranted, starting with correlation with recent breast imaging examinations. If none are available or if the finding is not reconciled, then diagnostic mammography and ultrasound are indicated for further evaluation.

All imaging, including FDG PET/CT, is less sensitive for detecting axillary nodal metastases compared with sentinel lymph node biopsy, the current gold standard. However, the specificity of FDG PET/CT has been reported as 0.93 [0.90–0.95 95% CI], which is superior to its sensitivity [0.64; 0.59–0.69 95% CI].[64] FDG PET/CT may have clinical utility for initial staging by detecting extra-axillary nodal metastases such as internal mammary and supraclavicular lymph nodes.[65,66] Internal mammary nodal metastases were equally detected by PET/CT and breast MRI in patients before neoadjuvant chemotherapy.[66] Identification of extra-axillary nodal metastases at initial staging has prognostic significance and can impact clinical management by altering adjuvant radiation therapy planning.[65]

PET/MRI

There is increasing interest in evaluating the clinical utility of FDG PET/MRI for patients with breast cancer for both primary disease, locoregional and distant metastatic staging.[67,68] One advantage over PET/CT is the significant reduction (50%–80%) in radiation dose with PET/MRI.[69,70] PET/MRI appears to have higher sensitivity for identifying liver and bone lesions than PET/CT.[70–72] However, PET/CT may be better for detecting small lung metastases than PET/MRI[70,73]; although the number of malignant nodules missed by PET/MRI was low (0.8%).[69] The diagnostic performance of PET/MRI for pulmonary metastases may improve as further technical development of motion-robust MRI sequences for lung imaging continue to evolve.

FES PET/CT

In 2020, the United States Food and Drug Administration approved FES for clinical use with PET imaging to detect ER-positive lesions in patients with recurrent or metastatic breast cancer as an adjunct to biopsy. This is a major achievement because FES has been studied in more than one thousand patients participating in research since 1988. A historical perspective on the discovery and development of FES was recently published.[74]

FES is a radiolabeled estrogen that can be used together with PET imaging to determine the location and ligand-binding function of ER throughout the body. Several studies have demonstrated concordance between FES PET imaging results and ER status in primary and metastatic breast cancer using tissue reference standards.[75–78] Proposed clinical applications of FES PET/CT include the detection of ER+ metastases,[75–78] evaluation of suspected recurrence in patients with a history of ER+ primary breast cancer,[79] problem-solving when conventional work-up is inconclusive,[80] and therapy selection.[81–84]

FES PET/CT can be performed for post- and pre-menopausal women, as well as men, with breast cancer. The recommended injected dose of FES is 6 mCi (222 MBq; 111–222 MBq; 3–6 mCi).[75] Uptake time before scanning is typically 60 minutes (50–70 minutes), similar to FDG.[75] Unlike FDG PET imaging preparation, fasting before injection and the limitation of physical activity is not required for FES PET/CT.[75] FES PET/CT can be performed while patients are taking aromatase inhibitors, but not with ER antagonists such as tamoxifen or fulvestrant due to competitive blocking of ER for FES binding.[85] Owing to the normal hepatobiliary clearance of FES, there is limited evaluation of liver lesions and abdominal lymph nodes located near bowel with high physiologic clearance activity.[75]

ONGOING RESEARCH

There are many exciting ongoing investigations in the area of molecular imaging for breast cancer. For example, radiopharmaceuticals for in vivo measurement of other clinically established tumor biomarkers beyond ER are being developed and evaluated in clinical trials. These investigational imaging agents include ^{18}F-fluorofuranylnorprogesterone (^{18}F-FFNP) for progesterone receptor, ^{89}Zr-trastuzumab or ^{89}Zr-pertuzumab for HER2, and ^{18}F-fluorothymidine (^{18}F-FLT) and ^{18}F-ISO-1 for proliferation.[86–88] Furthermore, new approaches involving radiomics, texture analysis, and deep learning may offer additional prognostic and predictive information.[89] Lastly, dedicated breast PET imaging devices and simultaneous breast PET/MRI protocols have been developed that may expand the utility of multimodality molecular imaging for primary breast tumor evaluation.[90,91]

CLINICS CARE POINTS

- FDG PET/CT can be used for systemic staging of breast cancer, evaluation of suspected disease recurrence, and assessment of treatment response.
- Potential causes for a false negative FDG PET/CT examination include ductal carcinoma in situ, invasive lobular carcinoma, and sub-centimeter cancers.
- Abnormal FDG uptake in the breast incidentally detected on PET/CT has a high likelihood of malignancy and warrants further evaluation.

DISCLOSURE

The University of Wisconsin School of Medicine and Public Health Department of Radiology receives research support from GE Healthcare.

REFERENCES

1. Bray F, Ferlay J, Soerjomataram I, et al. Global cancer statistics 2018: GLOBOCAN estimates of incidence and mortality worldwide for 36 cancers in 185 countries. CA Cancer J Clin 2018;68(6): 394–424.
2. Siegel RL, Miller KD, Jemal A. Cancer statistics, 2020. CA Cancer J Clin 2020;70(1):7–30.
3. Li CI, Daling JR. Changes in breast cancer incidence rates in the United States by histologic subtype and race/ethnicity, 1995 to 2004. Cancer Epidemiol Biomarkers Prev 2007;16(12):2773–80.
4. Howlader N, Altekruse SF, Li CI, et al. US incidence of breast cancer subtypes defined by joint hormone receptor and HER2 status. J Natl Cancer Inst 2014; 106(5):dju055.
5. Boellaard R, Delgado-Bolton R, Oyen WJ, et al. FDG PET/CT: EANM procedure guidelines for tumour imaging: version 2.0. Eur J Nucl Med Mol Imaging 2015;42(2):328–54.
6. Delbeke D, Coleman RE, Guiberteau MJ, et al. Procedure guideline for tumor imaging with 18F-FDG PET/CT 1.0. J Nucl Med 2006;47(5):885–95.
7. Giuliano AE, Connolly JL, Edge SB, et al. Breast cancer-major changes in the American Joint Committee on Cancer eighth edition cancer staging manual. CA Cancer J Clin 2017;67(4):290–303.

8. DeSantis CE, Ma J, Gaudet MM, et al. Breast cancer statistics, 2019. CA Cancer J Clin 2019;69(6): 438–51.

9. Gradishar WJ, Anderson BO, Abraham J, et al. Breast Cancer, Version 3.2020, NCCN Clinical Practice Guidelines in Oncology. J Natl Compr Canc Netw 2020;18(4):452–78.

10. Moy L, Newell MS, Mahoney MC, et al. ACR Appropriateness Criteria Stage I Breast Cancer: Initial workup and surveillance for local recurrence and distant metastases in asymptomatic women. J Am Coll Radiol 2016;13(11s):e43–52.

11. Hyland CJ, Varghese F, Yau C, et al. Use of 18F-FDG PET/CT as an initial staging procedure for stage II-III breast cancer: a multicenter value analysis. J Natl Compr Canc Netw 2020;18(11):1510–7.

12. Ko H, Baghdadi Y, Love C, et al. Clinical utility of 18F-FDG PET/CT in staging localized breast cancer before initiating preoperative systemic therapy. J Natl Compr Canc Netw 2020;18(9):1240–6.

13. Hong S, Li J, Wang S. 18FDG PET-CT for diagnosis of distant metastases in breast cancer patients. A meta-analysis. Surg Oncol 2013;22(2):139–43.

14. Sun Z, Yi YL, Liu Y, et al. Comparison of whole-body PET/PET-CT and conventional imaging procedures for distant metastasis staging in patients with breast cancer: a meta-analysis. Eur J Gynaecol Oncol 2015;36(6):672–6.

15. Hogan MP, Goldman DA, Dashevsky B, et al. Comparison of 18F-FDG PET/CT for systemic staging of newly diagnosed invasive lobular carcinoma versus invasive ductal carcinoma. J Nucl Med 2015;56(11): 1674–80.

16. Ulaner GA, Castillo R, Goldman DA, et al. 18)F-FDG-PET/CT for systemic staging of newly diagnosed triple-negative breast cancer. Eur J Nucl Med Mol Imaging 2016;43(11):1937–44.

17. Riedl CC, Slobod E, Jochelson M, et al. Retrospective analysis of 18F-FDG PET/CT for staging asymptomatic breast cancer patients younger than 40 years. J Nucl Med 2014;55(10):1578–83.

18. Groheux D, Hindié E, Delord M, et al. Prognostic impact of (18)FDG-PET-CT findings in clinical stage III and IIB breast cancer. J Natl Cancer Inst 2012; 104(24):1879–87.

19. Pak K, Seok JW, Kim HY, et al. Prognostic value of metabolic tumor volume and total lesion glycolysis in breast cancer: a meta-analysis. Nucl Med Commun 2020;41(8):824–9.

20. Miller KD, Nogueira L, Mariotto AB, et al. Cancer treatment and survivorship statistics, 2019. CA Cancer J Clin 2019;69(5):363–85.

21. Colleoni M, Sun Z, Price KN, et al. Annual hazard rates of recurrence for breast cancer during 24 years of follow-up: results from the International Breast Cancer Study Group Trials I to V. J Clin Oncol 2016;34(9):927–35.

22. Runowicz CD, Leach CR, Henry NL, et al. American Cancer Society/American Society of Clinical Oncology breast cancer survivorship care guideline. J Clin Oncol 2016;34(6):611–35.

23. Monticciolo DL, Newell MS, Moy L, et al. Breast cancer screening in women at higher-than-average risk: recommendations from the ACR. J Am Coll Radiol 2018;15(3 Pt A):408–14.

24. Xiao Y, Wang L, Jiang X, et al. Diagnostic efficacy of 18F-FDG-PET or PET/CT in breast cancer with suspected recurrence: a systematic review and meta-analysis. Nucl Med Commun 2016;37(11): 1180–8.

25. Pennant M, Takwoingi Y, Pennant L, et al. A systematic review of positron emission tomography (PET) and positron emission tomography/ computed tomography (PET/CT) for the diagnosis of breast cancer recurrence. Health Technol Assess 2010;14(50):1–103.

26. Pan L, Han Y, Sun X, et al. FDG-PET and other imaging modalities for the evaluation of breast cancer recurrence and metastases: a meta-analysis. J Cancer Res Clin Oncol 2010;136(7):1007–22.

27. Isasi CR, Moadel RM, Blaufox MD. A meta-analysis of FDG-PET for the evaluation of breast cancer recurrence and metastases. Breast Cancer Res Treat 2005;90(2):105–12.

28. Hildebrandt MG, Gerke O, Baun C, et al. [18F]Fluorodeoxyglucose (FDG)-positron emission tomography (PET)/computed tomography (CT) in suspected recurrent breast cancer: a prospective comparative study of dual-time-point FDG-PET/CT, contrast-enhanced CT, and bone scintigraphy. J Clin Oncol 2016;34(16):1889–97.

29. Early Breast Cancer Trialists' Collaborative Group. Long-term outcomes for neoadjuvant versus adjuvant chemotherapy in early breast cancer: meta-analysis of individual patient data from ten randomised trials. Lancet Oncol 2018;19(1):27–39.

30. Slanetz PJ, Moy L, Baron P, et al. ACR Appropriateness Criteria((R)) monitoring response to neoadjuvant systemic therapy for breast cancer. J Am Coll Radiol 2017;14(11s):S462–75.

31. Fowler AM, Mankoff DA, Joe BN. Imaging neoadjuvant therapy response in breast cancer. Radiology 2017;285(2):358–75.

32. Schwarz-Dose J, Untch M, Tiling R, et al. Monitoring primary systemic therapy of large and locally advanced breast cancer by using sequential positron emission tomography imaging with [18F]fluorodeoxyglucose. J Clin Oncol 2009;27(4):535–41.

33. Wang Y, Zhang C, Liu J, et al. Is 18F-FDG PET accurate to predict neoadjuvant therapy response in breast cancer? A meta-analysis. Breast Cancer Res Treat 2012;131(2):357–69.

34. Cheng X, Li Y, Liu B, et al. 18F-FDG PET/CT and PET for evaluation of pathological response to

neoadjuvant chemotherapy in breast cancer: a meta-analysis. Acta Radiol 2012;53(6):615–27.

35. Mghanga FP, Lan X, Bakari KH, et al. Fluorine-18 fluorodeoxyglucose positron emission tomography-computed tomography in monitoring the response of breast cancer to neoadjuvant chemotherapy: a meta-analysis. Clin Breast Cancer 2013;13(4): 271–9.

36. Tian F, Shen G, Deng Y, et al. The accuracy of (18)F-FDG PET/CT in predicting the pathological response to neoadjuvant chemotherapy in patients with breast cancer: a meta-analysis and systematic review. Eur Radiol 2017;27(11):4786–96.

37. Liu Q, Wang C, Li P, et al. The role of (18)F-FDG PET/CT and MRI in assessing pathological complete response to neoadjuvant chemotherapy in patients with breast cancer: a systematic review and meta-analysis. Biomed Res Int 2016;2016:3746232.

38. Sheikhbahaei S, Trahan TJ, Xiao J, et al. FDG-PET/CT and MRI for evaluation of pathologic response to neoadjuvant chemotherapy in patients with breast cancer: a meta-analysis of diagnostic accuracy studies. Oncologist 2016;21(8):931–9.

39. Chen L, Yang Q, Bao J, et al. Direct comparison of PET/CT and MRI to predict the pathological response to neoadjuvant chemotherapy in breast cancer: a meta-analysis. Sci Rep 2017;7(1):8479.

40. Li H, Yao L, Jin P, et al. MRI and PET/CT for evaluation of the pathological response to neoadjuvant chemotherapy in breast cancer: a systematic review and meta-analysis. Breast 2018;40:106–15.

41. Gu YL, Pan SM, Ren J, et al. Role of magnetic resonance imaging in detection of pathologic complete remission in breast cancer patients treated with neoadjuvant chemotherapy: a meta-analysis. Clin Breast Cancer 2017;17(4):245–55.

42. Han S, Choi JY. Prognostic value of (18)F-FDG PET and PET/CT for assessment of treatment response to neoadjuvant chemotherapy in breast cancer: a systematic review and meta-analysis. Breast Cancer Res 2020;22(1):119.

43. Eisenhauer EA, Therasse P, Bogaerts J, et al. New response evaluation criteria in solid tumours: revised RECIST guideline (version 1.1). Eur J Cancer 2009; 45(2):228–47.

44. Gennari A, Donati S, Salvadori B, et al. Role of 2-[18F]-fluorodeoxyglucose (FDG) positron emission tomography (PET) in the early assessment of response to chemotherapy in metastatic breast cancer patients. Clin Breast Cancer 2000;1(2): 156–61.

45. Dose Schwarz J, Bader M, Jenicke L, et al. Early prediction of response to chemotherapy in metastatic breast cancer using sequential 18F-FDG PET. J Nucl Med 2005;46(7):1144–50.

46. Couturier O, Jerusalem G, N'Guyen JM, et al. Sequential positron emission tomography using [18F]fluorodeoxyglucose for monitoring response to chemotherapy in metastatic breast cancer. Clin Cancer Res 2006;12(21):6437–43.

47. Du Y, Cullum I, Illidge TM, et al. Fusion of metabolic function and morphology: sequential [18F]fluorodeoxyglucose positron-emission tomography/computed tomography studies yield new insights into the natural history of bone metastases in breast cancer. J Clin Oncol 2007;25(23):3440–7.

48. Tateishi U, Gamez C, Dawood S, et al. Bone metastases in patients with metastatic breast cancer: morphologic and metabolic monitoring of response to systemic therapy with integrated PET/CT. Radiology 2008;247(1):189–96.

49. Al-Muqbel KM, Yaghan RJ. Effectiveness of 18F-FDG-PET/CT vs bone scintigraphy in treatment response assessment of bone metastases in breast cancer. Medicine (Baltimore) 2016;95(21):e3753.

50. Kinahan PE, Perlman ES, Sunderland JJ, et al. The QIBA Profile for FDG PET/CT as an imaging biomarker measuring response to cancer therapy. Radiology 2020;294(3):647–57.

51. Wahl RL, Jacene H, Kasamon Y, et al. From RECIST to PERCIST: evolving considerations for PET response criteria in solid tumors. J Nucl Med 2009; 50(Suppl 1):122S–50S.

52. Young H, Baum R, Cremerius U, et al. Measurement of clinical and subclinical tumour response using [18F]-fluorodeoxyglucose and positron emission tomography: review and 1999 EORTC recommendations. European Organization for Research and Treatment of Cancer (EORTC) PET Study Group. Eur J Cancer 1999;35(13):1773–82.

53. Lee CI, Gold LS, Nelson HD, et al. Comparative effectiveness of imaging modalities to determine metastatic breast cancer treatment response. Breast 2015;24(1):3–11.

54. Helland F, Hallin Henriksen M, Gerke O, et al. FDG-PET/CT versus contrast-enhanced CT for response evaluation in metastatic breast cancer: a systematic review. Diagnostics (Basel) 2019;9(3):106.

55. Riedl CC, Pinker K, Ulaner GA, et al. Comparison of FDG-PET/CT and contrast-enhanced CT for monitoring therapy response in patients with metastatic breast cancer. Eur J Nucl Med Mol Imaging 2017; 44(9):1428–37.

56. Mortazavi-Jehanno N, Giraudet AL, Champion L, et al. Assessment of response to endocrine therapy using FDG PET/CT in metastatic breast cancer: a pilot study. Eur J Nucl Med Mol Imaging 2012;39(3): 450–60.

57. Kruse V, VDW C, Maes A, et al. Stable metabolic disease on FDG-PET provides information on response to endocrine therapy for breast cancer. Q J Nucl Med Mol Imaging 2017;61(1):108–14.

58. Mortimer JE, Dehdashti F, Siegel BA, et al. Metabolic flare: indicator of hormone responsiveness in

advanced breast cancer. J Clin Oncol 2001;19(11): 2797–803.

59. Avril N, Rose CA, Schelling M, et al. Breast imaging with positron emission tomography and fluorine-18 fluorodeoxyglucose: use and limitations. J Clin Oncol 2000;18(20):3495–502.

60. Groheux D, Giacchetti S, Moretti JL, et al. Correlation of high 18F-FDG uptake to clinical, pathological and biological prognostic factors in breast cancer. Eur J Nucl Med Mol Imaging 2011;38(3):426–35.

61. Adejolu M, Huo L, Rohren E, et al. False-positive lesions mimicking breast cancer on FDG PET and PET/CT. AJR Am J Roentgenol 2012;198(3): W304–14.

62. Falomo E, Strigel RM, Bruce R, et al. Incidence and outcomes of incidental breast lesions detected on cross-sectional imaging examinations. Breast J 2018;24(5):743–8.

63. Bertagna F, Treglia G, Orlando E, et al. Prevalence and clinical significance of incidental F18-FDG breast uptake: a systematic review and meta-analysis. Jpn J Radiol 2014;32(2):59–68.

64. Liang X, Yu J, Wen B, et al. MRI and FDG-PET/CT based assessment of axillary lymph node metastasis in early breast cancer: a meta-analysis. Clin Radiol 2017;72(4):295–301.

65. Aukema TS, Straver ME, Peeters MJ, et al. Detection of extra-axillary lymph node involvement with FDG PET/CT in patients with stage II-III breast cancer. Eur J Cancer 2010;46(18):3205–10.

66. Jochelson MS, Lebron L, Jacobs SS, et al. Detection of internal mammary adenopathy in patients with breast cancer by PET/CT and MRI. AJR Am J Roentgenol 2015;205(4):899–904.

67. Lin CY, Lin CL, Kao CH. Staging/restaging performance of F18-fluorodeoxyglucose positron emission tomography/magnetic resonance imaging in breast cancer: a review and meta-analysis. Eur J Radiol 2018;107:158–65.

68. Kirchner J, Grueneisen J, Martin O, et al. Local and whole-body staging in patients with primary breast cancer: a comparison of one-step to two-step staging utilizing (18)F-FDG-PET/MRI. Eur J Nucl Med Mol Imaging 2018;45(13):2328–37.

69. Martin O, Schaarschmidt BM, Kirchner J, et al. PET/MRI versus PET/CT for whole-body staging: results from a single-center observational study on 1,003 sequential examinations. J Nucl Med 2020;61(8): 1131–6.

70. Melsaether AN, Raad RA, Pujara AC, et al. Comparison of whole-body (18)F FDG PET/MR imaging and whole-body (18)F FDG PET/CT in terms of lesion detection and radiation dose in patients with breast cancer. Radiology 2016;281(1):193–202.

71. Botsikas D, Bagetakos I, Picarra M, et al. What is the diagnostic performance of 18-FDG-PET/MR compared to PET/CT for the N- and M- staging of breast cancer? Eur Radiol 2019;29(4):1787–98.

72. Sawicki LM, Grueneisen J, Schaarschmidt BM, et al. Evaluation of ^{18}F-FDG PET/MRI, ^{18}F-FDG PET/CT, MRI, and CT in whole-body staging of recurrent breast cancer. Eur J Radiol 2016;85(2):459–65.

73. Sawicki LM, Grueneisen J, Buchbender C, et al. Comparative performance of ^{18}F-FDG PET/MRI and ^{18}F-FDG PET/CT in detection and characterization of pulmonary lesions in 121 oncologic patients. J Nucl Med 2016;57(4):582–6.

74. Katzenellenbogen JA. The quest for improving the management of breast cancer by functional imaging: the discovery and development of 16alpha-[(18)F]fluoroestradiol (FES), a PET radiotracer for the estrogen receptor, a historical review. Nucl Med Biol 2021;92:24–37.

75. Kurland BF, Wiggins JR, Coche A, et al. Whole-body characterization of estrogen receptor status in metastatic breast cancer with 16alpha-18F-fluoro-17beta-estradiol positron emission tomography: meta-analysis and recommendations for integration into clinical applications. Oncologist 2020;25:835–44.

76. Evangelista L, Guarneri V, Conte PF. 18F-Fluoroestradiol positron emission tomography in breast cancer patients: systematic review of the literature & meta-analysis. Curr Radiopharm 2016;9(3):244–57.

77. van Kruchten M, de Vries EG, Brown M, et al. PET imaging of oestrogen receptors in patients with breast cancer. Lancet Oncol 2013;14(11):e465–75.

78. Chae SY, Ahn SH, Kim SB, et al. Diagnostic accuracy and safety of 16alpha-[(18)F]fluoro-17beta-oestradiol PET-CT for the assessment of oestrogen receptor status in recurrent or metastatic lesions in patients with breast cancer: a prospective cohort study. Lancet Oncol 2019;20(4):546–55.

79. Chae SY, Son HJ, Lee DY, et al. Comparison of diagnostic sensitivity of [(18)F]fluoroestradiol and [(18)F] fluorodeoxyglucose positron emission tomography/computed tomography for breast cancer recurrence in patients with a history of estrogen receptor-positive primary breast cancer. EJNMMI Res 2020;10(1):54.

80. van Kruchten M, Glaudemans AW, de Vries EF, et al. PET imaging of estrogen receptors as a diagnostic tool for breast cancer patients presenting with a clinical dilemma. J Nucl Med 2012;53(2):182–90.

81. Mortimer JE, Dehdashti F, Siegel BA, et al. Positron emission tomography with 2-[18F]Fluoro-2-deoxy-D-glucose and 16alpha-[18F]fluoro-17beta-estradiol in breast cancer: correlation with estrogen receptor status and response to systemic therapy. Clin Cancer Res 1996;2(6):933–9.

82. van Kruchten M, Glaudemans A, de Vries EFJ, et al. Positron emission tomography of tumour [(18)F]fluoroestradiol uptake in patients with acquired hormone-resistant metastatic breast cancer prior to

oestradiol therapy. Eur J Nucl Med Mol Imaging 2015;42(11):1674–81.

83. Linden HM, Stekhova SA, Link JM, et al. Quantitative fluoroestradiol positron emission tomography imaging predicts response to endocrine treatment in breast cancer. J Clin Oncol 2006;24(18):2793–9.

84. Boers J, Venema CM, de Vries EFJ, et al. Molecular imaging to identify patients with metastatic breast cancer who benefit from endocrine treatment combined with cyclin-dependent kinase inhibition. Eur J Cancer 2020;126:11–20.

85. Linden HM, Kurland BF, Peterson LM, et al. Fluoroestradiol positron emission tomography reveals differences in pharmacodynamics of aromatase inhibitors, tamoxifen, and fulvestrant in patients with metastatic breast cancer. Clin Cancer Res 2011; 17(14):4799–805.

86. Kumar M, Salem K, Tevaarwerk AJ, et al. Recent advances in imaging steroid hormone receptors in breast cancer. J Nucl Med 2020;61(2):172–6.

87. Henry KE, Ulaner GA, Lewis JS. Clinical potential of human epidermal growth factor receptor 2 and human epidermal growth factor receptor 3 imaging in breast cancer. PET Clin 2018;13(3): 423–35.

88. Elmi A, McDonald ES, Mankoff D. Imaging tumor proliferation in breast cancer: current update on predictive imaging biomarkers. PET Clin 2018;13(3): 445–57.

89. Huang SY, Franc BL, Harnish RJ, et al. Exploration of PET and MRI radiomic features for decoding breast cancer phenotypes and prognosis. NPJ Breast Cancer 2018;4:24.

90. Fowler AM, Kumar M, Henze Bancroft L, et al. Measuring glucose uptake in primary invasive breast cancer using simultaneous time-of-flight breast PET/MRI: a method comparison study with prone PET/CT. Radiol Imaging Cancer 2021;3(1):e200091.

91. Narayanan D, Berg WA. Dedicated breast gamma camera imaging and breast PET: current status and future directions. PET Clin 2018;13(3):363–81.

18F-FDG-PET/CT Imaging for Gastrointestinal Malignancies

Brandon A. Howard, MD, PhD*, Terence Z. Wong, MD, PhD

KEYWORDS

• Cancer • Hepatobiliary • Esophagus • Stomach • Colon • Pancreas • Rectum • Anus

KEY POINTS

- The usefulness of 18F-FDG-PET/CT scanning varies depending on the type of gastrointestinal tumor.
- PET combined with contrast-enhanced computed tomography scanning is particularly valuable for evaluating gastrointestinal tumors.
- Although not the primary imaging modality for most gastrointestinal malignancies, 18F-FDG-PET/CT scanning can guide therapeutic decisions when used strategically.

INTRODUCTION

Gastrointestinal (GI) malignancies encompass a wide range of disease sites, each with its own unique challenges. In organizing this review, we have chosen to divide the GI system into the following disease site categories: esophagogastric, colon, hepatobiliary, pancreas, and rectal–anal. We summarize 2-deoxy-2-[18F] fluoro-D-glucose positron emission tomography/computed tomography scanning (FDG-PET/CT) applications for initial staging and follow-up of these different GI malignancies, with particular attention to the role that FDG-PET/CT scanning plays in the management of these patients. Neuroendocrine tumors and small bowel tumors are not primarily evaluated by FDG-PET/CT, and are discussed in greater detail elsewhere in this issue.

GENERAL CONSIDERATIONS

The usual patient preparation (fasting, glucose control, limiting exercise) is important for patients undergoing FDG-PET/CT imaging for GI malignancies. Oral contrast is frequently helpful for anatomic definition and lesion localization within the GI tract. Flavored, noncaloric barium preparations can be used, which the patients can sip during the FDG uptake phase. Neutral oral contrast such as water can also be used before imaging pancreatic lesions. Metformin can result in high FDG activity throughout the bowel, making it difficult to identify underlying lesions. Having patients discontinue metformin for 24 to 48 hours before FDG-PET/CT scanning can decrease this artifact,[1] but is usually not practical owing to the risk of hyperglycemia.

Intravenous contrast can also be beneficial for anatomic localization and diagnosis, especially for FDG-PET/CT evaluation of the liver and pancreas. Newer generation multidetector PET/CT scanners are capable of providing thin-slice multiphase CT scans in the arterial and portal venous phases of enhancement. If contrast-enhanced CT is not performed concurrently as part of the FDG-PET/CT study, it is important to correlate the FDG-PET findings with a separate contrast-enhanced CT or MR scan.

ESOPHAGEAL CANCER
Initial Staging

Esophageal cancer comprises squamous cell carcinoma (in the proximal two-thirds esophagus) and

Division of Nuclear Medicine and Radiotheranostics, Department of Radiology, Duke University Medical Center, DUMC Box 3949, 2301 Erwin Road, Durham, NC 27710, USA
* Corresponding author.
E-mail address: brandon.howard@duke.edu

Radiol Clin N Am 59 (2021) 737–753
https://doi.org/10.1016/j.rcl.2021.06.001

adenocarcinoma (distal third and esophagogastric junction [EGJ]). Its incidence has been increasing, owing to the greater frequency of adenocarcinoma arising in the squamous metaplasia of Barrett's esophagus, with an estimated 19,260 new cases and 15,530 deaths in the United States in 2021.[2] Except for cervical esophageal cancer, for which definitive chemoradiation is used, surgical resection with lymphadenectomy is the best curative therapy in patients without distant metastases. However, morbidity is high, and imaging is critical to help select only those patients who will benefit from esophagectomy. With conventional imaging, metastatic disease is found during surgery in as many as 60% of patients, and more accurate staging with advanced imaging is needed.

Although pathologic staging best correlates with survival, FDG-PET/CT scans, endoscopic ultrasound (EUS) examination, and CT scans have improved the accuracy of clinical staging.[3] FDG-PET/CT scanning from the skull base to the mid-thighs is currently recommended for initial staging of esophageal and EGJ cancers unless there is known metastatic disease.[4] FDG-PET/CT scanning is more sensitive than CT alone for detecting metastasis and therefore allows better patient selection for surgical resection.[5] In a prospective multicenter trial, FDG-PET/CT scanning found metastases in 41% and changed management in 38% of cases.[6] Limitations of FDG-PET/CT scanning include a decreased sensitivity for detection of liver metastases if the CT component is without intravenous contrast and potential false-positive findings.[7–10]

FDG-PET/CT scanning has limited ability to differentiate between clinical (c)T1, T2, and T3 tumors[5,11] and plays no role in T staging, except for possibly determining mediastinal invasion.[12] FDG-PET scanning has less usefulness in early stage (cT1) tumors because of a low prevalence of metastatic disease and risk of false-positive findings.[7,8] FDG-PET/CT scanning sensitivity compared with endoscopy in a screening setting was found to be 4% and it is not useful for this purpose.[13] Although focal FDG avidity in the esophagus is most often malignant, uptake in esophageal papilloma may be a false positive finding.[14] FDG-PET/CT scanning is helpful in delineating the target volume before radiation therapy; a small study determined that respiratory-gated CT scanning underestimated the size of the target volume by 20% when compared with FDG-PET/CT scanning.[15] The metabolic tumor volume (MTV) on a baseline FDG-PET/CT scan before neoadjuvant chemotherapy correlated with pathologic response in 61 patients with squamous cell and adenocarcinoma of the esophagus.[16]

For nodal staging, EUS examination is superior for assessment, having an 85% sensitivity,[17] with additional fine needle aspiration improving cN staging sensitivity and accuracy.[18] CT scan sensitivity is 30% to 60% using a node long axis of greater than 1 cm.[19,20] In a large meta-analysis of studies originating in Asia, the pooled sensitivity and specificity for the detection of regional lymph node metastasis was 66% and 96%, respectively.[21] In a retrospective review of 148 patients with esophageal cancer, FDG-PET scanning did not alter nodal staging in any patient who had undergone complete EUS–fine needle aspiration.[22]

In esophageal squamous cell carcinoma, FDG-PET/CT scanning performs similarly to EUS examination in discriminating N0 from N1 disease, while being slightly more sensitive but otherwise similar to EUS for distinguishing T1a or less disease from other tumors.[23] The most commonly involved lymph nodes in upper esophageal cancer are supraclavicular, retrotracheal, and paratracheal, whereas the most common in lower esophageal cancer are paraesophageal and gastrohepatic nodes.[24] FDG-PET/CT scanning is useful before endoscopy, helping to delineate nodal distribution before fine needle aspiration.[4]

In a novel study of 20 patients with mostly squamous cell histology, FDG-PET imaging was performed on the same day before surgical resection with lymph node dissection. Radioactivity in the harvested lymph nodes was measured using a well counter and correlated with pathology. Lymph node analysis from PET images yielded sensitivity, specificity, positive predictive value, and negative predictive value of 29%, 97%, 44%, and 94%, respectively. Ex vivo counts were more accurate, yielding 95%, 79%, 14%, and 99.8%, for these respective parameters. The authors suggested that FDG uptake in nodes may be helpful in navigation surgery for esophageal cancer.[25]

Mining PET data to find radiomic signatures predictive of outcomes is a burgeoning area of research in esophageal cancer. Yip and colleagues[26] found that PET-based textural features (entropy and run–length matrix) correlated with outcome after neoadjuvant chemotherapy, better than the standardized uptake value (SUV). Convolutional neural network analysis of FDG-PET/CT scans was used to predict lymphovascular invasion and perineural invasion in 798 patients with esophageal squamous carcinoma.[27] In 65 patients with esophageal cancer treated with chemoradiation and followed for 3 years, pretreatment FDG-PET scans and medical records were analyzed using a random forest machine learning approach;

the MTV was found to be the strongest predictor of response and survival.[28]

With the rapid technological changes in PET/CT scanners (time-of-flight resolution and advanced reconstruction techniques), previous assumptions regarding PET quantitation vis-à-vis the maximum (SUV_{max}), and data in older literature, will need to be reassessed. In particular, SUV has limitations, such as body composition, glucose level, uptake time, and reconstruction parameters, and sometimes can be misleading; there has been greater interest in qualitative scoring paradigms across a range of tumor types, and esophageal cancer is no exception.

Huang and colleagues[29] applied a qualitative 4-point scale to FDG-PET analysis: 1, no focal uptake; 2, focal uptake greater than surrounding tissue or blood pool but equal or less than the liver; 3, diffuse uptake greater than blood pool up to marginally greater than liver; and 4, focal uptake much greater than liver. Scores of 1 to 3 were viewed as negative and a score of 4 was positive. Taking into account multiple parameters derived from the postchemoradiation FDG-PET scan, including above and below the median values of the SUV_{max}, the percent change in SUV_{max}, and MTV, only the American Joint Commission on Cancer stage and qualitative 4-point scale to FDG-PET analysis score significantly correlated with overall survival on multivariable Cox regression analysis.[29] In a retrospective study of 128 patients with esophageal squamous cell cancer by Wang and colleagues[30] it was found that a tumor-to-liver SUV ratio was superior to SUV_{max} and tumor-to-blood pool ratio by receiver operating characteristic analysis in predicting tumor response and survival after chemoradiation.

Interim assessment

Several keys studies have revealed a potential role for FDG-PET/CT scans in identifying responders early (ie, 14 days) during neoadjuvant chemotherapy, thereby sparing nonresponding patients a toxic therapy without clinical benefit and allowing them to be resected sooner.[31,32] MUNICON II, a prospective trial of 56 patients with EGJ adenocarcinoma showed that event-free and overall survival was significantly shorter in metabolic nonresponders compared with metabolic responders, with a metabolic response defined as a 35% or greater decrease in the SUV on FDG-PET scanning 2 weeks into neoadjuvant chemotherapy. Metabolic responders continued neoadjuvant chemotherapy for up to 12 weeks, and nonresponders received salvage radiochemotherapy before resection.[33] In a study of 134 patients with squamous cell cancer by Li and

colleagues,[34] where FDG-PET was performed before and during neoadjuvant chemoradiation, SUV_{max} was found to be an independent prognostic factor for OS by Cox regression analysis, complementary to length of tumor and TNM stage. Other studies have shown similar results.[35–37]

In the ongoing phase II CALGB 8083 trial, patients with resectable esophageal and EGJ adenocarcinoma (n = 257) had their chemotherapy during neoadjuvant chemoradiation changed based on a greater or less than 35% decrease in SUV on FDG-PET scanning. Preliminary data indicate that this led to improved pathologic complete response rates in metabolic responders compared with nonresponders.[38]

Preoperative Assessment

Preoperative chemoradiation is a category 1 recommendation for locally advanced squamous cell carcinoma or adenocarcinoma of the thoracic esophagus or EGJ by the National Comprehensive Cancer Network (NCCN). FDG-PET/CT scanning from the skull base to mid-thigh is recommended in the NCCN guidelines for assessment after neoadjuvant or definitive chemoradiation in both squamous cell carcinoma and adenocarcinoma, in part to exclude the development of metastatic disease.[4] Many studies have shown that decreased uptake of FDG is predictive of survival in patients with locally advanced esophageal or EGJ cancer who undergo neoadjuvant treatment.[39,40] However, the exact cutoff values for absolute decrease and percent change in SUV between pretreatment and post-treatment scans varied widely between studies. In a report by Cerfolio and colleagues,[41] a decrease in SUV of more than 64% correlated with a complete pathologic response. Smith and colleagues[42] found that a decrease in SUV of more than 50% conferred a 12-month disease-free survival advantage over those patients who had a decrease in SUV of less than 50% (93% vs 43%). Kukar and colleagues,[43] in a retrospective study of 77 patients with adenocarcinoma who underwent PET scanning before and after neoadjuvant chemoradiation, found that pretherapy SUV, and change in SUV were significantly higher in patients who achieved complete pathologic response. A change in SUV of less than 45% was associated with residual disease. **Fig. 1** shows an EGJ adenocarcinoma with celiac nodal metastases that responded to neoadjuvant chemoradiation and correlated with a complete pathologic response. In many of these studies, the PET response did not correlate well with the pathologic response, with microscopic disease still present in metabolic responders. Accordingly, surgery is still recommended even if a strong postneoadjuvant therapy metabolic response is observed on PET.

Elevated FDG uptake in lymph nodes after neoadjuvant chemotherapy is highly specific (99%) but not sensitive (12%) in identifying nodal metastases.[44] As discussed elsewhere in this article, textural features of PET data are an emerging area of research[45] and may be predictive of outcomes in esophageal cancer. In a retrospective study by Simoni and colleagues,[46] 54 patients with adenocarcinoma and squamous cell carcinoma underwent FDG-PET/CT scanning before and after induction therapy, and then again after neoadjuvant chemoradiation and surgery. In addition to MTV and TLG, 3 radiomic features extracted from the pre-induction PET scan were correlated significantly with a pathologic response.

Although other studies have indicated limited usefulness of FDG-PET for the assessment of response to neoadjuvant therapy in esophageal cancer, many of these were likely confounded by false-positive PET findings, with FDG-PET scanning performed during or soon after preoperative therapy.[47,48] Radiation and chemoradiation may cause local inflammation in the esophagus, limiting the usefulness of FDG-PET scans in early response assessment of esophageal cancer. Accordingly, the NCCN guidelines recommend that FDG-PET/CT scanning should be performed at least 5 to 8 weeks after the completion of neoadjuvant chemoradiation.[4]

Post-treatment Follow-up

For patients with esophageal cancer who recur locoregionally and are treated with esophagectomy and/or chemoradiation, a CT scan is recommended as follow-up, but not an FDG-PET/CT scan, unless distant disease is suspected. For surveillance, a CT scan is recommended.[4] Although not recommended in the NCCN, FDG-PET/CT scanning may still be useful in follow-up: a meta-analysis by Goense and colleagues[49] of 486 patients with esophageal cancer after treatment with curative intent found FDG-PET/CT to detect recurrence with a pooled sensitivity and specificity of 96% and 78%, respectively.

GASTRIC CANCER
Initial Staging

Approximately 26,560 new cases of gastric cancer are estimated for 2021 in the United States, with 11,180 deaths.[2] The 5-year survival rate is 70% for localized tumors, 32% once spread locoregionally, and 6% with distant metastases.[2] Of gastric cancers, 95% are adenocarcinomas and classified as either proximal (about the cardia) or distal, and either diffuse or intestinal in histologic type. The diffuse type, typified by tumor cells scattered within a fibrous stroma, is mostly

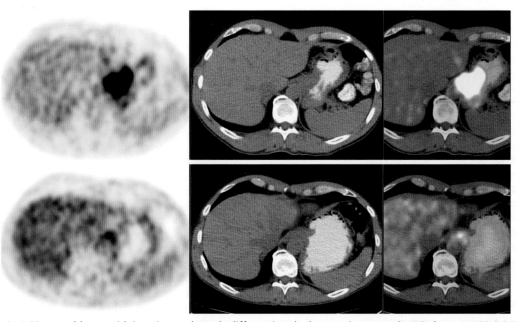

Fig. 1. A 50-year-old man with invasive moderately differentiated adenocarcinoma at the EGJ (*top row*: FDG-PET, CT scan, fused images). Metastatic gastrohepatic and celiac nodes were also noted (not shown). FDG-PET/CT scan after chemoradiation (*bottom row*) shows decrease in size of the primary mass and significant decrease in FDG activity (physiologic range). Esophagogastrectomy revealed no residual tumor at pathology.

associated with low-risk areas and gene mutations. Intestinal type is found in high-risk areas and is associated with *Helicobacter pylori* infection, smoking, and dietary factors including heavy alcohol intake. Tumors having an epicenter located more than 2 cm into proximal stomach are staged as gastric carcinomas, whereas those involving the EGJ with the epicenter less than 2 cm into the proximal stomach are staged as esophageal cancers.

Tumors in the lower two-thirds stomach are treated with subtotal gastrectomy; otherwise, total gastrectomy is recommended. For small, early gastric cancer confined to the mucosa, endoscopic resection is appropriate. Once it has invaded the submucosa (T1b), radical gastrectomy and lymphadenectomy are required. Locally advanced gastric cancer without distant metastases may be treated with surgical resection and perioperative chemotherapy. Despite advances in imaging and treatment, the 5-year survival is 25% to 30%, with EGJ (cardia) and diffuse-type noncardia gastric cancer having the worst prognosis.[50]

The current NCCN guidelines recommend CT scans of the chest, abdomen, and pelvis with oral and intravenous contrast as the primary modality for initial staging of gastric cancer, with FDG-PET/CT scans used for confirmation if there is no evidence of M1 disease.[51] EUS examination is used for assessing early stage disease, particularly depth of tumor invasion and local nodal involvement, although its accuracy is limited (46% and 67%, for these respective parameters). CT scanning is 43% to 83% accurate for T staging.[51] In a retrospective study of 229 patients with early stage gastric cancers by Yoon and associates,[52] FDG uptake was detected in only 18% of patients and found to depend on location (distal stomach with higher uptake), size, and depth of invasion. Diffuse and mucinous tumor types often demonstrate low FDG uptake, contributing to lower accuracy of FDG-PET scans compared with CT scans.[48,53] In a retrospective review of 105 patients with gastric cancer who underwent preoperative staging, 14% of tumors were not metabolically active, and intestinal subtype correlated with s higher SUV_{max} than nonintestinal, and FDG-PET scanning upstaged 19% of patients, with the majority a result of hitherto unknown distant metastases.[54]

The SUV_{max} of FDG in the primary tumor was found to be associated with the degree of differentiation, with the signet ring histology often being negative.[55] This finding is likely secondary to a decreased expression of GLUT1 in the signet ring cell subtype.[52] In a study of 341 patients with gastric cancer, FDG uptake was greatest in medullary and tubular subtypes, and lowest in signet ring, although when high uptake by SUV_{max} was observed in signet ring cell carcinoma, a greater likelihood of regional and distant metastatic disease was found.[56] The PET scan detection rates range from 40% to 90%, owing to this variable histology.[53,57,58] Accordingly, FDG-PET scanning may not be appropriate as initial evaluation for T1 disease.[51] FDG-PET scanning is less sensitive, but more specific compared with CT scans for local nodal involvement, and FDG-PET/CT scanning is more accurate in preoperative staging (68%) than PET scanning (47%) or CT scanning (53%) alone.[59]

When FDG avidity is observed, it is prognostically significant. In a large meta-analysis of 1,080 patients by Wu and coworkers,[60] high pretreatment SUV was prognostic, with hazard ratios of 1.7 for overall and recurrence-free survival. A high SUV_{max} and high MTV correlated with a higher risk of recurrence in advanced gastric cancer before curative surgery.[61] In a large study of 566 patients with gastric cancer by Song,[62] a nomogram was developed and found that tumor SUV_{max} and nodal SUV_{max} on preoperative PET/CT scans were independent predictors for lymph node metastases, with a further improvement in prediction found when albumin and carbohydrate antigen 19-9 were also used. In a study of 168 patients, Kwon and colleagues[63] found that FDG avidity of lymph nodes (defined as focal uptake on visual inspection and by MTV) was an independent predictor of recurrence-free survival, although avidity of the primary tumor was not—possibly reflecting confounding heterogeneous histology and background gastric wall uptake.

A pitfall of FDG-PET interpretation is inflammatory gastric activity, which can be focal as well as diffuse. Indeed, 1 study of 88 patients, performed in a Japanese PET/CT cancer screening program, found FDG uptake useful in predicting *H pylori* infection and subsequent atrophic gastritis (a risk factor for cancer). Uptake was higher in the gastric fundus than other areas of the stomach, but not significantly correlated with pathology.[64] Interestingly, of the 4 early gastric cancers detected, none had increased FDG uptake. Less common false positives include IgG4-related disease[65] and myofibroblastic sarcoma of the gastric cardia.[66]

Subsequent Treatment Strategy

In patients who cannot undergo surgery and receive primary chemotherapy or radiation, post-treatment assessment is usually performed with

CT scans, although FDG-PET/CT scanning is recommended in patients who have renal insufficiency or are allergic to iodinated contrast. FDG-PET/CT scanning may be used in follow-up for pathologic stage II to III disease or stage I to III disease after neoadjuvant or adjuvant therapy, although CT scanning every 6 to 12 months for the first 2 years, then every year for 5 years, is standard practice at many institutions.[51] EUS examination performed better than PET/CT scanning in gastric cancer restaging (89% vs 69% accuracy) before resection in a group of patients, 80 of whom then had neoadjuvant chemotherapy and 100 who proceeded directly to surgery.[67]

FDG-PET/CT scanning likely has value in the assessment of response after perioperative chemotherapy or preoperative chemoradiation (which is used in cT2 or higher, any N, M0 disease). In a study of 21 patients, the percent change in the SUV was the best-performing PET parameter after neoadjuvant therapy in distal esophageal and gastric adenocarcinomas; however, the pathologic response by histologic grading was still found to be a better predictor of survival than FDG uptake.[68] In a retrospective study by Schneider and colleagues[69] of 72 patients with gastric cancer or EGJ or gastric cardia (Siewert II or III) cancers, patients were enrolled who underwent FDG-PET before, and 14 days after the first of 3 cycles of neoadjuvant chemotherapy. Metabolic response was defined as a 35% or greater decrease in the SUV_{max}. The presence of a metabolic response did not correlate with pathologic response (ie, one-half had a major and one-half had minor pathologic regression), whereas in metabolic nonresponders, 90% had minor and 10% had major regression.

These results suggest that FDG-PET scans may identify patients who should immediately go to surgery or receive multimodality therapy.[69] In a prospective study of 20 patients with gastric cancer by Won and colleagues,[70] the authors demonstrated that a response similar to metabolic responders could be recovered in metabolic nonresponders if chemotherapy were switched after the postcycle 1 PET scan showing no metabolic response. Upon tumor recurrence, high FDG uptake by SUV_{max} on PET/CT scanning was found to correlate with worse 3-year postrecurrence survival in work by Kim and colleagues.[71]

HEPATOCELLULAR CARCINOMA

Hepatocellular carcinoma (HCC) is the sixth most common cancer in the world, with 42,220 new cases and 30,200 deaths in the United States in 2018.[72,73] The diagnosis of HCC is made when certain CT scan or MR imaging features (Liver Reporting & Data System 5) are encountered in high-risk patients (eg, cirrhosis, chronic hepatitis B, or prior HCC). For equivocal findings (Liver Reporting & Data System 2–4), a biopsy or additional imaging may be used.

FDG-PET/CT scanning is not recommended for routine initial imaging owing to its limited sensitivity, which likely results from lower tumor GLUT1 expression and a high concentration of glucose-6-phosphatase in normal liver, leading to rapid clearance of FDG and decreased contrast between normal parenchyma and well-differentiated HCC.[74] In a prospective study by Park and colleagues[75] of 99 patients with HCC, sensitivity for detection of HCC was only 61%, although it increased with tumor size and multiplicity and poorly differentiated histology, and the overall survival rate was lower in FDG-positive patients. FDG positivity in HCC has been reported between 38% and 70% with an overall sensitivity of 60%.[76]

FDG-PET scanning does have high specificity in HCC, and may be used to evaluate an equivocal imaging finding. An HCC detected by CT scanning/MR imaging with high FDG uptake by SUV likely is more biologically aggressive and less likely to respond to locoregional therapies.[77] A meta-analysis of 1,721 patients showed that FDG-PET/CT scanning may be useful in predicting overall and disease-free survival rates, but is of low sensitivity for HCC detection.[78]

FDG-PET has high sensitivity for detection of extrahepatic metastases, approaching 100%,[79] and detects recurrences earlier than conventional imaging.[80,81] In a small study of 34 patients with HCC who underwent FDG-PET/CT scanning before Y-90 radioembolization, FDG avidity in HCC was associated with a shorter time to progression within treated lesions and within more distant lesions in the liver, as well as a shorter progression-free survival rate after Y-90 radioembolization.[82]

An emerging role for FDG-PET/CT scanning in HCC is the workup for liver transplantation,[83] which is the ideal therapy for HCC because it can remove both the HCC and the underlying tumor-generating cirrhosis. The selection of patients with HCC for liver transplant has traditionally been performed by the Milan criteria, which require (1) 1 lesion smaller than 5 cm or up to 3 lesions smaller than 3 cm, (2) no extrahepatic disease, and (3) no vascular invasion. However, the Milan criteria are restrictive and do not include other factors that reflect tumor biology.

Although HCC vascular invasion is a major determinant of post-liver transplant outcomes, its detection requires invasive tissue sampling, which carries a higher risk in these patients. Several studies have shown that tumor differentiation independently predicts recurrence and survival after transplantation. FDG uptake is a sensitive and specific indicator for poorly differentiated tumors and has been found to be predictive of vascular invasion in HCC.[84,85]

A large Japanese multicenter study of 182 liver transplant recipients found that those patients who did not conform to the Milan criteria recurred at a much higher rate at 5 years relative to those who were within Milan criteria (38% vs 7%, respectively); however, there was a subgroup of patients outside of Milan criteria with a negative PET/CT scan and low alpha fetoprotein who did just as well as recipients who were within the Milan criteria. Many studies have shown FDG negativity in HCC before transplantation to be strongly predictive of high disease-free survival rates.[86–89] Consequently, there has been recent development of expanded liver transplant criteria that incorporate FDG-PET metabolic information, for example, the National Cancer Center Korea criteria.[90] FDG-PET/CT scanning is not routinely recommended for post-treatment assessment in HCC.[91]

BILIARY TRACT CANCERS
Gallbladder Cancer

Gallbladder cancer is a rare cancer, with approximately 9700 cases per year in the United States. The 5-year survival rate is 50% for stage 1 disease, and less than 10% for stage III and above.[92] It grows rapidly, invading the liver and spreading to lymph nodes, hematogenously, and intraperitoneally, and is often detected at a late stage. Complete resection is possible for early disease (T1–2, N0), and distant metastasis and N2 disease are contraindications to surgery. Management includes cholecystectomy with partial hepatectomy, chemotherapy, radiation therapy, and endoscopic stenting.[92]

FDG-PET/CT imaging of gallbladder cancer is not commonly performed, with ultrasound examination, CT scanning, and MR imaging being the mainstays for evaluation. A meta-analysis examining the diagnostic accuracy of FDG-PET/CT scanning for gallbladder cancer reported sensitivity of 87% (95% confidence interval, 82%–92%) and specificity of 78% (95% confidence interval, 68%–86%), with an area under the curve of 0.88. Recent retrospective studies indicate that FDG-PET scanning may be useful for detecting regional nodal or distant metastatic disease, which is occult on CT scanning in patients who would otherwise be resectable.[93–96] Leung and colleagues[97] studied 100 patients with 63

gallbladder cancers and found the sensitivity and specificity of FDG-PET scanning to be 56% and 94%, respectively. FDG-PET scanning found malignancy not seen on CT scanning in 3 patients, and confirmed benignity in 2 patients with suspicious CT findings. The impact was greater in patients without prior cholecystectomy and when evaluating findings suspicious for nodal disease on CT scanning.[97] Gallbladder inflammation and infection are potential false positives.[98,99]

Cholangiocarcinoma

Cholangiocarcinoma is the second most common primary hepatic cancer; most tumors arise at the liver hilum (Klatskin tumor), and the others arise in the distal common bile duct or intrahepatic ducts of the liver (intrahepatic cholangiocarcinoma). The 5-year survival rate for resectable disease ranges from 22% to 44%. Survival is related to size and number of tumors, lymph node metastasis, and invasion of the vasculature. Peritoneal spread is present in 10% to 20% of patients at presentation and precludes surgical resection.[100]

Lee and associates retrospectively reviewed the diagnostic and prognostic role of FDG-PET/CT scans in 76 patients with intrahepatic cholangiocarcinoma. FDG-PET/CT scanning was more sensitive for detecting nodal metastasis than CT scanning or MR imaging (74.5% vs 61.8%) and identified distant metastases occult on other modalities in 6 patients. Higher measures of FDG uptake (SUV$_{max}$, MTV, TLG) were correlated with significantly reduced survival.[101] Other retrospective studies indicate that PET scans may be useful for detecting regional nodal or distant metastatic disease, which is occult on CT scans, in patients who would have otherwise resectable disease.[93–95,102,103] FDG uptake on preoperative PET scan by MTV is associated with K-ras mutation.[104]

Extrahepatic cholangiocarcinoma includes common bile duct cancer and Klatskin tumor, and carries a high mortality. Surgical resection and lymph node dissection can confer long-term survival; however, this is only possible with accurate staging. FDG-PET/CT scanning is not routinely recommended for evaluation; however, recent reviews have demonstrated diagnostic and prognostic usefulness. In a retrospective review of 234 patients with extrahepatic cholangiocarcinoma by Kim and coworkers, FDG-PET/CT scanning was compared with contrast-enhanced CT scanning and MR imaging. FDG-PET/CT scanning was performed to characterize indeterminate primary tumor lesions or findings equivocal for nodal and distant metastases on other imaging.

The PET sensitivity for detection of primary tumor was inferior to CT scanning or MR imaging (78.6% vs 95.0%–97.0%), as it was for detection of nodal metastasis (44% vs 75%–78%). By multivariate analysis, the SUV_{max} of the primary tumor and metastatic disease was associated with poorer overall survival (hazard ratios of 1.75 and 8.1, respectively). When focusing on the periductal infiltrating subtype of extrahepatic cholangiocarcinoma, an SUV_{max} of greater than 5 in the primary tumor was associated with an increased risk of nodal and distant metastasis (odds ratios of 1.6 and 101, respectively) and a hazard ratio of 1.8 of poor overall survival.[105]

PANCREATIC CANCER
Initial Staging

Pancreatic ductal adenocarcinoma (PDAC) is the second most common GI cancer after colorectal cancer in the United States, with approximately 60,430 new diagnoses and 48,220 deaths expected in 2021.[2] It has remained one of the most lethal cancers in the world, with a dismal 5-year survival of 5%, primarily owing to advanced stage at presentation. The standard of care for resectable tumors is surgery followed by adjuvant chemotherapy; however, less than 20% are resectable at diagnosis. Selected patients at risk for positive margins will now undergo neoadjuvant therapy, which may downstage tumors so that they may be resected. In stage 1 disease, the tumor is confined to the pancreas; in stage 2, the tumor extends outside the pancreas but without vascular involvement; in stage 3 disease, there is vascular involvement; and in stage 4, there is distant metastatic disease.[106]

Multidetector, contrast-enhanced pancreas protocol CT scanning is the preferred initial imaging modality for PDAC. Typically, arterial and parenchymal phase images are acquired with thin slices and multiplanar reconstruction to define vascular anatomy that is critical for surgical planning. However, FDG-PET/CT scanning should be considered in high-risk patients to detect metastatic disease outside the pancreas. High-risk indicators include borderline resectable disease, marked elevation of carbohydrate antigen 19-9, large primary tumors, large regional lymph nodes, and severe clinical symptoms.[107]

At diagnosis, FDG-PET scanning can distinguish between benign and malignant pancreatic lesions, especially when combined with EUS examination, although inflammatory disease is a source of false positives.[108] A prospective study by Buchs and colleagues[109] of 45 patients showed 96% sensitivity but 67% specificity for detection with contrast-enhanced PET/contrast-enhanced CT scanning, which decreased to 72% and 33% when PET/CT scanning was performed without intravenous contrast. **Fig. 2** shows an example of a small ampullary adenocarcinoma on FDG-PET/CT scanning and the importance of contrast enhancement. In a prospective study of 108 PDAC patient PET scans, the accuracy rate was 80% for local invasion, 94% for distant metastasis, and 42% for lymph node spread.[110]

The benefit of FDG-PET/CT scanning in upstaging patients with PDAC has been shown in 1 study as an increased detection rate of metastatic disease with PET/CT scanning compared with CT scanning and PET scanning alone, with a sensitivity of 87% for PET/CT scanning and a change in clinical management of 11%.[111] However, the role of FDG-PET/CT scanning in this setting is still evolving. In a 2014 meta-analysis by Rijkers and colleagues[112] of 35 studies, PET/CT scanning yielded 90% sensitivity, 76% specificity, 89% positive predictive value, 78% negative predictive value, and 86% accuracy. FDG-PET scanning could differentiate between PDAC and chronic pancreatitis with 90% and 84% sensitivity and specificity, respectively.[112] In another large meta-analysis by Wang and associates,[113] pooled sensitivity and specificity of FDG-PET scanning were 91% and 81% for the primary tumor, 64% and 81% for nodal metastases, and 67% and 96% for liver metastases, respectively. A higher SUV was associated with lower overall survival (hazard ratio, 2.4). In a study of 105 patients with early stage (I–II) PDAC by Pimiento and colleagues,[114] FDG uptake before surgical resection when stratified into high or low based on the median SUV_{max} correlated with pathologic stage, overall survival, and recurrence-free survival.

Although conventional PET parameters such as SUV_{max}, MTV, and TLG show usefulness, given the unchanged poor survival of PDAC over the last 2 decades, new tools are needed. PET-based radiomic biomarkers may improve patient risk stratification, by better representing tumor biology and cellular heterogeneity, and revealing prognostic textural features in the images. Toyama and colleagues retrospectively reviewed pretreatment FDG-PET/CT scanning in 161 patients with PDAC and extracted 42 PET radiomic features using freely available software.[115,116] Of 10 PET features found to be predictive of overall survival in univariate Cox regression analysis, only gray-level zone length matrix gray-level nonuniformity, a marker of lesion heterogeneity, was a significant predictor by multivariate analysis. Applying a random forest machine learning approach to these features, gray-level zone length matrix gray-level

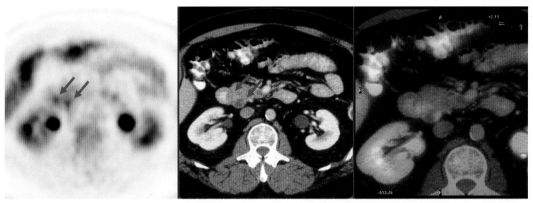

Fig. 2. Initial staging of a 58-year-old man with a pancreatic head mass. FDG-PET/contrast-enhanced CT scan shows 2 small foci of hypermetabolic activity (*red arrows*) suspicious for malignancy with adjacent nonavid cystic/necrotic component. Patient underwent Whipple procedure with pathology revealing poorly differentiated adenocarcinoma at the ampulla. Note the importance of oral and intravenous contrast for defining this lesion.

nonuniformity and TLG were able to stratify patients into 3 groups according to prognosis.[116]

Subsequent Treatment Strategy

FDG-PET/CT scanning is not routinely recommended in the post-treatment assessment of PDAC and its potential clinical benefit in post-therapy assessment is being investigated. Korn and colleagues prospectively studied 52 patients with metastatic PDAC who underwent PET scanning at baseline, 6 weeks, and 12 weeks after chemotherapy. Patients with a complete metabolic response lived significantly longer than those with a partial metabolic response.[117]

In the neoadjuvant setting, FDG-PET response by PET Response Criteria in Solid Tumors (PERCIST) after preoperative chemotherapy correlated with pathologic response better than RECIST in a study of 42 patients with PDAC. A decrease in MTV of less than 50% independently predicted relapse-free survival (hazard ratio, 3.9) and overall survival (hazard ratio, 14).[118] Wang and coworkers[119] retrospectively reviewed 32 patients who underwent FDG-PET/CT scanning within 6 months after resection, and found that patients with PET-positive findings in locoregional nodes and distant sites had a significantly worse overall survival.

COLON CANCER

It is estimated that 104,270 people in the United States will be diagnosed with colon cancer in 2021, with 52,980 deaths.[2] The incidence and mortality of colon cancer has been declining over the past several years, indicating the effectiveness of screening.

Initial Staging

Adenocarcinoma of the colon typically has high metabolic activity on FDG-PET scans. Tumors with mucinous features, however, may not have significant FDG uptake (Fig. 3). Owing to the variable and potentially high physiologic FDG activity within the bowel, small primary tumors may be difficult to identify on FDG-PET/CT scans. Oral contrast can be helpful in characterizing these lesions. The NCCN guidelines do not recommend FDG-PET/CT scanning as a first-line modality for staging colon cancer.[120] T staging is determined by the tumor penetration into the muscularis mucosa, muscularis propria, and adjacent surrounding tissues. This is best established with a CT scan, and FDG-PET scanning does not contribute to this assessment. N staging is related to the number of metastatic nodes, primarily determined by CT scan or MR imaging. The sensitivity and specificity of nodal assessment is highly dependent on the threshold size used in the evaluation. In a study by Rollven and colleagues,[121] a size threshold of 1 cm resulted in high specificity (90%) but low sensitivity (28%) for detecting metastatic nodes. Alternatively, using a threshold of 0.5 cm resulted in high sensitivity (90%) but low specificity (31%). CT morphologic features such as short/long axis ratio, enhancement, heterogeneity, border features, and clustering of nodes have also been found to be important in determining if nodes are metastatic.[122] The additional information from FDG-PET scanning does not improve the accuracy of nodal assessment over a CT scan alone for colorectal cancer.[123] This is likely because both CT and FDG-PET scans have a low sensitivity for small nodes.

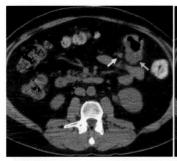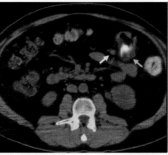

Fig. 3. Moderately differentiated mucinous adenocarcinoma in the transverse colon (*green arrow*). Although intensely hypermetabolic on FDG-PET, low-density regions of the primary tumor have low FDG uptake, in keeping with mucinous histology. The tumor invaded the visceral peritoneum and contained one tumor deposit on pathology. The adjacent subcentimeter round node (*yellow arrow*) was not FDG-avid and 0/26 nodes were involved at surgery.

Although FDG-PET/CT scanning may not contribute routinely to T and N staging for colorectal cancer, it can provide added sensitivity for detecting distant metastatic disease in patients with advanced or high-risk tumors.[124] FDG-PET/CT scanning may be useful for clarifying equivocal findings on CT scans or MR imaging (eg, lung nodules, liver lesions) and can provide added assurance that no unsuspected metastatic disease is present before surgery. Although CT scanning remains the modality of choice for primary staging of colon cancer, the selective use of FDG-PET/CT scanning can change patient management in 30% of cases.[124] Given the potential impact that FDG-PET/CT scanning can have on patients with colon cancer and with the current advances in PET/CT technology, it has recently been suggested that additional applications be reconsidered in future guidelines.[125]

Response to Therapy

Several studies have indicated that FDG-PET/CT scanning obtained early in the course of chemotherapy may be useful for predicting response to treatment.[126,127] A review by de Geus-Oei and colleagues[128] summarized the findings of several small studies that showed promise for early response assessment. However, the response criteria and timing of the scans in these studies were heterogeneous, and no standardized early response algorithm has been tested in a large clinical study. More research is needed in this area before it can be applied in routine clinical practice.

After liver ablation procedures, FDG-PET/CT scanning can be used to accurately detect residual disease soon after treatment, allowing retreatment as needed.[128,129] Neither contrast-enhanced CT scanning nor MR imaging are effective in identifying residual tumor in this scenario.

Evaluation for Recurrence

Although FDG-PET/CT scanning is the most sensitive imaging modality to detect recurrent colon cancer, it is not currently recommended as the primary modality. The current NCCN guidelines recommend follow-up with serum carcinoembryonic antigen, colonoscopy, and contrast-enhanced CT scan.[120] If disease is suspected by carcinoembryonic antigen, FDG-PET/CT scanning can be used to follow-up if the CT scan is negative. FDG-PET/CT scanning can also be used in the event of metastatic disease, to determine resectability. Monteil and colleagues[130] randomized 376 patients with colorectal cancer to FDG-PET/CT scanning every 6 months versus conventional surveillance for 36 months after curative surgery. Patients followed by FDG-PET/CT scanning had earlier detection and treatment of recurrent disease, but there was no difference in overall survival between the 2 groups, and follow-up by FDG-PET/CT scanning was more expensive.[130]

RECTAL AND ANAL CANCERS
Initial Staging

Although often grouped together, rectal and anal cancers are substantially different in terms of histology, staging, and patterns of nodal spread (**Table 1**). Anatomically, the rectum and anus are separated by the dentate line, which is not visible on a CT scan. Rectal staging is based on depth of invasion and number of nodes, similar to colon cancer. MR imaging is the preferred imaging modality for initially staging rectal cancer, and FDG-PET/CT scanning is not usually indicated.[131,132]

In contrast, anal cancer staging is based on size and the location of metastatic nodes, and FDG-PET/CT scanning can be helpful in newly diagnosed patients.[133] One of the most important distinguishing features is that, unlike rectal cancer, anal cancer spreads regionally to the inguinal and femoral nodes. It is particularly important to recognize this distinction when evaluating patients with anal cancer by FDG-PET/CT scanning, because the presence of metastatic inguinal

Table 1
Differences in TNM staging between rectal and anal cancer, based on the American Joint Commission on Cancer Staging, 8th edition

	Rectal Cancer	Anal Cancer
Typical histology	Adenocarcinoma	Squamous cell carcinoma
T staging	Depth of invasion	Size of tumor
N staging	Number of nodes Presence of tumor deposits	Location of nodes

Regional nodes	Rectal (superior, middle, inferior); Inferior
	  mesenteric; internal iliac; mesorectal;
	  presacral, lateral sacral, sacral promontory
		Mesorectal; internal iliac;
		  external iliac; inguinal

M staging	Distant metastases With or without peritoneal carcinomatosis	Distant metastases

Data from Pedersen CK, Babu AS. Understanding the Lymphatics: Review of the N Category in the Updated TNM Staging of Cancers of the Digestive System. *AJR Am J Roentgenol.* Jul 2020;215(1):58-68.

nodes substantially alters treatment (radiation treatment planning). Metastatic inguinal nodes are considered regional for anal cancer, but considered distant metastases for rectal cancer. The evaluation of inguinal nodes by FDG-PET/CT can be challenging, because this site is often involved by inflammatory/reactive pathology. In addition, HIV-positive patients are at higher risk for anal cancer and can have nonspecific metabolically active adenopathy. Patients with anal cancer with inguinal node metastases have a much poorer prognosis. Because both size and FDG activity can be nonspecific in inguinal nodes, additional considerations (asymmetry with contralateral nodes, roundness, CT morphology, enhancement, and border characteristics) are often helpful for assessing these nodes. An example of a patient being staged for anal cancer is shown in **Fig. 4**. In this case, a left inguinal node with moderate FDG activity raises concern for inguinal metastasis, and should be included in the radiation

treatment plan unless biopsied and proven to be benign.

Evaluation for Recurrence

For patients suspected of having recurrent rectal cancer (increasing carcinoembryonic antigen), further evaluation includes a physical examination, colonoscopy, and CT scanning. FDG-PET/CT scanning, especially with a contrast-enhanced CT scan, is the most sensitive imaging test for detecting recurrent disease and may be performed initially or as a follow-up to a negative CT scan.[131] In patients with known metastatic disease and/or liver lesions, the additional information from FDG-PET/CT scanning can help to determine surgical options.

In patients with anal cancer, follow-up is based on physical examination, anoscopy, and CT scanning or MR imaging.[133] FDG-PET/CT scanning does not play a role, although it may be supportive in assessing metastatic disease.

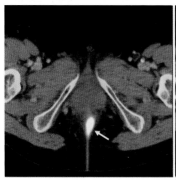 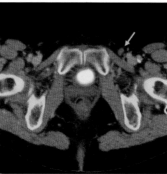

Fig. 4. Importance of inguinal nodes in staging anal cancer. Moderately differentiated invasive squamous cell carcinoma of the anus (*yellow arrow*). Left inguinal node has benign features on CT scan but moderate FDG activity on PET (*green arrow*). If metastatic, this would reflect N1 disease and would change the radiation therapy treatment plan. Biopsy was negative for metastasis.

SUMMARY

GI malignancies affect a broad range of disease sites, each with different treatment and management issues. The role of FDG-PET/CT scanning varies significantly by disease site, and it is important for the interpreting physician to appreciate these differences. In many cases, FDG-PET/CT scanning is not the primary imaging modality for evaluating patients with GI cancers, but when used strategically and in combination with other clinical modalities, FDG-PET/CT can have a substantial impact on patient care.

CLINICS CARE POINTS

- GI malignancies are a diverse group of diseases, and the contributions of FDG-PET/CT for diagnosing and guiding therapy vary widely among the different disease sites.

- The combination of FDG-PET and CT with oral and intravenous contrast can be particularly valuable for evaluating GI tumors.

- For many GI malignancies, combined FDG-PET/CT is a sensitive imaging modality for detecting recurrent disease.

DISCLOSURE

The authors have nothing to disclose.

REFERENCES

1. Hamidizadeh R, Eftekhari A, Wiley EA, et al. Metformin discontinuation prior to FDG PET/CT: a randomized controlled study to compare 24- and 48-hour bowel activity. Radiology 2018;289(2):418–25.

2. Siegel RL, Miller KD, Fuchs HE, et al. Cancer statistics, 2021. CA Cancer J Clin 2021;71(1):7–33.

3. Kim TJ, Kim HY, Lee KW, et al. Multimodality assessment of esophageal cancer: preoperative staging and monitoring of response to therapy. Radiographics 2009;29(2):403–21.

4. National Comprehensive Cancer Network. Esophageal and esophagogastric junction cancers (Version 2.2021). Available at: https://www.nccn.org/professionals/physician_gls/pdf/esophageal_blocks.pdf. Accessed May 6, 2021.

5. Tirumani H, Rosenthal MH, Tirumani SH, et al. Esophageal carcinoma: current concepts in the role of imaging in staging and management. Can Assoc Radiol J May 2015;66(2):130–9.

6. Chatterton BE, Ho Shon I, Baldey A, et al. Positron emission tomography changes management and prognostic stratification in patients with oesophageal cancer: results of a multicentre prospective study. Eur J Nucl Med Mol Imaging 2009;36(3):354–61.

7. Cuellar SL, Carter BW, Macapinlac HA, et al. Clinical staging of patients with early esophageal adenocarcinoma: does FDG-PET/CT have a role? J Thorac Oncol 2014;9(8):1202–6.

8. Little SG, Rice TW, Bybel B, et al. Is FDG-PET indicated for superficial esophageal cancer? Eur J Cardiothorac Surg 2007;31(5):791–6.

9. Walker AJ, Spier BJ, Perlman SB, et al. Integrated PET/CT fusion imaging and endoscopic ultrasound in the pre-operative staging and evaluation of esophageal cancer. Mol Imaging Biol 2011;13(1):166–71.

10. Findlay JM, Bradley KM, Maile EJ, et al. Pragmatic staging of oesophageal cancer using decision theory involving selective endoscopic ultrasonography, PET and laparoscopy. Br J Surg 2015;102(12):1488–99.

11. Amin MB, Greene FL, Edge SB, et al. The eighth edition AJCC cancer staging manual: continuing to build a bridge from a population-based to a more "personalized" approach to cancer staging. CA Cancer J Clin 2017;67(2):93–9.

12. Munden RF, Macapinlac HA, Erasmus JJ. Esophageal cancer: the role of integrated CT-PET in initial staging and response assessment after preoperative therapy. J Thorac Imaging 2006;21(2):137–45.

13. Sekiguchi M, Terauchi T, Kakugawa Y, et al. Performance of 18-fluoro-2-deoxyglucose positron emission tomography for esophageal cancer screening. World J Gastroenterol 2017;23(15):2743–9.

14. Iwamuro M, Okamoto Y, Kawano S, et al. Esophageal papilloma detected by positron emission tomography. Intern Med 2020;59(7):1003–4.

15. Scarsbrook A, Ward G, Murray P, et al. Respiratory-gated (4D) contrast-enhanced FDG PET-CT for radiotherapy planning of lower oesophageal carcinoma: feasibility and impact on planning target volume. BMC Cancer 2017;17(1):671.

16. Domachevsky L, Kashtan H, Brenner B, et al. Baseline 18F-FDG PET/CT as predictor of the pathological response to neoadjuvant therapy in esophageal cancer: a retrospective study. Medicine (Baltimore) 2018;97(49):e13412.

17. Puli SR, Reddy JB, Bechtold ML, et al. Staging accuracy of esophageal cancer by endoscopic ultrasound: a meta-analysis and systematic review. World J Gastroenterol 2008;14(10):1479–90.

18. Vazquez-Sequeiros E, Norton ID, Clain JE, et al. Impact of EUS-guided fine-needle aspiration on lymph node staging in patients with esophageal carcinoma. Gastrointest Endosc 2001;53(7):751–7.

19. Block MI, Patterson GA, Sundaresan RS, et al. Improvement in staging of esophageal cancer

with the addition of positron emission tomography. Ann Thorac Surg 1997;64(3):770–6 [discussion 776-7].

20. Kato H, Kuwano H, Nakajima M, et al. Comparison between positron emission tomography and computed tomography in the use of the assessment of esophageal carcinoma. Cancer 2002; 94(4):921–8.

21. Jiang C, Chen Y, Zhu Y, et al. Systematic review and meta-analysis of the accuracy of 18F-FDG PET/CT for detection of regional lymph node metastasis in esophageal squamous cell carcinoma. J Thorac Dis 2018;10(11):6066–76.

22. Keswani RN, Early DS, Edmundowicz SA, et al. Routine positron emission tomography does not alter nodal staging in patients undergoing EUS-guided FNA for esophageal cancer. Gastrointest Endosc 2009;69(7):1210–7.

23. Jeong DY, Kim MY, Lee KS, et al. Surgically resected T1- and T2-stage esophageal squamous cell carcinoma: T and N staging performance of EUS and PET/CT. Cancer Med 2018;7(8):3561–70.

24. Garcia B, Goodman KA, Cambridge L, et al. Distribution of FDG-avid nodes in esophageal cancer: implications for radiotherapy target delineation. Radiat Oncol 2016;11(1):156.

25. Yoshimura S, Takahashi M, Aikou S, et al. One-by-one comparison of lymph nodes between 18F-FDG uptake and pathological diagnosis in esophageal cancer. Clin Nucl Med 2020;45(10):741–6.

26. Yip SS, Coroller TP, Sanford NN, et al. Relationship between the temporal changes in positron-emission-tomography-imaging-based textural features and pathologic response and survival in esophageal cancer patients. Front Oncol 2016;6: 72.

27. Yeh JC, Yu WH, Yang CK, et al. Predicting aggressive histopathological features in esophageal cancer with positron emission tomography using a deep convolutional neural network. Ann Transl Med 2021;9(1):37.

28. Desbordes P, Ruan S, Modzelewski R, et al. Predictive value of initial FDG-PET features for treatment response and survival in esophageal cancer patients treated with chemo-radiation therapy using a random forest classifier. PLoS One 2017;12(3): e0173208.

29. Huang YC, Li SH, Lu HI, et al. Post-chemoradiotherapy FDG PET with qualitative interpretation criteria for outcome stratification in esophageal squamous cell carcinoma. PLoS One 2019;14(1): e0210055.

30. Wang C, Zhao K, Hu S, et al. The PET-derived tumor-to-liver standard uptake ratio (SUV TLR) is superior to tumor SUVmax in predicting tumor response and survival after chemoradiotherapy in

patients with locally advanced esophageal cancer. Front Oncol 2020;10:1630.

31. Ott K, Weber WA, Lordick F, et al. Metabolic imaging predicts response, survival, and recurrence in adenocarcinomas of the esophagogastric junction. J Clin Oncol 2006;24(29):4692–8.

32. Weber WA, Ott K, Becker K, et al. Prediction of response to preoperative chemotherapy in adenocarcinomas of the esophagogastric junction by metabolic imaging. J Clin Oncol 2001;19(12): 3058–65.

33. zum Büschenfelde CM, Herrmann K, Schuster T, et al. 18)F-FDG PET-guided salvage neoadjuvant radiochemotherapy of adenocarcinoma of the esophagogastric junction: the MUNICON II trial. J Nucl Med 2011;52(8):1189–96.

34. Li Y, Zschaeck S, Lin Q, et al. Metabolic parameters of sequential 18F-FDG PET/CT predict overall survival of esophageal cancer patients treated with (chemo-) radiation. Radiat Oncol 2019;14(1): 35.

35. Gabrielson S, Sanchez-Crespo A, Klevebro F, et al. 18F FDG-PET/CT evaluation of histological response after neoadjuvant treatment in patients with cancer of the esophagus or gastroesophageal junction. Acta Radiol 2019;60(5):578–85.

36. Sánchez-Izquierdo N, Perlaza P, Pagès M, et al. Assessment of response to neoadjuvant chemoradiotherapy by 18F-FDG PET/CT in patients with locally advanced esophagogastric junction adenocarcinoma. Clin Nucl Med 2020;45(1):38–43.

37. Tandberg DJ, Cui Y, Rushing CN, et al. Intratreatment response assessment with 18F-FDG PET: correlation of semiquantitative PET features with pathologic response of esophageal cancer to neoadjuvant chemoradiotherapy. Int J Radiat Oncol Biol Phys 2018;102(4):1002–7.

38. Goodman KA, Niedzwiecki D, Hall N, et al. Initial results of CALGB 80803 (Alliance): A randomized phase II trial of PET scan-directed combined modality therapy for esophageal cancer. J Clin Oncol 2017;35(4_suppl):1.

39. Swisher SG, Erasmus J, Maish M, et al. 2-Fluoro-2-deoxy-D-glucose positron emission tomography imaging is predictive of pathologic response and survival after preoperative chemoradiation in patients with esophageal carcinoma. Cancer 2004; 101(8):1776–85.

40. Smithers BM, Couper GC, Thomas JM, et al. Positron emission tomography and pathological evidence of response to neoadjuvant therapy in adenocarcinoma of the esophagus. Dis Esophagus 2008;21(2):151–8.

41. Cerfolio RJ, Bryant AS, Talati AA, et al. Change in maximum standardized uptake value on repeat positron emission tomography after chemoradiotherapy in patients with esophageal cancer

identifies complete responders. J Thorac Cardio-vasc Surg 2009;137(3):605–9.

42. Smith JW, Moreira J, Abood G, et al. The influence of (18)fluorodeoxyglucose positron emission to-mography on the management of gastroesopha-geal junction carcinoma. Am J Surg 2009;197(3):308–12.

43. Kukar M, Alnaji RM, Jabi F, et al. Role of repeat 18F-fluorodeoxyglucose positron emission tomog-raphy examination in predicting pathologic response following neoadjuvant chemoradiother-apy for esophageal adenocarcinoma. JAMA Surg 2015;150(6):555–62.

44. Fencl P, Belohlavek O, Harustiak T, et al. FDG-PET/CT lymph node staging after neoadjuvant chemo-therapy in patients with adenocarcinoma of the esophageal-gastric junction. Abdom Radiol (Ny) 2016;41(11):2089–94.

45. Zwanenburg A, Vallières M, Abdalah MA, et al. The image biomarker standardization initiative: stan-dardized quantitative radiomics for high-throughput image-based phenotyping. Radiology 2020;295(2):328–38.

46. Simoni N, Rossi G, Benetti G, et al. (18)F-FDG PET/CT metrics are correlated to the pathological response in esophageal cancer patients treated with induction chemotherapy followed by neoadju-vant chemo-radiotherapy. Front Oncol 2020;10:599907.

47. Gillham CM, Lucey JA, Keogan M, et al. 18)FDG uptake during induction chemoradiation for oeso-phageal cancer fails to predict histomorphologi-cal tumour response. Br J Cancer 2006;95(9):1174–9.

48. Wieder HA, Krause BJ, Herrmann K. PET and PET-CT in esophageal and gastric cancer. Methods Mol Biol 2011;727:59–76.

49. Goense L, van Rossum PS, Reitsma JB, et al. Diag-nostic performance of (1)(8)F-FDG PET and PET/CT for the detection of recurrent esophageal can-cer after treatment with curative intent: a system-atic review and meta-analysis. J Nucl Med 2015;56(7):995–1002.

50. De Raffele E, Mirarchi M, Cuicchi D, et al. Evolving role of FDG-PET/CT in prognostic evaluation of resectable gastric cancer. World J Gastroenterol 2017;23(38):6923–6.

51. National Comprehensive Cancer Network. Gastric cancer (version 2.2021). Available at: https://www.nccn.org/professionals/physician_gls/pdf/gastric_blocks.pdf. Accessed May 6, 2021.

52. Yoon JK, Byun C, Jo KS, et al. Clinicopathologic parameters associated with the FDG-avidity in staging of early gastric cancer using 18F-FDG PET. Medicine (Baltimore) 2019;98(31):e16690.

53. Stahl A, Ott K, Weber WA, et al. FDG PET imaging of locally advanced gastric carcinomas: correlation with endoscopic and histopathological findings. Eur J Nucl Med Mol Imaging 2003;30(2):288–95.

54. Bosch KD, Chicklore S, Cook GJ, et al. Staging FDG PET-CT changes management in patients with gastric adenocarcinoma who are eligible for radical treatment. Eur J Nucl Med Mol Imaging 2020;47(4):759–67.

55. Maman A, Sahin A, Ayan AK. The relationship of SUV value in PET-CT with tumor differentiation and tumor markers in gastric cancer. Eur J Med 2020;52(1):67–72.

56. Arslan E, Aksoy T, Gundogan C, et al. Metabolic characteristics and diagnostic contribution of (18)F-FDG PET/CT in gastric carcinomas. Mol Imaging Radionucl Ther 2020;29(1):25–32.

57. Yamada A, Oguchi K, Fukushima M, et al. Evalua-tion of 2-deoxy-2-[18F]fluoro-D-glucose positron emission tomography in gastric carcinoma: relation to histological subtypes, depth of tumor invasion, and glucose transporter-1 expression. Ann Nucl Med 2006;20(9):597–604.

58. Atay-Rosenthal S, Wahl RL, Fishman EK. PET/CT findings in gastric cancer: potential advantages and current limitations. Imaging Med 2012;4(2):241–50.

59. Chen J, Cheong JH, Yun MJ, et al. Improvement in preoperative staging of gastric adenocarcinoma with positron emission tomography. Cancer 2005;103(11):2383–90.

60. Wu Z, Zhao J, Gao P, et al. Prognostic value of pre-treatment standardized uptake value of F-18-fluoro-deoxyglucose PET in patients with gastric cancer: a meta-analysis. BMC Cancer 2017;17(1):275.

61. Kwon HR, Pahk K, Park S, et al. Prognostic value of metabolic information in advanced gastric cancer using preoperative (18)F-FDG PET/CT. Nucl Med Mol Imaging 2019;53(6):386–95.

62. Song BI. Nomogram using F-18 fluorodeoxyglu-cose positron emission tomography/computed to-mography for preoperative prediction of lymph node metastasis in gastric cancer. World J Gastro-intest Oncol 2020;12(4):447–56.

63. Kwon HW, An L, Kwon HR, et al. Preoperative nodal (18)F-FDG avidity rather than primary tumor avidity determines the prognosis of patients with advanced gastric cancer. J Gastric Cancer 2018;18(3):218–29.

64. Kobayashi S, Ogura M, Suzawa N, et al. (18)F-FDG uptake in the stomach on screening PET/CT: value for predicting Helicobacter pylori infection and chronic atrophic gastritis. BMC Med Imaging 2016;16(1):58.

65. Otsuka R, Kano M, Hayashi H, et al. Probable IgG4-related sclerosing disease presenting as a gastric submucosal tumor with an intense tracer uptake on PET/CT: a case report. Surg Case Rep 2016;2(1):33.

66. Niu R, Wang JF, Zhang DC, et al. Low-grade myo-fibroblastic sarcoma of gastric cardia on 18F-FDG positron emission tomography/computed tomography: an extremely rare case report. Medicine (Baltimore) 2018;97(4):e9720.

67. Redondo-Cerezo E, Martinez-Cara JG, Jimenez-Rosales R, et al. Endoscopic ultrasound in gastric cancer staging before and after neoadjuvant chemotherapy. A comparison with PET-CT in a clinical series. United Eur Gastroenterol J 2017;5(5): 641–7.

68. Manoharan V, Lee S, Chong S, et al. Serial imaging using [18F]Fluorodeoxyglucose positron emission tomography and histopathologic assessment in predicting survival in a population of surgically resectable distal oesophageal and gastric adenocarcinoma following neoadjuvant therapy. Ann Nucl Med 2017;31(4):315–23.

69. Schneider PM, Eshmuminov D, Rordorf T, et al. 18) FDG-PET-CT identifies histopathological non-responders after neoadjuvant chemotherapy in locally advanced gastric and cardia cancer: cohort study. BMC Cancer 2018;18(1):548.

70. Won E, Shah MA, Schöder H, et al. Use of positron emission tomography scan response to guide treatment change for locally advanced gastric cancer: the Memorial Sloan Kettering Cancer Center experience. J Gastrointest Oncol 2016;7(4): 506–14.

71. Kim SH, Song BI, Kim HW, et al. Prognostic value of restaging F-18 fluorodeoxyglucose positron emission tomography/computed tomography to predict 3-year post-recurrence survival in patients with recurrent gastric cancer after curative resection. Korean J Radiol 2020;21(7):829–37.

72. Bray F, Ferlay J, Soerjomataram I, et al. Global cancer statistics 2018: GLOBOCAN estimates of incidence and mortality worldwide for 36 cancers in 185 countries. CA Cancer J Clin 2018;68(6): 394–424.

73. Siegel RL, Miller KD, Jemal A. Cancer statistics, 2018. CA Cancer J Clin 2018;68(1):7–30.

74. Lee SM, Kim HS, Lee S, et al. Emerging role of (18) F-fluorodeoxyglucose positron emission tomography for guiding management of hepatocellular carcinoma. World J Gastroenterol 2019;25(11): 1289–306.

75. Park JW, Kim JH, Kim SK, et al. A prospective evaluation of 18F-FDG and 11C-acetate PET/CT for detection of primary and metastatic hepatocellular carcinoma. Evaluation Studies Research Support, Non-U.S. Gov't. J Nucl Med 2008;49(12):1912–21.

76. Khan MA, Combs CS, Brunt EM, et al. Positron emission tomography scanning in the evaluation of hepatocellular carcinoma. J Hepatol 2000; 32(5):792–7.

77. Fattovich G, Stroffolini T, Zagni I, et al. Hepatocellular carcinoma in cirrhosis: incidence and risk factors. Gastroenterology 2004;127(5 Suppl 1): S35–50.

78. Sun DW, An L, Wei F, et al. Prognostic significance of parameters from pretreatment (18)F-FDG PET in hepatocellular carcinoma: a meta-analysis. Abdom Radiol (Ny) 2016;41(1):33–41.

79. Sugiyama M, Sakahara H, Torizuka T, et al. 18F-FDG PET in the detection of extrahepatic metastases from hepatocellular carcinoma. J Gastroenterol 2004;39(10):961–8.

80. Paudyal B, Oriuchi N, Paudyal P, et al. Early diagnosis of recurrent hepatocellular carcinoma with 18F-FDG PET after radiofrequency ablation therapy. Oncol Rep 2007;18(6):1469–73.

81. Lu RC, She B, Gao WT, et al. Positron-emission tomography for hepatocellular carcinoma: Current status and future prospects. World J Gastroenterol 2019;25(32):4682–95.

82. Abuodeh Y, Naghavi AO, Ahmed KA, et al. Prognostic value of pre-treatment F-18-FDG PET-CT in patients with hepatocellular carcinoma undergoing radioembolization. World J Gastroenterol 2016; 22(47):10406–14.

83. Yaprak O, Acar S, Ertugrul G, et al. Role of pre-transplant 18F-FDG PET/CT in predicting hepatocellular carcinoma recurrence after liver transplantation. World J Gastrointest Oncol 2018;10(10): 336–43.

84. Bailly M, Venel Y, Orain I, et al. 18F-FDG PET in liver transplantation setting of hepatocellular carcinoma: predicting histology? Clin Nucl Med 2016;41(3): e126–9.

85. Lin CY, Liao CW, Chu LY, et al. Predictive Value of 18F-FDG PET/CT for Vascular Invasion in Patients With Hepatocellular Carcinoma Before Liver Transplantation. Clin Nucl Med 2017;42(4):e183–7.

86. Lee SD, Kim SH, Kim YK, et al. 18)F-FDG-PET/CT predicts early tumor recurrence in living donor liver transplantation for hepatocellular carcinoma. Transpl Int 2013;26(1):50–60.

87. Kornberg A, Freesmeyer M, Barthel E, et al. 18F-FDG-uptake of hepatocellular carcinoma on PET predicts microvascular tumor invasion in liver transplant patients. Am J Transplant 2009;9(3): 592–600.

88. Kornberg A, Kupper B, Tannapfel A, et al. Patients with non-[18 F]fludeoxyglucose-avid advanced hepatocellular carcinoma on clinical staging may achieve long-term recurrence-free survival after liver transplantation. Liver Transpl 2012;18(1):53–61.

89. Hong G, Suh KS, Suh SW, et al. Alpha-fetoprotein and (18)F-FDG positron emission tomography predict tumor recurrence better than Milan criteria in living donor liver transplantation. J Hepatol 2016; 64(4):852–9.

90. Lee SD, Lee B, Kim SH, et al. Proposal of new expanded selection criteria using total tumor size and (18)F-fluorodeoxyglucose - positron emission tomography/computed tomography for living donor liver transplantation in patients with hepatocellular carcinoma: The National Cancer Center Korea criteria. World J Transpl 2016;6(2):411–22.

91. National Comprehensive Cancer Network. Hepatobiliary cancers (Version 2.2021). Available at: https://www.nccn.org/professionals/physician_gls/pdf/hepatobiliary_blocks.pdf. Accessed May 6, 2021.

92. Shaikh F, Awan O, Khan SA. 18F-FDG PET/CT imaging of gallbladder adenocarcinoma - a pictorial review. Cureus 2015;7(8):e298.

93. Petrowsky H, Wildbrett P, Husarik DB, et al. Impact of integrated positron emission tomography and computed tomography on staging and management of gallbladder cancer and cholangiocarcinoma. J Hepatol 2006;45(1):43–50.

94. Corvera CU, Blumgart LH, Akhurst T, et al. 18F-fluorodeoxyglucose positron emission tomography influences management decisions in patients with biliary cancer. J Am Coll Surg 2008;206(1):57–65.

95. Lee SW, Kim HJ, Park JH, et al. Clinical usefulness of 18F-FDG PET-CT for patients with gallbladder cancer and cholangiocarcinoma. J Gastroenterol 2010;45(5):560–6.

96. Lamarca A, Barriuso J, Chander A, et al. 18)F-fluorodeoxyglucose positron emission tomography ((18)FDG-PET) for patients with biliary tract cancer: Systematic review and meta-analysis. J Hepatol 2019;71(1):115–29.

97. Leung U, Pandit-Taskar N, Corvera CU, et al. Impact of pre-operative positron emission tomography in gallbladder cancer. HPB (Oxford) 2014;16(11):1023–30.

98. Ramia JM, Muffak K, Fernandez A, et al. Gallbladder tuberculosis: false-positive PET diagnosis of gallbladder cancer. World J Gastroenterol 2006;12(40):6559–60.

99. Kitazono MT, Colletti PM. FDG PET imaging of acute cholecystitis. Clin Nucl Med 2006;31(1):23–4.

100. Khan SA, Davidson BR, Goldin RD, et al. Guidelines for the diagnosis and treatment of cholangiocarcinoma: an update. Gut 2012;61(12):1657–69.

101. Lee Y, Yoo IR, Boo SH, et al. The role of F-18 FDG PET/CT in intrahepatic cholangiocarcinoma. Nucl Med Mol Imaging 2017;51(1):69–78.

102. Kim JY, Kim MH, Lee TY, et al. Clinical role of 18F-FDG PET-CT in suspected and potentially operable cholangiocarcinoma: a prospective study compared with conventional imaging. Am J Gastroenterol 2008;103(5):1145–51.

103. Ruys AT, Bennink RJ, van Westreenen HL, et al. FDG-positron emission tomography/computed tomography and standardized uptake value in the primary diagnosis and staging of hilar cholangiocarcinoma. HPB (Oxford) 2011;13(4):256–62.

104. Ikeno Y, Seo S, Iwaisako K, et al. Preoperative metabolic tumor volume of intrahepatic cholangiocarcinoma measured by (18)F-FDG-PET is associated with the KRAS mutation status and prognosis. J Transl Med 2018;16(1):95.

105. Kim NH, Lee SR, Kim YH, et al. Diagnostic performance and prognostic relevance of FDG positron emission tomography/computed tomography for patients with extrahepatic cholangiocarcinoma. Korean J Radiol 2020;21(12):1355–66.

106. Zins M, Matos C, Cassinotto C. Pancreatic adenocarcinoma staging in the era of preoperative chemotherapy and radiation therapy. Radiology 2018;287(2):374–90.

107. National Comprehensive Cancer Network. Pancreatic adenocarcinoma (version 2.2021). Available at: https://www.nccn.org/professionals/physician_gls/pdf/pancreatic_blocks.pdf. Accessed May 6, 2021.

108. Ergul N, Gundogan C, Tozlu M, et al. Role of (18)F-fluorodeoxyglucose positron emission tomography/computed tomography in diagnosis and management of pancreatic cancer; comparison with multidetector row computed tomography, magnetic resonance imaging and endoscopic ultrasonography. Rev Esp Med Nucl Imagen Mol 2014;33(3):159–64.

109. Buchs NC, Bühler L, Bucher P, et al. Value of contrast-enhanced 18F-fluorodeoxyglucose positron emission tomography/computed tomography in detection and presurgical assessment of pancreatic cancer: a prospective study. J Gastroenterol Hepatol 2011;26(4):657–62.

110. Asagi A, Ohta K, Nasu J, et al. Utility of contrast-enhanced FDG-PET/CT in the clinical management of pancreatic cancer: impact on diagnosis, staging, evaluation of treatment response, and detection of recurrence. Pancreas 2013;42(1):11–9.

111. Farma JM, Santillan AA, Melis M, et al. PET/CT fusion scan enhances CT staging in patients with pancreatic neoplasms. Ann Surg Oncol 2008;15(9):2465–71.

112. Rijkers AP, Valkema R, Duivenvoorden HJ, et al. Usefulness of F-18-fluorodeoxyglucose positron emission tomography to confirm suspected pancreatic cancer: a meta-analysis. Eur J Surg Oncol 2014;40(7):794–804.

113. Wang Z, Chen JQ, Liu JL, et al. FDG-PET in diagnosis, staging and prognosis of pancreatic carcinoma: a meta-analysis. World J Gastroenterol 2013;19(29):4808–17.

114. Pimiento JM, Davis-Yadley AH, Kim RD, et al. Metabolic activity by 18F-FDG-PET/CT is prognostic for stage I and II pancreatic cancer. Clin Nucl Med 2016;41(3):177–81.

115. Nioche C, Orlhac F, Boughdad S, et al. A freeware for tumor heterogeneity characterization in PET, SPECT, CT, MRI and US to accelerate advances in radiomics. J Nucl Med 2017;58(supplement 1):1316.

116. Toyama Y, Hotta M, Motoi F, et al. Prognostic value of FDG-PET radiomics with machine learning in pancreatic cancer. Sci Rep 2020;10(1):17024.

117. Korn RL, Von Hoff DD, Borad MJ, et al. 18F-FDG PET/CT response in a phase 1/2 trial of nab-paclitaxel plus gemcitabine for advanced pancreatic cancer. Cancer 2017;17(1):23.

118. Yokose T, Kitago M, Matsusaka Y, et al. Usefulness of (18) F-fluorodeoxyglucose positron emission tomography/computed tomography for predicting the prognosis and treatment response of neoadjuvant therapy for pancreatic ductal adenocarcinoma. Cancer Med 2020;9(12):4059–68.

119. Wang L, Dong P, Wang W, et al. Early recurrence detected by 18F-FDG PET/CT in patients with resected pancreatic ductal adenocarcinoma. Medicine (Baltimore) 2020;99(11):e19504.

120. National Comprehensive Cancer Network. Colon cancer (Version 2.2021). Available at: https://www.nccn.org/professionals/physician_gls/pdf/colon_blocks.pdf. Accessed May 6, 2021.

121. Rollven E, Abraham-Nordling M, Holm T, et al. Assessment and diagnostic accuracy of lymph node status to predict stage III colon cancer using computed tomography. Cancer 2017;17(1):3.

122. Yang Z, Zhang X, Fang M, et al. Preoperative diagnosis of regional lymph node metastasis of colorectal cancer with quantitative parameters from dual-energy CT. AJR Am J Roentgenol Jul 2019; 213(1):W17–25.

123. Kwak JY, Kim JS, Kim HJ, et al. Diagnostic value of FDG-PET/CT for lymph node metastasis of colorectal cancer. World J Surg 2012;36(8):1898–905.

124. Petersen RK, Hess S, Alavi A, et al. Clinical impact of FDG-PET/CT on colorectal cancer staging and treatment strategy. Am J Nucl Med Mol Imaging 2014;4(5):471–82.

125. Maffione AM, Rubello D, Caroli P, et al. Is it time to introduce PET/CT in colon cancer guidelines? Clin Nucl Med 2020;45(7):525–30.

126. Hendlisz A, Golfinopoulos V, Garcia C, et al. Serial FDG-PET/CT for early outcome prediction in patients with metastatic colorectal cancer undergoing chemotherapy. Ann Oncol 2012;23(7):1687–93.

127. Liu FY, Yen TC, Wang JY, et al. Early prediction by 18F-FDG PET/CT for progression-free survival and overall survival in patients with metastatic colorectal cancer receiving third-line cetuximab-based therapy. Clin Nucl Med 2015;40(3):200–5.

128. de Geus-Oei LF, Vriens D, van Laarhoven HW, et al. Monitoring and predicting response to therapy with 18F-FDG PET in colorectal cancer: a systematic review. J Nucl Med 2009;50(Suppl 1):43s–54s.

129. Vandenbroucke F, Vandemeulebroucke J, Ilsen B, et al. Predictive value of pattern classification 24 hours after radiofrequency ablation of liver metastases on CT and positron emission tomography/ CT. J Vasc Interv Radiol 2014;25(8):1240–9.

130. Monteil J, Le Brun-Ly V, Cachin F, et al. Comparison of 18FDG-PET/CT and conventional follow-up methods in colorectal cancer: a randomised prospective study. Dig Liver Dis 2021;53(2):231–7.

131. National Comprehensive Cancer Network. Rectal cancer (Version 1.2021). Available at: https://www.nccn.org/professionals/physician_gls/pdf/rectal_blocks.pdf. Accessed May 6, 2021.

132. Pedersen CK, Babu AS. Understanding the lymphatics: review of the N category in the updated TNM staging of cancers of the digestive system. AJR Am J Roentgenol 2020;215(1):58–68.

133. National Comprehensive Cancer Network. Anal carcinoma (version 1.2021).

Precision Nuclear Medicine
The Evolving Role of PET in Melanoma

Chadwick L. Wright, MD, PhD[a],*, Eric D. Miller, MD, PhD[b], Carlo Contreras, MD[c], Michael V. Knopp, MD, PhD[a]

KEYWORDS

- Positron emission tomography • Computed tomography • Immuno-oncology • Immunotherapy
- Melanoma

KEY POINTS

- FDG PET/CT is highly sensitive and well suited for the non-invasive detection and monitoring of metastatic melanoma lesions.
- Tumor response assessment with conventional anatomic imaging approaches may be challenging in those melanoma patients treated with targeted or immune-oncology therapeutics.
- Recent advances in digital PET technology may enable new clinical approaches to assess whole-body tumor burden with higher image definition, faster image acquisition times, and at lower radiotracer doses.

INTRODUCTION

Melanoma remains the most deadly form of skin cancer, with an incidence that has risen faster than nearly any other cancer in the last 50 years.[1–3] For stage I cutaneous malignant melanoma, the 5-year survival rate is 90%, whereas it is 15% to 20% for stage IV melanoma with distant metastatic disease.[4] In the metastatic setting, it can spread to distant organs of the body through vascular and/or lymphatic spread. In addition, disease recurrence occurs in 50% to 80% of melanoma patients with locoregional metastatic involvement and almost all patients with distant metastases.[5] An estimated 100,350 new cases of cutaneous melanoma were projected in 2020 with 6850 deaths. While the number of cases has been increasing, mortality rates are declining most likely due to promising new systemic therapies for the treatment of locally advanced and metastatic disease. In recent years, the development and clinical use of new IO therapeutics (ie,

targeted small-molecule inhibitors and immunotherapy) have improved survival in melanoma patients. From 2013 until 2017, in men and women (ages 20–64 years), the overall mortality from melanoma dropped by 7% annually. During that same time for patients 65 years of age and older, mortality rates were declining by 5% to 6% per year, while prior to 2013, mortality rates were increasing.[6] Imaging to assess for malignant/metastatic disease is a vital component of the work-up of patients with newly diagnosed lymph node-positive or recurrent melanoma so that the most appropriate therapy can be selected and delivered. Similarly, imaging plays a critical role in subsequently assessing the treatment response in patients with recurrent malignancy and/or metastatic disease.

Positron emission tomography with computed tomography (PET/CT) is clinically used for the detection and assessment of malignant/metastatic lesions in patients with melanoma as well as

Conflicts of Interest: None.
[a] Department of Radiology, Wright Center of Innovation in Biomedical Imaging, The Ohio State University Wexner Medical Center, 395 W. 12th Avenue, Suite 460, Columbus, OH 43210, USA; [b] Department of Radiation Oncology, James Cancer Center, The Ohio State University Wexner Medical Center, 460 W. 10th Avenue, 2nd Floor, Columbus, OH 43210, USA; [c] Division of Surgical Oncology, Department of Surgery, The Ohio State University Wexner Medical Center, 2050 Kenny Road, Tower 4th Floor, Columbus, OH 43221, USA
* Corresponding author.
E-mail address: wright.491@osu.edu

Radiol Clin N Am 59 (2021) 755–772
https://doi.org/10.1016/j.rcl.2021.05.007
0033-8389/21/© 2021 Elsevier Inc. All rights reserved.

many other cancers.[7] In the case of melanoma, ^{18}F-fluorodeoxyglucose (FDG) PET/CT imaging enables a whole-body assessment of physiologic and pathophysiologic glucose metabolism in order to identify metabolically reprogrammed cancer lesions, which demonstrate increased FDG uptake relative to the normal tissues nearby. FDG PET/CT can also provide insight into therapeutic responses of tumors to cytotoxic chemotherapy. Whereas conventional diagnostic imaging approaches with CT and magnetic resonance imaging (MRI) use anatomic changes in tumor size as the measure of treatment response, FDG PET/CT can provide additional functional insight by evaluating the metabolic activity of the tumor as another measure of treatment response. In particular, FDG PET/CT enables visual/qualitative assessment of glucose utilization throughout the body as well as semiquantitative measurement for evaluation of the metabolic response to therapy.[8] The most widely used PET method for quantifying FDG activity is the standardized uptake value (SUV).[8] In general, FDG PET/CT demonstrates high sensitivity and specificity for detecting and staging melanoma lesions when compared with CT and its improved accuracy can impact clinical and therapeutic management of melanoma patients.[9]

The purpose of this review is to provide an overview of the current perspectives and future opportunities for PET imaging in the management of melanoma. Herein, we describe the current role of FDG PET/CT in the clinical management of melanoma including initial staging, treatment monitoring during therapy, restaging following therapy, and the subsequent detection of recurrent malignancy/metastatic disease. We also provide an overview of new developments in PET imaging technology including new and emerging imaging technologies, novel imaging approaches, and emerging concepts. Finally, we provide a brief perspective on clinical trials investigating the use of PET in melanoma patients to assess the response to therapies focusing primarily on immunotherapy.

ROLE OF FDG PET IN MANAGEMENT OF MELANOMA
Initial Staging

In order to determine the most optimal therapeutic plan for a newly diagnosed melanoma patient, the detection and localization of all sites of malignant/metastatic disease are essential.[10] While the primary melanoma site and locoregional metastases may be detected on clinical examination, the detection of distant disease (including visceral metastases) is often more challenging and may not

present until the disease is quite advanced and causing clinical symptoms. Furthermore, melanoma spreads distantly in an often atypical pattern with a high frequency of metastatic spread to the spleen, adrenal glands, and small bowel when compared to other malignancies.[11] FDG PET/CT adds value as part of the comprehensive diagnostic evaluation of patients with advanced-stage or high-risk melanoma. Early studies evaluating the ability of FDG PET to detect distant metastatic disease are limited by the inclusion of patients with all stages of melanoma (ie, stages I–IV). In general, these studies showed FDG PET sensitivity ranging from 84% to 94%, and specificity ranging from 83% to 97%, compared to CT sensitivity of 55% to 58% and specificity of 70% to 84%.[12,13] Rodriguez Rivera and colleagues performed a meta-analysis on the use of FDG PET in patients with only stage III cutaneous melanoma.[14] In this meta-analysis, the overall sensitivity and specificity of FDG PET in detecting metastatic disease were 89% and 89%, respectively, with a change in stage and/or management noted in 22% of patients. A systematic review from Krug and colleagues evaluating the utility of FDG PET for initial staging of cutaneous malignant melanoma included 2905 patients and patients with both early-stage and advanced disease.[15] The pooled sensitivity and specificity for detection of metastasis by FDG PET was 83% and 85%, respectively, with disease management changes in 33% of patients. FDG PET was determined to be most helpful in patients with stages III and IV disease and especially in the detection of deep soft tissue, lymph node, and visceral metastases. Similarly, the diagnostic accuracy of FDG PET/CT was even higher for stages III and IV malignant melanoma when compared to stages I and II.[16]

While the majority of evidence is retrospective with multiple systematic reviews and meta-analyses, there is limited prospective evidence highlighting the utility of FDG PET in the initial staging of patients with cutaneous melanoma. In fact, a prospective nonrandomized clinical trial of 144 patients with early-stage cutaneous melanoma showed no benefit with the addition of FDG PET to standard clinical work-up.[17] Bastiaannet and colleagues performed a prospective comparison of FDG PET alone to CT in melanoma patients with palpable lymph node metastases.[18] While FDG PET and CT tended to upstage patients by identifying the presence of distant metastases at similar rates in the study, FDG PET was able to identify more metastatic sites including the presence of bone and subcutaneous metastases when compared to CT alone. Hybrid FDG PET/CT imaging was then demonstrated to have a higher sensitivity than either FDG PET alone or CT in a separate meta-analysis evaluating multiple tumor histologies including melanoma.[19]

Another prospective multicenter registry study was performed in Ontario evaluating the clinical utility of FDG PET/CT in patients with potentially resectable localized high-risk melanoma or recurrent disease being considered for metastasectomy.[20] Of 319 patients included in this study, 18% were upstaged to M1 status following FDG PET/CT, which had a subsequent impact on surgical management of these patients. Another study demonstrated the clinical impact on patient management when using FDG PET/CT for melanoma patients being evaluated for metastectomy. In this study, half of the patients were subsequently spared surgery due to the detection of additional unresectable metastases and about 25% of patients had no change in the intended management plan.[10] Therefore, FDG PET/CT can play an important role in initial surgical staging for those melanoma patients evaluated for potential metastectomy. For the detection of intracranial metastatic melanoma lesions, FDG PET performs poorly when compared with contrast-enhanced MRI and CT[21], although larger metastatic lesions may be detectable on FDG PET.

Sentinel lymph node biopsy is standard of care for initial staging of melanoma patients. It has been reported that the false-negative rate of sentinel lymph node biopsy is 6% to 29% and therefore new imaging approaches may be helpful in further detecting and quantifying metastatic nodal involvement.[22] The status of the sentinel lymph node is the single most important predictor of survival in node-negative melanoma.[23] To this end, FDG PET has a sensitivity of 17%, a positive predictive value of 50%, and a negative predictive value of 82%.[24] A systematic review of pooled data from eight studies showed that FDG PET, in comparison to sentinel lymph node biopsy (SLNB), has a positive likelihood ratio (LR) of 1.33, a negative LR of 1.00, and a diagnostic odds ratio of 1.2.[15] The Cochrane Collaboration has analyzed four studies evaluating PET/CT prior to SLNB, and found that PET/CT has a sensitivity of 10% and a specificity of 97%, which is inferior to a combination of ultrasound with fine needle aspirate of lymph nodes of concern prior to SLNB.[25] It should be noted that these earlier studies likely utilized analogue photomultiplier tube-based PET detector imaging systems and these reported poor performance characteristics for PET detection of metastatic lymph nodes should not be surprising. Immunohistochemical evaluation of the excised sentinel lymph node(s) is capable of detecting isolated metastatic tumor cells, which would be below the detection limit of conventional analogue PET (cPET) and cPET/CT systems. As such, FDG cPET and FDG cPET/CT systems did not improve the detection of metastatic lymph nodes when compared with sentinel lymph node biopsy. More recently, the use of combined modality imaging with integrated FDG PET/MRI with diffusion weighted imaging also did not reliably differentiate metastatic lymph nodes from benign lymph nodes when correlated with sentinel lymph node biopsy. It is proposed that very small metabolic tumor volumes within metastatic lymph nodes may account for this historical poor sensitivity of FDG PET and therefore higher definition PET imaging approaches with smaller voxel volumes may improve the detection of subcentimeter metastatic deposits.[22]

Given the limited prospective clinical evidence, imaging guidelines from the National Comprehensive Cancer Network (NCCN) suggest that cross-sectional imaging, including FDG PET/CT, should be considered in those melanoma patients with stage III disease for baseline staging and in patients with stage IV or recurrent disease.[26]

Treatment Monitoring During Therapy and Restaging Following Completion of Therapy

As metastatic melanoma patients have poor prognoses,[27] diagnostic imaging again serves as the noninvasive approach for evaluating treatment response to various oncologic therapies. In particular, FDG PET/CT readily assists in routine detection and response assessment of distant extracranial melanoma metastasis.[13,28] In the current era of immunotherapy/immune checkpoint inhibitor-based immuno-oncology (IO) treatments for melanoma patients, the imaging assessment of response to IO treatment has become more complex.[29] These IO therapeutics have introduced new challenges for the interpretation of therapeutic response when compared with historical conventional cytotoxic chemotherapeutics. For example, small molecular IO inhibitors may improve patient survival while demonstrating minimal anatomic tumor size changes on follow-up diagnostic imaging. Due to the unconventional or delayed anatomic tumor responses of IO therapies on CT and/or MRI imaging, this challenge highlights the importance of adapting or developing new immune-related imaging response criteria strategies in patients treated with IO as opposed to cytotoxic chemotherapy. In the IO treatment setting, pseudo-progression is a phenomenon that presents as an initial enlargement of tumor size followed by a subsequent reduction in size. These initially enlarging tumors may result from immune-mediated tumor infiltrates and consequently these tumor infiltrates can increase FDG uptake on early PET imaging. It is important to recognize these early potential tumor pseudo-progression events in melanoma patients on IO therapies and to help to distinguish it from actual tumor disease progression on follow-up imaging. Some other imaging findings that can suggest therapy-related inflammatory response are reactive uptake in the lymph node drainage basins for malignant/metastatic lesions as well as diffusely increased FDG uptake in the spleen. These observations have resulted in the development of the immune-related Response Evaluation Criteria in Solid Tumor (irRECIST).[9]

It is important to note that traditional methods to evaluate treatment response have focused on WHO, RECIST, and EORTC criteria, which were developed for cytotoxic therapy regimens as opposed to IO regimens.[30] Per RECIST 1.1 criteria, PET/CT studies cannot independently be used for treatment response assessment because the attenuation-correction CT component of the PET/CT image acquisition is often deemed of inferior diagnostic quality when compared to dedicated diagnostic CT imaging owing to the lower radiation dose and lack of intravenous contrast administration on the attenuation-correction CT imaging for PET.[31] Consequently, the majority of the seminal, prospective, therapeutic trials evaluating systemic therapies for stages III and IV melanoma (such as the Checkmate and KEYNOTE series) did not evaluate the role of PET in assessing clinical outcomes. Multiple clinical trials are now underway to address the role of PET in melanoma detection and response assessment. **Table 1** highlights the current clinical trials that are assessing PET imaging at various time points and with various PET radiopharmaceuticals in melanoma patients treated with different IO therapeutics. **Table 2** highlights the current international clinical trials incorporating PET imaging into the response assessment during IO therapy or the surveillance period following IO therapy for melanoma.

It has been proposed that FDG PET may be able to detect and assess early metabolic responses in melanoma lesions to IO therapies as well as quantify changes in the whole-body metabolic tumor burden. On the other hand, persistently stable or increasing FDG avidity in tumor lesions treated with IO therapeutics may be an indicator of tumor resistance. It is likely that current and future clinical trials will also need to identify, characterize, and distinguish response patterns on FDG PET/CT for tumor response as well as nontarget tissue/organ toxicities that may develop during IO therapy.

Such toxicities include dermatitis, inflammatory endocrinopathies, inflammatory esophageal/gastrointestinal manifestations, pneumonitis, hepatitis, etc. Many of these potential toxicities may be easily detectable on FDG PET/CT imaging in clinically asymptomatic patients undergoing routine imaging assessment.[9]

More specifically, PET/CT may play a more important role in determining the functional/metabolic impacts of these IO therapies, especially when correlated with conventional anatomic imaging findings with CT and MRI. A systematic review and meta-analysis by Ayati and colleagues highlights the utility of various baseline PET parameters (ie, SUV_{peak}, metabolic tumor volume, and total lesion glycolysis) as predictors of the final response to IO in patients with metastatic melanoma. Furthermore, PET-based response assessments using these various PET parameters improved sensitivity and specificity when compared to conventional imaging-based response criteria.[32] PERCIST, PERCIMT, PECRIT, and EORTC 1999 criteria are other imaging assessment tools that have emerged which integrate PET/CT but are less frequently incorporated into clinical trials than RECIST.[33] These PET criteria integrate various PET-specific metrics to determine treatment response, including features of target versus nontarget lesions, and the maximum voxel value of standardized uptake value (SUV_{max}).[28,34]

New PET response assessment concepts and strategies for patients treated with IO therapeutics have led to a renewed interest in early interval PET imaging to better predict clinical response. On the interim FDG PET/CT imaging during IO, the presence of stable-appearing anatomic disease and relatively increased FDG avidity (ie, pseudo-progression) can represent early tumor inflammatory response (ie, favorable outcome), which will eventually demonstrate imaging findings on subsequent scans that are more consistent with tumor treatment/regression. In fact, evolving and new response assessment strategies, which integrate both anatomic and functional/metabolic metrics, may be more predictive of early and/or eventual response to IO.[34]

Cho and colleagues performed a prospective study in patients with advanced melanoma treated with IO by serially monitoring treatment response via FDG PET/CT at days 21 to 28 and again at 4 months after the initiation of IO therapy.[34] These authors used a combination of anatomic and functional imaging data collected at the early time points to develop criteria predictive of response to IO with 100% sensitivity, 93% specificity, and 95% accuracy. A similar study was performed by

Table 1
Clinical trials investigating PET at various time points and with various PET radiopharmaceuticals in melanoma patients treated with different IO therapeutics as registered at www.clinicaltrials.gov at the time of submission

Study ID	Radiopharmaceutical(s)	IO Therapy	Primary Endpoint	Imaging Time Points
NCT03356470	FDG and FLT	Nivolumab or Pembrolizumab	Correlate baseline and posttreatment molecular imaging biomarkers of response to immunotherapy	Baseline and 10–12 wk posttherapy
NCT03089606	FDG and [^{11}C]AMT	Pembrolizumab	Association of SUV_{max} with objective response rate	Baseline and 12 wk posttherapy
NCT03888950	FDG	Nivolumab or Pembrolizumab	Quantify changes in FDG uptake by PERCIST criteria	Baseline, days 21–31, and 3 mo posttherapy
NCT04272658	FDG	Nivolumab or Pembrolizumab or combo Ipilimumab/Nivolumab	Differentiate progression vs pseudoprogression using 4D body-to-whole dynamic acquisition	Not specified
NCT03584334	FDG	Nivolumab or Pembrolizumab	Threshold of FDG retention index to distinguish progression vs pseudo-progression	Baseline, 7 wk, and 3 mo posttherapy
NCT02716077	FDG	Pembrolizumab	Disease-free survival	Not specified
NCT04221438	FLT	Encorafenib and Binimetinib	Change in SUV_{max}	Baseline and 8–9 wk posttherapy
NCT04462406	FDG	Nivolumab or Pembrolizumab or combo with Ipilimumab	Event-free survival – active surveillance following negative PET or positive PET but negative biopsy	Baseline and 12 mo posttherapy
NCT03520634	[^{18}F]PD-L1	Nivolumab	Determine optimal dose of tracer and timing of imaging	Baseline and 6 wk posttherapy
NCT02591654	FLT	Pembrolizumab	Prevalence of lesion detection	Baseline and 6 wk posttherapy

Sachpekidis and colleagues who evaluated the utility of interim FDG PET/CT performed following two cycles (6 weeks) of IO with response assessment based on tumor metabolic activity rather than anatomic tumor dimensions.[35] A subsequent study from the same group demonstrated a threshold of four new FDG-avid tumor lesions on subsequent posttreatment FDG PET/CT imaging was a reliable indicator of IO treatment failure. Furthermore, as these new FDG-avid tumor lesions demonstrated diameters exceeding 1 cm in size, the sensitivity and specificity for treatment failure approached 90%.[30] Similarly, modifications to the traditional PERCIST response assessment for patients treated with IO (ie, immunotherapy-modified PERCIST or imPERCIST) have demonstrated that new lesions, even in the setting of partial metabolic response or stable metabolic response, are metastatic in 55% of cases. Therefore, the detection of any new lesion should be considered indeterminate as opposed to immediately progressive disease and closely monitored

Table 2
Clinical trials integrating and investigating incorporating PET imaging into the response assessment during IO therapy or the surveillance period following IO therapy for melanoma patients as registered at www.clinicaltrials.gov at the time of submission

Study ID	Brief Description	Country Enrolling Patients
NCT03356470	Comparing FDG PET and FLT PET, along with blood and tissue biomarkers	United States
NCT03888950	Evaluate whether FDG PET predicts therapeutic response after two cycles of PD-1 directed therapy	France
NCT04272658	Determine the value of 4D body-to-whole dynamic acquisition in FDG PET for immunotherapy monitoring	France
NCT03584334	Using FDG PET to distinguish tumor progression vs pseudo-progression in patients with melanoma or non-small cell lung cancer	France
NCT02716077	Early evaluation of response to pembrolizumab in patients with melanoma	United States
NCT04478318	Determine the minimum FDG PET scan duration on a total-body vs conventional scanner	United States
NCT04462406	Determine how FDG PET may allow early discontinuation of PD-1 directed therapy in unresectable stages IIIB–IV melanoma	United States
NCT03116412	Prospective randomized multicenter trial to assess the role of imaging during follow-up after resection of stages IIb-c and III melanoma	Sweden
NCT03554083	Determine the role of FDG PET in assessing response to neoadjuvant combination targeted and immunotherapy for patients with high-risk stage III melanoma	United States
NCT02621021	Determine the role of FDG PET in assessing response to talimogene laherparepvec with or without radiation for patients with advanced melanoma, Merkel cell carcinoma, or other solid tumors with skin metastasis	United States
NCT02575404	Determine the role of FDG PET in assessing response to GR-MD-02 plus pembrolizumab for patients with advanced melanoma, non-small cell lung cancer, or head and neck squamous cell cancer	United States
NCT04165967	Determine the role of FDG PET in assessing response to adoptive tumor-infiltrating lymphocyte transfer plus nivolumab for patients with metastatic melanoma that failed immunotherapy	Switzerland
NCT03311308	Correlate hypoxia measurements in tumor via FDG PET in advanced melanoma patients treated with pembrolizumab with or without metformin	United States
NCT03161756	Determine the role of FDG PET in assessing response to denosumab plus nivolumab with or without ipilimumab for patients with metastatic melanoma	Australia
NCT04207086	Determine the role of FDG PET in assessing response to neoadjuvant pembrolizumab plus levatinib for patients with resectable stages III/IV melanoma	Australia
NCT03475134	Determine the role of FDG PET and ^{68}Ga-NODAGA-RGD PET in assessing response to tumor-infiltrating lymphocyte therapy plus nivolumab rescue for patients with unresectable locally advanced or metastatic melanoma	Switzerland
NCT02858921	Determine the role of FDG PET in assessing response to neoadjuvant dabrafenib, trametinib, and/or pembrolizumab for patients with BRAF mutant resectable stage III melanoma	Australia

on follow-up imaging or biopsied as clinically indicated.[36]

In 2017, the PET/CT Criteria for early prediction of Response to Immune checkpoint inhibitor Therapy (PECRIT) and PET Response Evaluation Criteria for Immunotherapy (PERCIMT) were developed and proposed.[8] In 2017, the revised Response Evaluation Criteria in Solid Tumor (RECIST) criteria for the evaluation of immunotherapy response (iRECIST) were also proposed.[8] Annovazzi and colleagues assessed the predictive value of FDG PET/CT performed 3 to 4 months after initiation of IO and compared various PET metrics and response criteria.[37] This retrospective study cohort consisted of patients treated with IO using either ipilimumab or with PD-1 inhibitors. Interestingly, for patients treated with ipilimumab, the metabolic tumor volume combined with PERCIMT criteria was the most reliable predictor for best overall response at 6 months, while for patients treated with PD-1 inhibitors, multiple PET metrics were found to be reliable predictors of response. Other authors have suggested that even earlier imaging time points following initiation of IO may be potentially predictive of IO treatment response (eg, 2 weeks following initiation of anti-PD1 therapy for advanced melanoma). The ability to quickly and reliably assess IO treatment efficacy or treatment resistance would enable the clinical determination of when to stop an ineffective IO therapy and switch to another therapy, thus reducing the financial burden and risk of future immune-related adverse events (irAEs) in those patients with treatment-resistant disease.[9,38,39] FDG PET/CT is again useful in detecting the presence and resolution of irAEs. A retrospective review of 147 patients treated with IO for advanced melanoma who underwent either contrast-enhanced CT scan or FDG PET/CT, irAEs were detected with imaging in 31% of patients. Follow-up imaging was also helpful in monitoring for the resolution of irAEs.[40]

Within the NeoCombi trial, which evaluated the role of perioperative dabrafenib and trametinib therapy in resectable stages IIIB–C melanoma patients, 18 patients had evidence of a metabolic complete response on preoperative PET/CT.[41] In addition, 11 of these 18 had both a complete response by RECIST criteria and a pathologic complete response in the resection specimen, whereas six patients with a metabolic complete response on PET/CT did not have a pathologic complete response in the resected specimen. In a different single institution phase Ib trial, a subset of six patients with resectable stages III/IV melanoma underwent pretreatment FDG PET/CT followed by just one dose of neoadjuvant pembrolizumab, follow-up FDG PET/CT 3 weeks later, and then surgical resection. In this subset of patients, a 20% decrease in tumor diameter using RECIST at 3 weeks following single-dose pembrolizumab was associated with treatment response in the surgical specimen but the change in FDG-avidity at 3 weeks following the single-dose IO administration was not yet predictive.[42] While complete resolution of metastatic melanoma lesions on posttreatment imaging is the most comforting in terms of patient prognosis, data from a retrospective analysis of 104 patients treated with PD-1-directed IO for metastatic melanoma showed that CT imaging alone might be too conservative to predict treatment success. In this study, patients with a complete metabolic response on FDG PET/CT and a partial response on CT had comparable progression-free survival to patients with a complete response on CT.[21] An example of using FDG PET/CT to monitor response to IO in metastatic melanoma is shown in **Fig. 1**.

In addition to assessing the tumor response to systemic IO therapies, FDG PET/CT has been shown to be a useful imaging modality for assessing extracranial metastasis following stereotactic body radiation therapy (SBRT).[27] Youland and colleagues reported on 80 extracranial metastases in 48 patients treated with SBRT who completed pretreatment and posttreatment FDG PET/CT, which were evaluated using PERCIST (version 1.0). This study also suggested that the optimal interval between completion of SBRT and obtaining the first posttreatment FDG PET/CT scan should be more than 2 months in order to minimize radiation therapy-related inflammation observed at earlier time points. In this SBRT treatment study, an initial increase in tumor SUV corrected for lean body mass was observed in 14 metastatic lesions resulting in a classification of progressive disease. However, in this study, this increase in SUV was not associated with risk of metastasis control failure, progression-free survival, or overall survival. Response assessment following SBRT is sometimes challenging due to resultant treatment-related fibrosis and scarring in the target lesion(s) as well as the surrounding tissues. Postradiation inflammatory changes in adequately treated tumor lesions and surrounding tissues can contribute to increased FDG activity in these regions on PET/CT imaging immediately following therapy. As noted, such transient increases in FDG avidity in posttreatment lesions/tissues can be minimized by performing restaging FDG PET/CT imaging 2 to 3 months after completion of SBRT.[27]

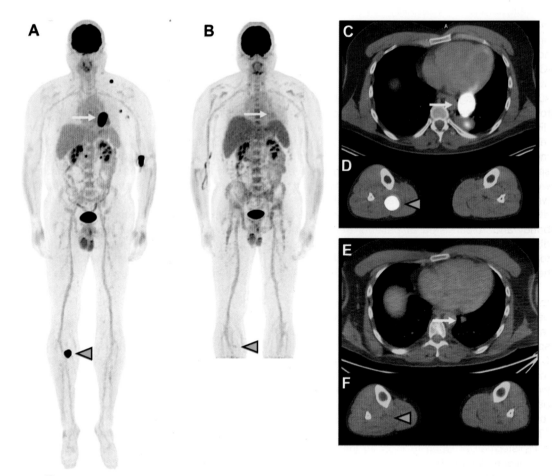

Fig. 1. ^{18}F-FDG-PET/CT for assessing response to immune checkpoint therapy (ipilimumab/nivolumab) in a 44-year-old-man with metastatic melanoma of unknown primary. Selected images prior to therapy are shown in panels *A* [maximal intensity projection (MIP) image], *C* and *D* (fusion images of the chest and lower extremities), while selected images obtained approximately 4 months later, after starting therapy, are shown in panels *B* (MIP), *E* and *F* (fusion images of the chest and lower extremities). The MIP images (*A*, *B*) demonstrate resolution of increased FDG uptake associated with multiple metastases with the fusion images demonstrating response in a left lower lobe mass (*yellow arrow*, *C* and *E*) and in a right proximal calf lesion (*blue arrowhead*, *D* and *F*). (*Courtesy of* Jonathan McConathy, MD, PhD, at the University of Alabama at Birmingham (UAB).)

Detection of Recurrent Malignancy and Metastatic Disease

Approximately 50% of patients treated for melanoma will relapse and these relapse events present as local recurrence (20%), locoregional nodal metastases (50%), and distant metastases (30%).[7] Surveillance imaging recommendations are also confounded by the fact that while most melanomas recur within 2 years of initial treatment, a significant proportion of patients may remain disease-free for decades. According to the NCCN guidelines, periodic assessment in the posttreatment setting for stages IIb–IV melanoma patients should be considered for 5 years using appropriate radiographic, CT, MRI, and FDG PET/CT approaches. FDG PET can detect malignant/metastatic lesions in posttreatment and clinically asymptomatic melanoma patients. It should be noted that FDG PET/CT is generally not considered in the surveillance imaging recommendations for most cancers despite its capability to detect recurrent malignancy/metastases.[43]

Consensus for surveillance imaging following completion of definitive treatment for melanoma is lacking, with limited evidence highlighting the utility of FDG-PET/CT as a routine cancer surveillance methodology. Prior to the development of IO-based therapies for melanoma, few effective systemic therapies for melanoma were available and this greatly reduced the clinical opportunities for investigating imaging surveillance approaches in these patients. However, in the current era of IO-based therapies for melanoma, there is now renewed interest in the prompt detection of recurrent/relapsed melanoma as it may result in earlier initiation of new IO treatments. This new clinical paradigm justifies a reassessment of the utility and timing of surveillance imaging for the detection of asymptomatic recurrent malignancy and metastatic disease. Bleicher and colleagues performed a retrospective study of 580 patients with stage II melanoma treated definitively.[44] In this retrospective analysis, over 25% of recurrences were found on follow-up surveillance imaging, with over 40% of the recurrences in stage IIC disease detected on surveillance imaging. While bone and brain metastases were typically discovered following the onset of clinical symptoms, follow-up surveillance imaging was also helpful in detecting extracranial metastases.

Several studies have reported on the use of follow-up surveillance FDG PET/CT in melanoma patients after curative resection. Following the resection of stages IIIB/C melanoma, one retrospective study examined surveillance FDG PET/CT imaging at 6-month intervals and described that PET/CT was an effective approach to detecting recurrent disease in asymptomatic melanoma patients during the first year following surgical resection.[45] Lewin and colleagues reported on 170 patients with stage III melanoma who completed follow-up surveillance FDG PET/CT with stage IIIA patients completing scans at 6 and 18 months and stage IIIB/C patients completing scans at 6-month intervals for the first 2 years and an additional scan at 36 months following completion of therapy.[46] Recurrent disease was detected in 38% of patients, with 69% of relapses being asymptomatic. False-positive FDG PET/CT findings also occurred in 7% of patients. Positive predictive values (PPV) of individual scans were 56% to 83%, while negative scans had predictive values (NPV) of 89% to 96% for true nonrecurrence. A negative FDG PET/CT at 18 months had negative predictive values of 80% to 84% for true nonrecurrence at any time over the 47-month follow-up period of this study. Overall, 52% of patients with recurrence underwent curative-intent resection. In this setting for stage III melanoma patients, a negative FDG PET/CT study is the most predictive finding. At present, conventional imaging surveillance approaches for recurrent melanoma have not yet demonstrated improved outcomes or suggested healthcare cost-saving/economic benefit.

In a separate study from Denmark, where FDG PET/CT was included as standard-of-care follow-up at 6, 12, and 24 months following treatment for stage IIB (and greater) melanoma patients,

Vensby and colleagues reported on the value of FDG PET/CT following surgical resection in 238 patients.[7] In 526 FDG PET/CT studies, 25% were positive for recurrent disease, 69% were negative, and 5% had equivocal findings. Sensitivity was 89%, specificity was 92%, and PPV and NPV were 78% and 97%, respectively. The authors found no statistically significant difference in diagnostic accuracy in patients completing scans with or without clinical concern for recurrent disease. This study highlighted the high NPV of FDG PET/CT as part of follow-up surveillance despite the limitation of a false positivity rate of 9%.

A retrospective study from Mayo Clinic reported on 299 patients with stages III–IV melanoma followed with surveillance FDG PET/CT imaging following resection.[47] Overall, 52% of patients developed recurrent disease with the first recurrence presenting as clinically occult in 60% of patients. Both patients with clinically occult as well as those with clinically evident recurrent malignant/metastatic disease underwent curative-intent salvage therapy at similar rates (66% vs 75%, $P = .240$). FDG PET/CT again had high sensitivity (88%), specificity (90%), and NPV (99%), but this study's PPV of 37% emphasized the need for histologic confirmation of suspected recurrent malignancy/metastasis based on abnormal PET findings. An example of restaging melanoma with FDG PET/CT is shown in **Fig. 2**.

Stahlie and colleagues reported on an expanded cohort of a pilot study evaluating the utility of follow-up FDG PET/CT surveillance in asymptomatic high-risk stage III melanoma patients following surgical resection.[48] FDG PET/CT was completed every 6 months for 2 years following resection with the final scan completed at 3 years. Overall, 34% of patients developed a recurrence with 20% detected on the first follow-up FDG PET/CT study and no false positives were reported. Sensitivity and specificity of detecting recurrence in asymptomatic patients were 92% and 100%, respectively, with PPV of 100% and NPV of 99%. It should be noted that multiple studies have reported a wide range of metrics for sensitivity, specificity, NPV, and PPV for follow-up surveillance FDG PET/CT in melanoma and this is likely due to a variety of different inclusion criteria as well as variable follow-up imaging intervals.

Although the early detection of recurrent/metastatic melanoma may enable earlier therapeutic interventions, prospective randomized clinical trials are still needed to demonstrate that early detection and intervention prolongs survival.[7] In high-risk patients, the NPV of FDG PET/CT for detecting melanoma disease relapse is high (97%) but not

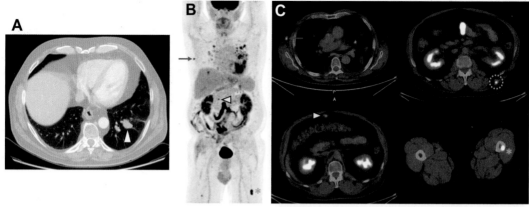

Fig. 2. ¹⁸F-FDG-PET/CT detects multiple metastases in a 71-year-old-man with recurrent melanoma. (*A*) An axial imaging from a diagnostic chest CT demonstrates a suspicious left lower lobe nodule which was subsequently biopsied bronchoscopically and shown to be a melanoma metastasis. The remainder of the diagnostic CT examination of the chest, abdomen, and pelvis demonstrated an equivocal omental nodule but no definite metastatic disease. Based on these results, the patient began evaluation for a wedge resection of this metastasis, which included restaging with FDG PET/CT. (*B*) The maximal intensity projection (MIP) imaging from an FDG-PET study demonstrates multiple metastases as well as inflammation in the lungs. (*C*) Fused PET/CT images demonstrate metastases with increased FDG uptake in the right axilla (*red arrow*), omentum (*yellow arrow*), left back musculature (*dotted green circle*), and left femur (*blue asterisk*). Surgical biopsy confirmed the right axillary lymph node metastasis, and the patient was treated with systemic therapy rather than metastectomy. (*Courtesy of* Jonathan McConathy, MD, PhD, at the University of Alabama at Birmingham (UAB).)

perfect and FDG PET/CT was more likely to miss cutaneous disease recurrences, which reiterates the importance of routine visual clinical skin inspection.[7,43] A meta-analysis performed by Xing and colleagues investigated the utility of various imaging methods for the staging and surveillance of melanoma patients.[49] FDG PET/CT had the highest sensitivity (86%), specificity (91%), and diagnostic odds ratio (67) for detecting distant metastatic disease with a PPV of 80% for patients considered at high risk of distant spread. The practical concerns for FDG PET/CT surveillance in melanoma patients include false-positive PET findings, which can lead to patient anxiety, additional follow-up imaging, and even direct tissue sampling for histopathologic assessment.[46,50] It has been recommended that surveillance by FDG PET/CT should be prospectively compared with other imaging/clinical approaches as well as with no surveillance at all.[46]

RECENT ADVANCES IN PET: NEW TECHNOLOGIES, APPROACHES, AND ANALYTICS

Although FDG PET/CT in oncology patients is typically interpreted qualitatively, it also has the ability to accurately quantify physiologic and pathophysiologic processes. This is an opportunity for radiologists and nuclear medicine physicians to develop, refine, and validate new PET approaches and analytical strategies for more personalized and precise nuclear medicine practices. In particular, current nuclear medicine and PET practices must advance to further improve (1) lesion detectability and disease burden quantification, (2) lesion characterization to distinguish between benign versus malignant processes, and (3) diagnostic confidence with existing or new imaging biomarkers in order to best align multidisciplinary therapeutic management and minimize treatment-related toxicity.

New PET/CT imaging and analytical approaches for improving the accurate detection and characterization of small cutaneous and subcutaneous melanoma recurrences, metastatic nodal involvement (especially in nodes <15 mm), and subcentimeter distant metastatic lesions remain an unmet clinical need. Addressing this need for melanoma is essential because improved lesion detectability allows for identifying melanoma lesions at the smallest and often earliest stage. Likewise, improved characterization of otherwise indeterminate lesions into either benign or malignant will likely contribute to reduced patient anxiety, fewer diagnostic imaging studies or biopsies, and shorter time from scan to treatment. Similarly, consistent and accurate quantification of whole-body disease burden will allow oncologists to more effectively personalize therapies.[51]

A recent technical innovation introduced solid-state digital photon counting PET detectors into the latest generation of digital PET/CT (dPET/CT) systems and these have replaced the conventional analogue photomultiplier tube-based PET detectors (cPET).[52,53] Intraindividual comparison observations with dPET/CT systems have highlighted improved performance with the improved visualization of subcentimeter radiotracer-avid lesions on the dPET, which were not as visually conspicuous on cPET. There also improved delineation of normal physiologic radiotracer activity within normal small tissues and organs (eg, orbits, pituitary gland, and adrenal glands) on dPET when compared with cPET. These new dPET detectors also allowed for radically new PET imaging systems (eg, total body PET), image acquisition approaches, and image reconstruction methods to be developed. The authors have performed greater than 200 intraindividual comparison studies between dPET/CT and cPET/CT systems in oncology patients (NCT02283125) and we will highlight some initial experiences with dPET/CT as well as new opportunities enabled by dPET detector technology that will help to address the unmet clinical needs for melanoma patients.[54] Specifically, dPET technologies enable improved PET image quality with higher definition PET reconstructions, lower radiotracer doses for diagnostic PET imaging (in accordance with ALARA), and shorter PET image acquisitions times for patients with symptomatic disease burden.[53]

Higher Definition PET and Lesion Detectability

A current challenge for nuclear medicine physicians and radiologists who interpret PET/CT studies is the detection and visualization of small metastatic lesions (<15 mm). It is important to understand that the size of the lesion, its FDG-avidity, and the patient's body-mass index are notable biological factors that significantly contribute to a lesion's detectability on PET. In terms of technical factors that influence lesion detectability on PET, partial volume effects are particularly important and sometimes make it very challenging to distinguish tumor-specific radiotracer uptake from normal background activity. Other technical factors that influence lesion detectability include the radiotracer dose, radiotracer injection-to-PET scan time, PET image acquisition time, and PET image reconstruction. In general, cPET systems employ standard definition PET image reconstructions with voxel lengths of 3 to 4 mm (matrix sizes between 144–200) for standard-of-care diagnostic imaging protocols. On the other hand, dPET systems enable higher definition PET reconstructions with smaller voxel lengths of 1 to 2 mm (matrix sizes exceeding 200–400) and possibly even smaller. Higher definition dPET reconstructions lead to decreased PET voxel volumes, reduced partial volume effects, increased visual conspicuity of radiotracer-avid lesions for the interpreting physician, and more precise quantification of the lesion's radiotracer avidity. Higher definition dPET reconstructions are again especially helpful for visualizing and assessing small lesions. In current clinical dPET/CT system implementations, higher definition PET imaging is feasible without prolonged PET image acquisition times but do require optimized PET reconstruction approaches when compared with standard definition cPET approaches.[51,54] It has become evident that cPET and dPET image reconstruction optimization can greatly enhance the nuclear medicine physician's ability to visualize and quantify small FDG avid lesions.[51,53] Such reconstruction optimization approaches for improved detection and visualization of melanoma lesions on dPET have been described.[55]

Improved PET Characterization of Indeterminate Lesions

Indeterminate lesions detected on anatomic diagnostic CT or MRI or even low-dose attenuation-correction CT imaging represent another unmet clinical need that dPET technologies may help to address. In general, FDG cPET imaging has been used to further characterize indeterminate lesions detected on anatomic imaging as benign or malignant but its diagnostic performance often relies on lesion size. Indeterminate lesions are also detected on FDG PET/CT given that FDG uptake is not cancer-specific and may relate to the patient's underlying tumor biology, acute or chronic inflammation (eg, postvaccination, postoperative changes, and during/after radiation or IO therapy), acute or chronic infectious processes, and altered radiotracer biodistribution. In such cases of indeterminate PET findings, correlation with the patient's history and symptoms, physical examination, additional imaging, and direct tissue sampling may be needed to determine if a finding is benign or malignant. The development of new dPET imaging approaches with FDG or other disease-specific PET radiopharmaceuticals may help address this clinical dilemma of indeterminate PET findings and especially when these findings are associated with smaller lesions on anatomic imaging.[51]

The utilization of higher definition dPET image reconstruction is one approach to improve lesion characterization. Again, higher definition reconstruction allows for more precise localization of radiotracer activity within the smaller voxel volumes, reduces partial volume effects, and more accurately quantifies the radiopharmaceutical activity within small lesions (Figs. 3 and 4). This reduction of partial volume effects with higher definition reconstructions may also make small lesions more visually conspicuous on PET and demonstrate higher quantitative PET metrics (ie, higher SUV_{max} values). Similarly, the use of higher definition reconstructions for large heterogeneous lesions may allow for the improved visualization and identification of regions of high-grade tumor versus low-grade tumor within a partially necrotic mass.

Likewise, quantitative PET assessment of FDG uptake within a lesion also has been used to better characterize the visually detected FDG-avid lesion. Multiple quantitative PET assessment approaches have been developed and utilized in order to provide objective metrics for comparison of lesions within and between patients. The most clinically utilized quantitative FDG PET parameter is the maximum SUV (SUV_{max}). Advanced and evolving PET image feature analytics and approaches are also promising for melanoma patients. Beyond SUV metrics like SUV_{max}, SUV_{mean}, and SUV_{peak}, there are FDG PET metrics like the MTV (metabolic tumor volume) and TLG (total lesion glycolysis), which provide a comprehensive whole-body assessment of tumor metabolic disease burden.[56] In addition, an assessment of tumor lesion heterogeneity in melanoma patients using FDG PET imaging has been described and FDG-PET tumor heterogeneity is associated with overall survival in those patients treated with immunotherapy.[56,57] Given that melanoma lesions can be highly heterogeneous in terms of the tumor cells and the tumor microenvironment, more precise PET imaging assessment of tumor heterogeneity may provide insights into treatment resistance, disease progression, or recurrence.[57]

In addition, bone marrow-to-liver SUV_{max} ratio (BLR) and the spleen-to-liver ratio (SLR) have been described as potential FDG-PET imaging biomarkers in melanoma patients being treated with IO. With continued advances in imaging analytics and quantitative imaging biomarker approaches, multiple pretreatment tumor imaging biomarkers may help to guide therapy selection as well as response assessment to therapies. These approaches apply to individual tumor lesions, whole-body tumor burden, and even normal hematopoietic tissues/organs (eg, bone marrow and spleen). In terms of normal hematopoietic tissue/organ assessments in melanoma patients

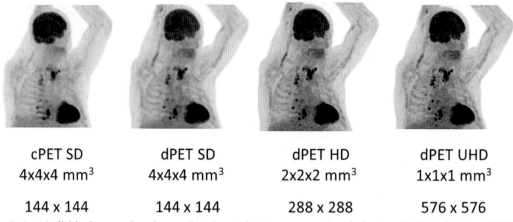

cPET SD	dPET SD	dPET HD	dPET UHD
$4\times4\times4\ mm^3$	$4\times4\times4\ mm^3$	$2\times2\times2\ mm^3$	$1\times1\times1\ mm^3$
144 × 144	144 × 144	288 × 288	576 × 576

Fig. 3. Intraindividual comparison in a patient imaged using a conventional photomultiplier-tube-based PET/CT (cPET) (Gemini 64 ToF, Philips) system and a digital photon-counting PET/CT (dPET) (Vereos, Philips) system with different reconstruction matrix/voxel volume sizes. This case demonstrates the capabilities of higher definition dPET to improve lesion detectability in subcentimeter metastatic nodal lesions without significant impact on background image quality. The patient was intravenously administered a standard dose of 478 MBq of FDG and then underwent imaging on the dPET/CT system at 53 minutes and the cPET/CT system at 81 minutes post injection. Both cPET and dPET emission scans were acquired with 90 seconds per bed position. There are multiple FDG-avid lesions in the base of neck and thoracic regions, which are visually more conspicuous on dPET imaging and become even more suspicious with higher definition dPET reconstructions. Left to right: Maximum-intensity projection images from standard definition cPET (SD, matrix size = 144 × 144, voxel length = 4 mm, voxel volume = 4 × 4 × 4 mm^3), standard definition dPET (SD, matrix size = 144 × 144, voxel length = 4 mm, voxel. volume = 4 × 4 × 4 mm^3), high definition dPET (HD, 288 × 288, 2 mm, 2 × 2 × 2 mm^3), and ultra-high definition dPET (UHD, 576 × 576, 1 mm, 1 × 1 × 1 mm^3).

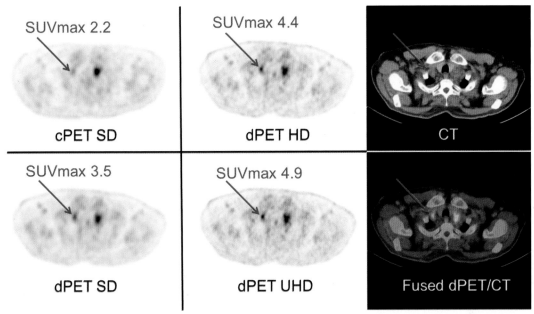

Fig. 4. Intraindividual comparison in a patient imaged using a cPET/CT (Gemini 64 ToF, Philips) system and a dPET/CT (Vereos, Philips) system with different reconstruction matrix/voxel volume sizes. This case further demonstrates the capabilities of higher definition dPET reconstructions to reduce partial volume effects, more precisely localize FDG activity especially within small lesions, and increase the visual conspicuity of FDG-avid lesions. In addition, higher definition dPET reconstructions enable more precise measurement of SUV_{max} in small lesions (ie, <15 mm in short axis). The patient was intravenously administered a standard dose of 478 MBq of FDG and then underwent imaging on the dPET/CT system at 53 minutes and the cPET/CT system at 81 minutes post injection. Both cPET and dPET emission scans were acquired with 90 seconds per bed position. *Left and middle*: Axial images taken at the level of a right supraclavicular lymph node (*red arrows*) are shown with associated SUV_{max} value. Although there is an FDG-avid soft tissue lesion mass noted in the left supraclavicular region on both cPET and dPET, there is a small lymph node in the right supraclavicular regions (red *arrow*) which is visually more conspicuous on dPET images when compared with cPET and becomes more suspicious with higher definition dPET reconstructions. *Right*: Corresponding attenuation correction CT image and fused dPET/CT image at the level of the right supraclavicular lymph node.

treated with immunotherapy, it has been shown that those patients with high pretreatment BLR and SLR were associated with poorer outcomes.[56]

Another new dPET-enabled approach for improved lesion characterization is dynamic PET perfusion imaging (DPPI) at the time of radiopharmaceutical injection and throughout the early uptake period (eg, 0–20 min postinjection). Early dynamic PET imaging of target lesions allows for further qualitative and quantitative assessment of the lesion's immediate perfusion (hypoperfused vs isoperfused vs hyperperfused) and early radiotracer uptake kinetics, which may help to distinguish viable tumor from inflammatory change when correlated with the later whole-body PET imaging (eg, 60–70 min postinjection of FDG). In the future, these dPET-enabled approaches using higher definition reconstructions and/or DPPI to better characterize both indeterminate and malignant lesions before and after therapy may further improve diagnostic confidence, treatment stratification, and imaging response assessment.[54] Early dynamic FDG cPET/CT of the chest/abdomen only in melanoma patients undergoing immunotherapy failed to find any single FDG PET parameter that was predictive of which patients would derive clinical benefit from IO and which would not.[8] To date, no study has described dynamic FDG dPET assessment in melanoma patients treated with conventional cytotoxic therapy or immunotherapy.

Another approach to improve lesion characterization is the use of respiratory-gated PET imaging to reduce respiratory motion artifact (ie, blurring of discrete FDG-avid lesions) as well as to better visualize and quantify small tumor lesions in the thorax and upper abdomen. In fact, tumor SUV_{max} values in the chest and abdomen using breathholding FDG PET imaging approaches can be 30% to 40% higher than with free-breathing PET.[58] When the burden of melanoma metastatic disease is limited (ie, oligometastatic), accurate detection and characterization of malignant/metastatic lesion allows for potential surgical resection and/or targeted external radiation therapy, which confers survival benefits to melanoma patients at the cost of procedure-related morbidity.[45]

Reducing PET Radiotracer Dose and Imaging Faster with dPET

Digital PET systems also facilitate significant radiopharmaceutical dose reductions for whole-body PET imaging with no significant impact on overall image quality, background quality, lesion conspicuity, and quantification when compared with cPET systems. In keeping with ALARA, this new capability for whole-body dPET imaging at significantly reduced radiopharmaceutical doses translates into new clinical and research paradigms for patients to undergo multiple serial dPET/CT studies during a treatment or follow-up surveillance period with only a fraction of the total radiation dose needed for traditional cPET/CT imaging. Likewise, dPET/CT systems allow for even faster whole-body PET imaging at standard radiopharmaceutical doses without affecting image quality, lesion detectability, and quantification. This new capability of dPET/CT systems to facilitate faster whole-body PET imaging will also further minimize patient motion/misregistration artifacts as well as reduce the table time needed for PET imaging in patients with symptomatic lesions. Our team has again demonstrated the feasibility of greater than 50% radiopharmaceutical dose reductions or faster whole-body dPET acquisition times by greater than 50% without affecting PET image quality and quantification (**Fig. 5**).[54]

Need for Increased Integration of Advanced PET Imaging and PET Image Analytics Within Clinical Trials

For large prospective multicenter clinical trials, PET image acquisition and image reconstruction approaches can vary between and even within institutions. At present, there remains a need to continue to standardize PET image acquisition, image reconstruction, and image analytics within multicenter therapeutic clinical trials to minimize variability in PET image quality, quantitative PET metrics, and PET image features for the purpose of response assessment. To this end, harmonization efforts for multicenter PET imaging trials routinely use standardized PET phantoms to establish site-specific SUV quantification correction factors for participating institutions and can readily be implemented into future therapeutic clinical trials for melanoma. This is especially true as institutions begin to replace cPET/CT systems

with newer dPET/CT systems with improved performance characteristics. As new and emerging PET radiopharmaceuticals are also integrated into clinical trials, consideration needs to be made to develop, validate, and establish standardization approaches for each radiopharmaceutical in the multicenter clinical trial setting.[51]

Radiomics is the process of identifying, extracting, and quantifying image features from diagnostic images that can provide new insights into disease processes. As such, routine diagnostic imaging (ie, CT, MRI, and PET) may contain additional information with disease and therapeutic relevance that may not be currently appreciated in clinical practice. The development and validation of new imaging analytics and software tools are needed for PET/CT in order to begin extracting, quantifying, and correlating simultaneous PET and CT imaging features with patient-specific tumor characteristics and disease-specific treatment outcomes. Image feature tools will likely facilitate new precision nuclear medicine practices for PET in terms of lesion segmentation, lesion characterization, and quantification of whole-body disease burden. Radiomics and image feature analysis for PET/CT will also play a major role in developing future imaging response assessments to cancer-specific therapies (eg, IO). A current challenge for PET/CT radiomics is the extent to which PET/CT imaging features are influenced by the various PET radioisotopes, PET radiopharmaceuticals and subsequent biodistribution, range of radiopharmaceutical doses administered, PET image acquisition, attenuation correction CT image acquisition, and PET and CT image reconstruction techniques. As already mentioned, PET/CT standardization and harmonization within multicenter clinical trials will be required to minimize image feature variability between patients and institutions in order to facilitate robust radiomic analyses and discover new imaging biomarkers with insights into disease characterization and management.[51]

The current growth and development of advanced PET imaging technologies, PET radiopharmaceuticals, and PET imaging analytics is taking place simultaneously with growth and development in translational medicine technologies for the exquisitely sensitive detection of cancer-specific markers from biological samples in cancer patients. Liquid biopsy-driven PET/CT imaging approaches for the detection, localization, and treatment of recurrent malignant/metastatic disease in asymptomatic patients are already being developed, for example, the use of S-100B as a blood-based liquid biomarker for melanoma recurrence in asymptomatic patients. Of all of the

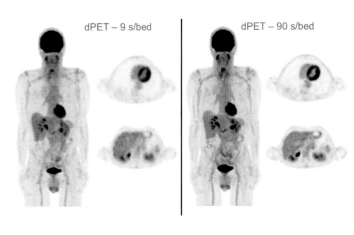

dPET – 9 s/bed   dPET – 90 s/bed

Fig. 5. Intraindividual comparison in a patient imaged using a dPET/CT (Vereos, Philips) system and acquired with different dPET image acquisition times (ie, standard = 90 seconds per bed position, and ultra-fast = 9 seconds per bed position). This case demonstrates the capabilities of dPET technology to facilitate ultra-fast PET imaging with markedly reduce PET image acquisition times (1/10th of the standard acquisition time) while generating visually comparable image quality. The patient was intravenously administered a standard dose of 484 MBq of FDG and then underwent ultra-fast imaging (left – 9 seconds per bed with a total PET acquisition <2 minutes) on the dPET/CT system at 53 minutes post injection followed by standard imaging (right – 90 seconds per bed with a total PET acquisition ~16 minutes) at 57 minutes post injection. For each acquisition, a maximum intensity projection image from SD dPET using optimized reconstruction methodologies is shown along with representative axial dPET SD images taken at the levels of the heart and liver. The ultra-fast whole-body dPET image acquisition produced visually comparable image quality when compared with the standard whole-body dPET image acquisition. In addition, the physiologic FDG activity is qualitatively and quantitatively similar on the ultra-fast and standard dPET acquisitions at the levels of the heart and liver. FDG uptake in the normal liver has an SUV_{mean} = 1.9 for both dPET acquisitions.

S-100B biomarker tests performed in one study, ~3% triggered an FDG PET/CT examination. In those patients for whom FDG PET detected recurrent disease, 23% were otherwise asymptomatic and only had abnormal S-100B. Although not yet perfect, this liquid biopsy biomarker screening strategy contributed to the subsequent detection of recurrent melanoma in otherwise asymptomatic patients.[59] Future prospective clinical trials that correlate and compare serial liquid biopsy biomarkers of disease recurrence with concurrent imaging studies are needed, especially in the surveillance setting (ie, liquid biopsy-driven imaging vs standardized scheduled surveillance imaging).

SUMMARY

Throughout the body with the exception of the brain, FDG PET plays an important clinical role in the staging of melanoma, therapeutic response assessment, detection of treatment resistance/failure, detection of treatment-related toxicities, and detection of disease progression. With increasing use of IO therapeutics in melanoma as well as other cancer patients, it remains a clinical challenge to assess and quantify treatment response by conventional anatomic imaging alone. Melanoma lesions tends to demonstrate high glucose utilization and therefore FDG PET/CT is highly sensitive and ideally suited for detecting, monitoring, and quantifying these lesions.[4]

New PET imaging technologies and approaches, new PET image reconstruction techniques and image analytics, and possibly new PET radiopharmaceuticals will likely provide additional insights into the underlying tumor biology before, during, and after therapy regardless of anatomic changes in tumor size, extent, and burden. Although treatment-related pseudo-progression can cause some confusion on early treatment imaging, more research and clinical trial validation are needed to establish optimal time points for FDG PET/CT imaging in the setting of IO therapy for melanoma.[9] Newer immune-related response criteria have been developed to begin addressing these new treatment-related effects. In addition, future studies will likely need to incorporate both early-treatment as well as long-term FDG PET/CT imaging (eg, 1-year follow-up after completion of IO) when therapy has been stopped in patients who have radiographically stable residual lesions in order to determine if it can provide useful prognostic information. At present, FDG PET findings of a complete metabolic response to immunotherapy are the most predictive biomarker for predicting long-term patient benefit and may allow for consideration of maintenance IO therapy discontinuation.[21]

PET/CT image features may serve as an early imaging biomarker of tumor response to therapy or even tumor resistance in order to help guide treating physicians. PET may also provide treating physicians with high-yield tissue targets when pursuing residual tumor biopsies. Given that the optimal duration for IO therapy for various cancers remains unknown, new imaging strategies need to be developed and clinically validated to determine when complete pathologic response has been achieved versus persistent residual viable tumor. In the presence of stable but residual soft tissue lesions after long-term maintenance IO therapy, PET may allow for therapy to be stopped (and therefore minimize any immune-related toxicities or adverse events) and the patients to be monitored in a surveillance setting. It has been argued that surveillance imaging is only effective if it leads to effective therapeutic strategies and survival benefits as opposed to lead-time bias. Further prospective clinical trials in surveillance FDG PET/CT imaging are therefore needed to support its role in follow-up surveillance for asymptomatic melanoma patients.

In the future, radiologists and nuclear medicine physicians will need to better understand the impact of IO therapeutics on their patients, develop strategies for assessing treatment response during IO, determine if early predictive biomarkers of treatment response or even treatment resistance exist, and recognizing early imaging features suggestive of treatment-related toxicities. It should be noted that different IO therapeutics may even have different capabilities for early PET prediction of response to therapy.[38] As our knowledge and understanding of melanoma and IO therapeutics grows, we will need to develop new tools and reporting structures to better guide medical decision-making. FDG PET has an important clinical role in the staging, therapeutic response assessment, and clinical management of melanoma patients. More recently, PET technology, imaging approaches, image reconstruction, and image analytics have advanced, whereas the role of FDG as the primary PET radiotracer in melanoma patients has not changed. As highlighted in this review, there are some challenges but many exciting opportunities to advance FDG PET into new precision nuclear medicine strategies for patients with melanoma.

CLINICS CARE POINTS

- In clinical care, FDG PET/CT has an important role in the non-invasive staging of melanoma as well as subsequent therapy response assessment and even the detection of disease progression.
- Targeted immuno-oncology therapeutics presents new challenges for response assessment

using conventional anatomic imaging alone which necessitates new and advanced molecular imaging approaches with PET.

- New digital PET technologies may enable novel approaches for imaging melanoma patients with higher image definition, lower radiotracer doses, and faster image acquisition times.

ACKNOWLEDGMENTS

C.L. Wright and M.V. Knopp acknowledge research support: Wright Center of Innovation in Biomedical Imaging and ODSA TECH 09-028, 10-012, and 13-060 and the National Institutes of Health R01CA195513 and 5U24CA180803. C.L. Wright also acknowledges research time support: NCI UG1CA233331.

REFERENCES

1. Erdmann F, Lortet-Tieulent J, Schüz J, et al. International trends in the incidence of malignant melanoma 1953-2008–are recent generations at higher or lower risk? Int J Cancer 2013;132(2):385–400.
2. Linos E, Swetter SM, Cockburn MG, et al. Increasing burden of melanoma in the United States. J Invest Dermatol 2009;129(7):1666–74.
3. Olsen CM, Green AC, Pandeya N, et al. Trends in Melanoma Incidence Rates in Eight Susceptible Populations through 2015. J Invest Dermatol 2019; 139(6):1392–5.
4. Plouznikoff N, Arsenault F. Clinical relevance of 18F-FDG PET/CT lower-limb imaging in patients with malignant cutaneous melanoma. Nucl Med Commun 2017;38(12):1103–8.
5. Mena E, Sanli Y, Marcus C, et al. Precision medicine and PET/computed tomography in melanoma. PET Clin 2017;12(4):449–58.
6. Siegel RL, Miller KD, Jemal A. Cancer statistics, 2020. CA Cancer J Clin 2020;70(1):7–30.
7. Vensby PH, Schmidt G, Kjær A, et al. The value of FDG PET/CT for follow-up of patients with melanoma: a retrospective analysis. Am J Nucl Med Mol Imaging 2017;7(6):255–62.
8. Sachpekidis C, Anwar H, Winkler JK, et al. Longitudinal studies of the (18)F-FDG kinetics after ipilimumab treatment in metastatic melanoma patients based on dynamic FDG PET/CT. Cancer Immunol Immunother 2018;67(8):1261–70.
9. Wong ANM, McArthur GA, Hofman MS, et al. The advantages and challenges of using FDG PET/CT for response assessment in melanoma in the era of targeted agents and immunotherapy. Eur J Nucl Med Mol Imaging 2017;44(Suppl 1):67–77.

10. Forschner A, Olthof SC, Gückel B, et al. Impact of (18)F-FDG-PET/CT on surgical management in patients with advanced melanoma: an outcome based analysis. Eur J Nucl Med Mol Imaging 2017;44(8):1312–8.

11. Trout AT, Rabinowitz RS, Platt JF, et al. Melanoma metastases in the abdomen and pelvis: Frequency and patterns of spread. World J Radiol 2013;5(2):25–32.

12. Holder WD Jr, White RL, Zuger JH, et al. Effectiveness of positron emission tomography for the detection of melanoma metastases. Ann Surg 1998;227(5):764–71.

13. Swetter SM, Carroll LA, Johnson DL, et al. Positron emission tomography is superior to computed tomography for metastatic detection in melanoma patients. Ann Surg Oncol 2002;9(7):646–53.

14. Rodriguez Rivera AM, Alabbas H, Ramjaun A, et al. Value of positron emission tomography scan in stage III cutaneous melanoma: a systematic review and meta-analysis. Surg Oncol 2014;23(1):11–6.

15. Krug B, Crott R, Lonneux M, et al. Role of PET in the initial staging of cutaneous malignant melanoma: systematic review. Radiology 2008;249(3):836–44.

16. Schröer-Günther MA, Wolff RF, Westwood ME, et al. F-18-fluoro-2-deoxyglucose positron emission tomography (PET) and PET/computed tomography imaging in primary staging of patients with malignant melanoma: a systematic review. Syst Rev 2012;1:62.

17. Wagner JD, Schauwecker D, Davidson D, et al. Inefficacy of F-18 fluorodeoxy-D-glucose-positron emission tomography scans for initial evaluation in early-stage cutaneous melanoma. Cancer 2005;104(3):570–9.

18. Bastiaannet E, Wobbes T, Hoekstra OS, et al. Prospective comparison of [18F]fluorodeoxyglucose positron emission tomography and computed tomography in patients with melanoma with palpable lymph node metastases: diagnostic accuracy and impact on treatment. J Clin Oncol 2009;27(28):4774–80.

19. Gao G, Gong B, Shen W. Meta-analysis of the additional value of integrated 18FDG PET-CT for tumor distant metastasis staging: comparison with 18FDG PET alone and CT alone. Surg Oncol 2013;22(3):195–200.

20. Singnurkar A, Wang J, Joshua AM, et al. 18F-FDG-PET/CT in the staging and management of melanoma: a prospective multicenter Ontario PET Registry Study. Clin Nucl Med 2016;41(3):189–93.

21. Tan AC, Emmett L, Lo S, et al. FDG-PET response and outcome from anti-PD-1 therapy in metastatic melanoma. Ann Oncol 2018;29(10):2115–20.

22. Schaarschmidt BM, Grueneisen J, Stebner V, et al. Can integrated 18F-FDG PET/MR replace sentinel lymph node resection in malignant melanoma? Eur J Nucl Med Mol Imaging 2018;45(12):2093–102.

23. Morton DL, Thompson JF, Cochran AJ, et al. Final trial report of sentinel-node biopsy versus nodal observation in melanoma. N Engl J Med 2014;370(7):599–609.

24. Wagner JD, Schauwecker D, Davidson D, et al. Prospective study of fluorodeoxyglucose–positron emission tomography imaging of lymph node basins in melanoma patients undergoing sentinel node biopsy. J Clin Oncol 1999;17(5):1508–15.

25. Dinnes J, Ferrante di Ruffano L, Takwoingi Y, et al. Ultrasound, CT, MRI, or PET-CT for staging and restaging of adults with cutaneous melanoma. Cochrane Database Syst Rev 2019;7(7):CD012806.

26. Coit DG, Thompson JA, Albertini MR, et al. Cutaneous Melanoma, Version 2.2019, NCCN clinical practice guidelines in oncology. J Natl Compr Canc Netw 2019;17(4):367–402.

27. Youland RS, Packard AT, Blanchard MJ, et al. 18F-FDG PET response and clinical outcomes after stereotactic body radiation therapy for metastatic melanoma. Adv Radiat Oncol 2017;2(2):204–10.

28. Wahl RL, Jacene H, Kasamon Y, et al. From RECIST to PERCIST: Evolving Considerations for PET response criteria in solid tumors. J Nucl Med 2009;50(Suppl 1):122S–50S.

29. Seymour L, Bogaerts J, Perrone A, et al. iRECIST: guidelines for response criteria for use in trials testing immunotherapeutics. Lancet Oncol 2017;18(3):e143–52.

30. Anwar H, Sachpekidis C, Winkler J, et al. Absolute number of new lesions on (18)F-FDG PET/CT is more predictive of clinical response than SUV changes in metastatic melanoma patients receiving ipilimumab. Eur J Nucl Med Mol Imaging 2018;45(3):376–83.

31. Eisenhauer EA, Therasse P, Bogaerts J, et al. New response evaluation criteria in solid tumours: revised RECIST guideline (version 1.1). Eur J Cancer 2009;45(2):228–47.

32. Ayati N, Sadeghi R, Kiamanesh Z, et al. The value of (18)F-FDG PET/CT for predicting or monitoring immunotherapy response in patients with metastatic melanoma: a systematic review and meta-analysis. Eur J Nucl Med Mol Imaging 2020;48(2):428–48.

33. Amrane K, Le Goupil D, Quere G, et al. Prediction of response to immune checkpoint inhibitor therapy using 18F-FDG PET/CT in patients with melanoma. Medicine (Baltimore) 2019;98(29):e16417.

34. Cho SY, Lipson EJ, Im HJ, et al. Prediction of Response to Immune Checkpoint Inhibitor Therapy Using Early-Time-Point 18F-FDG PET/CT Imaging in Patients with Advanced Melanoma. J Nucl Med 2017;58(9):1421–8.

35. Sachpekidis C, Anwar H, Winkler J, et al. The role of interim (18)F-FDG PET/CT in prediction of response

to ipilimumab treatment in metastatic melanoma. Eur J Nucl Med Mol Imaging 2018;45(8):1289–96.

36. Ito K, Teng R, Schöder H, et al. (18)F-FDG PET/CT for monitoring of ipilimumab therapy in patients with metastatic melanoma. J Nucl Med 2019;60(3): 335–41.

37. Annovazzi A, Vari S, Giannarelli D, et al. Comparison of 18F-FDG PET/CT criteria for the prediction of therapy response and clinical outcome in patients with metastatic melanoma treated with ipilimumab and PD-1 inhibitors. Clin Nucl Med 2020;45(3):187–94.

38. Seith F, Forschner A, Weide B, et al. Is there a link between very early changes of primary and secondary lymphoid organs in 18F-FDG-PET/MRI and treatment response to checkpoint inhibitor therapy? J Immunother Cancer 2020;8(2):e000656.

39. Seith F, Forschner A, Schmidt H, et al. 18F-FDG-PET detects complete response to PD1-therapy in melanoma patients two weeks after therapy start. Eur J Nucl Med Mol Imaging 2018;45(1):95–101.

40. Tirumani SH, Ramaiya NH, Keraliya A, et al. Radiographic profiling of immune-related adverse events in advanced melanoma patients treated with ipilimumab. Cancer Immunol Res 2015;3(10):1185–92.

41. Long GV, Saw RPM, Lo S, et al. Neoadjuvant dabrafenib combined with trametinib for resectable, stage IIIB–C, BRAFV600 mutation-positive melanoma (NeoCombi): a single-arm, open-label, single-centre, phase 2 trial. Lancet Oncol 2019;20(7): 961–71.

42. Huang AC, Orlowski RJ, Xu X, et al. A single dose of neoadjuvant PD-1 blockade predicts clinical outcomes in resectable melanoma. Nat Med 2019;25(3):454–61.

43. Lee HH, Paeng JC, Cheon GJ, et al. Recurrence of Melanoma After Initial Treatment: Diagnostic Performance of FDG PET in Posttreatment Surveillance. Nucl Med Mol Imaging 2018;52(5):327–33.

44. Bleicher J, Swords DS, Mali ME, et al. Recurrence patterns in patients with Stage II melanoma: The evolving role of routine imaging for surveillance. J Surg Oncol 2020;122(8):1770–7.

45. Madu MF, Timmerman P, Wouters MWJM, et al. PET/CT surveillance detects asymptomatic recurrences in stage IIIB and IIIC melanoma patients: a prospective cohort study. Melanoma Res 2017;27(3):251–7.

46. Lewin J, Sayers L, Kee D, et al. Surveillance imaging with FDG-PET/CT in the post-operative follow-up of stage 3 melanoma. Ann Oncol 2018;29(7):1569–74.

47. Leon-Ferre RA, Kottschade LA, Block MS, et al. Association between the use of surveillance PET/CT and the detection of potentially salvageable occult recurrences among patients with resected high-risk melanoma. Melanoma Res 2017;27(4):335–41.

48. Stahlie EHA, van der Hiel B, Stokkel MPM, et al. The use of FDG-PET/CT to detect early recurrence after resection of high-risk stage III melanoma. J Surg Oncol 2020;122(7):1328–36.

49. Xing Y, Bronstein Y, Ross MI, et al. Contemporary diagnostic imaging modalities for the staging and surveillance of melanoma patients: a meta-analysis. J Natl Cancer Inst 2011;103(2):129–42.

50. Nijhuis AAG, Dieng M, Khanna N, et al. False-Positive Results and Incidental Findings with Annual CT or PET/CT Surveillance in Asymptomatic Patients with Resected Stage III Melanoma. Ann Surg Oncol 2019;26(6):1860–8.

51. Wright CL, Maly JJ, Zhang J, et al. Advancing Precision Nuclear Medicine and Molecular Imaging for Lymphoma. PET Clin 2017;12(1):63–82.

52. Zhang J, Maniawski P, Knopp MV. Performance evaluation of the next generation solid-state digital photon counting PET/CT system. EJNMMI Res 2018;8(1):97.

53. Wright CL, Binzel K, Zhang J, et al. Advanced Functional Tumor Imaging and Precision Nuclear Medicine Enabled by Digital PET Technologies. Contrast Media Mol Imaging 2017;2017:5260305.

54. Wright CL, Washington IR, Bhatt AD, et al. Emerging Opportunities for Digital PET/CT to advance locoregional therapy in head and neck cancer. Semin Radiat Oncol 2019;29(2):93–101.

55. Aljared A, Alharbi AA, Huellner MW. BSREM Reconstruction for Improved Detection of In-Transit Metastases With Digital FDG-PET/CT in Patients With Malignant Melanoma. Clin Nucl Med 2018;43(5): 370–1.

56. Seban RD, Nemer JS, Marabelle A, et al. Prognostic and theranostic 18F-FDG PET biomarkers for anti-PD1 immunotherapy in metastatic melanoma: association with outcome and transcriptomics. Eur J Nucl Med Mol Imaging 2019;46(11):2298–310.

57. Sanli Y, Leake J, Odu A, et al. Tumor Heterogeneity on FDG PET/CT and immunotherapy: an imaging biomarker for predicting treatment response in patients with metastatic melanoma. AJR Am J Roentgenol 2019;1–9. https://doi.org/10.2214/AJR.18.19796.

58. Barwolf R, Zirnsak M, Freesmeyer M. Breath-hold and free-breathing F-18-FDG-PET/CT in malignant melanoma-detection of additional tumoral foci and effects on quantitative parameters. Medicine (Baltimore) 2017;96(2):e5882.

59. Deckers EA, Wevers KP, Muller Kobold AC, et al. S-100B as an extra selection tool for FDG PET/CT scanning in follow-up of AJCC stage III melanoma patients. J Surg Oncol 2019;120(6):1031–7.

PET Imaging for Head and Neck Cancers

Charles Marcus, MD[a,*], Sara Sheikhbahaei, MD[b], Veeresh Kumar N. Shivamurthy, MD[c], Greg Avey, MD[d], Rathan M. Subramaniam, MBBS, BMedSc, MClinEd, MPH, PhD, MBA, FRANZCR, FSNMMI, FAUR[e]

KEYWORDS

- FDG PET • PET/CT • Head and neck cancer • Neoplasm • Staging

KEY POINTS

- ^{18}F-FDG PET/CT has value in the evaluation and management of head and neck cancers with advantages over conventional anatomic imaging.
- ^{18}F-FDG PET/CT plays a significant role in the assessment of treatment response in head and neck cancers with high negative predictive value thereby reducing unnecessary invasive diagnostic procedures.
- Alternative PET tracers can provide additional information such as tumor hypoxia which can guide treatment planning.

INTRODUCTION

Head and neck cancers (HNCs) are a group of cancers involving the different structures in the head and neck region. In clinical practice, the most common location of these cancers is the oropharynx (34%), larynx (28%), and oral cavity (18%). Other locations include the hypopharynx, nasal cavity, nasopharynx, paranasal sinuses, salivary glands, and skin. Approximately 53,260 new cases of oral cavity and oropharynx cancer were estimated to be diagnosed in the United States in 2020, accounting for 2.9% of all new cancer diagnoses. The estimated number of deaths due to these cancers is approximately 10,750, accounting for 1.8% of all cancer deaths. In 2017, an estimated 383,415 people were living with oral cavity and pharyngeal cancers in the United States. The survival of these patients depends on the stage of disease, with 5-year survival ranging from 85.1% in patients with

localized disease to 40.1% in those with distant disease. This variance in outcomes emphasizes the importance of accurate and timely diagnosis and staging, where imaging plays a crucial role.[1] Most HNCs are squamous cell carcinoma by histopathology and termed head and neck squamous cell carcinomas (HNSCCs).[2] This article focuses on the role of ^{18}F-FDG PET/CT and PET/MR imaging in the evaluation and management of HNCs. A brief discussion on alternative PET radiotracers and their potential role in HNC evaluation is also presented.

STAGING HEAD AND NECK CANCERS

With recent advances in the understanding of the biology of different tumors of the head and neck, there have been changes in the primary tumor (T), local lymph node disease (N), and metastasis (M) staging of these tumors, as proposed by the

The authors have nothing to disclose.
[a] Department of Nuclear Medicine and Molecular Imaging, Emory University Hospital, Atlanta, GA, USA;
[b] Department of Radiology, Johns Hopkins Medical Institutions, 601 N. Caroline Street, JHOC 3235, Baltimore, MD 21287, USA; [c] Epilepsy Center, St. Francis Hospital and Medical Center, Trinity Health of New England, 114 Woodland Street, Hartford, CT 06105, USA; [d] Department of Radiology, University of Wisconsin School of Medicine and Public Health, 600 Highland Ave #3284, Madison, WI 53792, USA; [e] Dean's Office, Otago Medical School, University of Otago, 201 Great King Street, Dunedin 9016, New Zealand
* Corresponding author. Division of Nuclear Medicine and Molecular Imaging, Department of Radiology and Imaging Services, 1364 Clifton Road Northeast, 1st Floor #E163, Atlanta, GA 30322.
E-mail address: charlesmarcus1986@gmail.com

Radiol Clin N Am 59 (2021) 773–788
https://doi.org/10.1016/j.rcl.2021.05.005

most recent (eighth) edition of the *AJCC Cancer Staging Manual* by the American Joint Committee on Cancer (AJCC). For example, the human papillomavirus (HPV) status of HNSCC tumors has been found to have a significant impact on the behavior of cancers, and the vast majority of HNSCCs in the United States are attributed to HPV-related cancers. These tumors are more susceptible to chemoradiation and have better outcomes than HPV-negative tumors. This factor is incorporated into the most recent staging system.[3] When assessing these tumors, the important features to evaluate on imaging pertinent to the staging system include tumor size in the greatest dimension, maximum depth of invasion (evaluated primarily on MR imaging), invasion of tumor into adjacent structures, number of nodes involved, size of the involved node, features of extranodal extension, whether the nodes are ipsilateral or contralateral to the tumor, and findings of distant metastases, The depth of invasion, in addition to the tumor size, is included in the updated system, whereas prior versions included only the maximal tumor size.[4] In routine anatomic imaging, size criteria and abnormal morphology are used to identify pathologic lymph nodes. Although diagnostic accuracy is lower in small lymph nodes that do not meet size criteria, ^{18}F-FDG PET/CT can be useful in identifying metastatic disease in these small nodes.[5]

ROLE OF PET IN THE EVALUATION OF HEAD AND NECK CANCERS

In the initial workup of the HNC primary site, CT of the soft tissues of the neck or MR imaging of the neck is indicated to delineate the primary tumor. MR imaging may be preferred over CT in certain specific indications, such as assessing skull base extension, cranial nerve involvement, bone involvement of tumor in patients with dental implants, and resultant artifact, that make CT evaluation suboptimal. CT can add useful information to MR imaging findings in evaluating bone or cartilage involvement. The imaging techniques should extend to the base of the neck for optimal nodal evaluation. In patients where no obvious primary tumor has been identified, ^{18}F-FDG PET/CT is recommended before further evaluation or biopsy to potentially identify the primary site for targeted tissue sampling. Sampling of metastatic nodes may be necessary for diagnostic purposes, and some of these nodes can be cystic. As with the nodes often commonly encountered with HPV-associated tumors, image-guided biopsy is recommended to increase the yield.[6] In patients with extensive nodal disease or nodes involving the lower neck, aggressive tumor histology, and patients undergoing definitive radiation therapy, ^{18}F-FDG PET/CT can be useful in detecting additional nodal or distant disease. For surgical treatment planning, ^{18}F-FDG PET/CT is recommended for surgical planning of the contralateral neck in tumors that cross or are near the midline. In the evaluation of distant metastases in locally advanced HNCs, ^{18}F-FDG PET/CT is recommended. In the early follow-up of these patients, ^{18}F-FDG PET/CT can be performed in addition to or in place of anatomic imaging when evaluating recurrent, residual disease or second primary malignancy to guide treatment. Posttreatment response assessment with ^{18}F-FDG PET/CT following definitive radiation or chemoradiation therapy is recommended 3 to 6 months after treatment to reduce false-positive findings secondary to inflammation early in the follow-up. In late follow-up (>6 months), ^{18}F-FDG PET/CT is not routinely indicated unless there are clinical symptoms or concerning signs for recurrent disease. However, surveillance ^{18}F-FDG PET/CT can detect recurrent malignancy or a second primary tumor in approximately 10% of patients 1 year after treatment (NCCN guidelines v 2.2020).[7]

IMAGING FINDINGS
Staging

^{18}F-FDG PET/CT has been shown to be useful in pretreatment staging and evaluation, especially for detecting clinically negative metastases including clinically negative neck disease, with a significant impact on treatment strategies.

Staging: Primary Tumor

In HNC primary tumor evaluation, recent studies have shown that ^{18}F-FDG PET/CT may have advantages over CT and MR imaging with higher diagnostic accuracy. The limitations of primary tumor evaluation by ^{18}F-FDG PET/CT should be considered. Precise tumor size estimation, small-volume tumors, infiltration of surrounding soft tissues, depth of invasion, perineural spread, or bone marrow involvement may be better evaluated on MR imaging.[8] However, in small tumors (T1-T2), a prospective study has shown that ^{18}F-FDG PET/CT demonstrates higher sensitivity than MR imaging (83% vs 63%) in identifying these small tumors, with good interobserver variability. It should be noted that the use of contrast-enhanced diagnostic CT studies of the head and neck performed with these PET/CT studies provides better evaluation, especially for small tumors.[9] Streak or susceptibility artifact related to hardware or dental implants is commonly encountered in imaging

HNCs and can have a significant impact on the accurate evaluation of these primary tumors. 18F-FDG PET/CT has been shown to provide better evaluation of primary tumors in these patients than provided by MR imaging, with superior correlation with the pathologic tumor volume at resection. While reviewing images of these patients, careful evaluation of the non-attenuation-corrected PET images separately can provide a better picture of abnormal metabolic activity.[10]

Staging: Nodal Disease

It has been well established that 18F-FDG PET/CT provides added advantage to clinical examination and routine anatomic imaging in evaluating nodal metastases in HNC. An important finding published in the recent past is the advantage of 18F-FDG PET/CT in the evaluation of clinically negative HNSCC (T2-T4) in a prospective multicenter trial (ACRIN 6685). Using an optimal maximum standardized uptake value (SUVmax) cutoff of 1.8, the negative predictive value was estimated to be 94%, resulting in changes in surgical management in 22% of the patients, with additional nodal-level dissection in 14% and fewer dissection in 5% of these patients.[11] Approximately 10% of patients who undergo therapeutic or planned neck dissections can develop complications such as postoperative infection, seroma, flap-necrosis, etc. The advantage of 18F-FDG PET/CT described above can lead to a decrease in perioperative morbidity, with higher morbidity often associated with more extensive neck dissections and radiation. Given these improved outcomes, the 18F-FDG PET/CT approach has been found to be cost-effective per quality-adjusted life-year.[12] The overall diagnostic performance of 18F-FDG PET/CT in the detection of nodal metastases in HNC is good, with pooled sensitivity and specificity of 84% and 84%, respectively, per neck-side and 84% and 96% per nodal-level analyses, respectively, in a meta-analysis of 742 patients with HNC.[13] The outcome and survival of patients with HNC are affected by the risk of lymph node metastases, and hence, accurate early detection of cervical nodal metastases is crucial in these patients[14] (**Fig. 1**).

Staging: Distant Metastasis

In addition to the advantages of using 18F-FDG PET/CT for local tumor and nodal disease evaluation as described above, one of the most useful applications of this modality is detecting distant disease that is often not detected by conventional imaging techniques. Distant disease is associated with poor outcomes, and timely detection is extremely important for aggressive tailored treatment planning strategies to improve the prognosis in these patients.[15] The risk of distant metastases is higher in certain HNCs than in others. For example, the highest rates of distant metastases at primary evaluation were associated with nasopharyngeal cancers (9%), followed by those of the hypopharynx (7%), oropharynx (4%), larynx (3%), and oral cavity (2%). In cancers excluding the nasopharynx, the overall rate of distant metastases was approximately 3%. Overall, the most common site of distant metastases appears to be the lung (54%), followed by bone. However, in nasopharyngeal cancers, the most common site

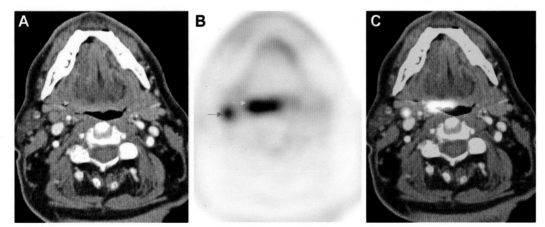

Fig. 1. Axial contrast-enhanced CT (*A*), axial 18F-FDG PET (*B*), and axial fused 18F-FDG PET/CT (*C*) 70-year-old man with a newly diagnosed HPV-associated T2 squamous cell carcinoma of the oropharynx with clinical negative cervical nodal disease. The staging 18F-FDG PET/CT demonstrates the hypermetabolic mass in the right tongue base (*yellow arrows*) with an 18F-FDG-avid right level IIa lymph node (SUVmax 9.2) (*blue arrows*) consistent with metastatic nodal disease.

of distant metastases is the bone (50%), followed by lung (33%) and liver (27%). Factors associated with distant metastases are nodal status, especially N3 disease, advanced T-stage, older age, poorly differentiated tumors, etc. In oropharyngeal cancers with known HPV status, HPV-negative tumors are associated with a higher chance of distant metastases than HPV-positive tumors (4% vs 2%; $P<.05$). In patients with risk factors of distant metastases and nasopharyngeal cancers with a higher risk of bone metastases, PET/CT is useful in the staging evaluation.[16] A meta-analysis including 1147 patients with HNC demonstrated a sensitivity of 83% and specificity of 96% in detecting distant metastases. The corresponding values for conventional imaging methods were 44% and 96%, respectively. These results show the advantage of using ^{18}F-FDG PET/CT over conventional imaging methods to detect distant metastatic disease[17] (Fig. 2).

TREATMENT PLANNING

In recent years, ^{18}F-FDG PET/CT findings have been increasingly used to plan image-guided radiation therapy for optimal tumor control and treatment response while maintaining minimal radiation to the adjacent normal background tissues, given the vital structures in the neck such as cranial nerves, blood vessels, salivary gland, spinal cord, etc. In up to 10% of patients, ^{18}F-FDG PET/CT findings can alter primary tumor and nodal disease volumes and detect additional metastatic disease or synchronous malignancies, resulting in changes in radiation treatment planning.[18,19] ^{18}F-FDG PET/CT-based nodal disease volume, in comparison with CT nodal volume, has shown improved regional disease control, and in turn, a positive impact on patient outcome.[20] Image-guided radiation treatment planning techniques are constantly evolving, and newer methods are being proposed to improve tumor control. For example, ^{18}F-FDG PET/CT-based intensity-modulated arc therapy, compared with more widely used static intensity-modulated radiation therapy dose-based painting by numbers, has shown improved dose to surrounding normal tissues at risk with better treatment efficacy and shorter delivery time.[21] In the recent past, integration and coordination of different medical specialties have improved the evaluation of oncologic patients.

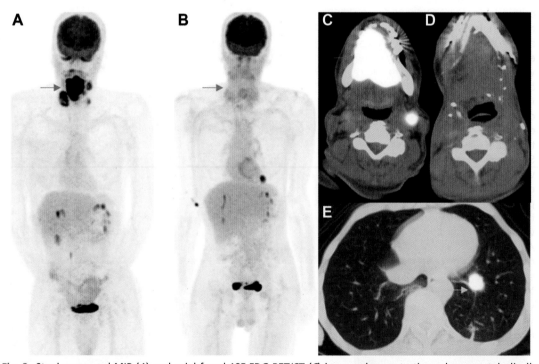

Fig. 2. Staging coronal MIP (A) and axial fused 18F-FDG PET/CT (C) images demonstrating a large metabolically active mass involving the floor of mouth (blue arrows) with bilateral metastatic cervical lymphadenopathy. Post treatment coronal MIP (B) and axial fused 18F-FDG PET/CT (D, E) images after surgical resection, neck dissection and flap reconstruction followed by chemoradiation demonstrating complete metabolic response to treatment. However, a new spiculated metabolically active left lower lobe lung nodule was noted (yellow arrows). Biopsy of the lung nodule demonstrated metastatic squamous cell carcinoma from head and neck cancer.

Comparing images of radiation treatment planning prior to treatment with follow-up, 18F-FDG PET/CT has been suggested to improve the diagnostic accuracy of differentiating disease recurrence versus postradiation inflammation.[22] An ongoing clinical trial (UPGRADE-RT) evaluates the implementation of 18F-FDG PET/CT-guided de-escalation of radiation therapy dose to small lymph nodes that do not meet size criteria assessed by 18F-FDG PET/CT in HNC patients to evaluate the risk of disease recurrence while improving quality of life with reduced complications related to radiation to important normal structures in the head and neck.[23]

TREATMENT RESPONSE ASSESSMENT

18F-FDG PET/CT plays an important role in the imaging evaluation of response to treatment within 6 months of completion of treatment, especially in patients undergoing organ-preserving systemic therapy alone or combined with radiation therapy. To reduce false-positive findings related to post-treatment inflammation, the optimal time for performing these scans is 3 to 6 months (NCCN guidelines v 2.2020).[7] Posttreatment 18F-FDG PET/CT performed up to 12 months after treatment completion in patients with OPSCC can detect residual or recurrent disease in almost half the patients. However, false-positive findings can also be seen in one-third of the patients. The greatest value appears to be a high negative predictive value in patients undergoing surgery (100%) or chemoradiation (97%). Lower positive predictive value and specificity is seen in patients undergoing chemoradiation in comparison with patients undergoing primary surgery, likely related to post-treatment inflammation. 18F-FDG PET/CT with SUVmax values greater than 5 are associated with a higher rate of residual or recurrent disease.[24] In a meta-analysis including 1293 HNSCC patients, the pooled sensitivity, specificity, positive predictive, and negative predictive values were 85%, 93%, 58%, and 98%, respectively. As shown by these results, a significantly higher negative predictive value has an impact on the clinical evaluation of these patients, resulting in fewer unnecessary diagnostic or therapeutic interventions. The authors found lower sensitivity (75% vs 89%; P = .01) and specificity (87% vs 95%; P<.005) in HPV-positive tumors. The reason behind these findings is not clearly understood, but proposed theories include better response to radiation therapy in comparison with HPV-negative tumors, resulting in longer duration for developing radioresistant tumor cells and increased inflammatory response secondary to T-cell-mediated immunity causing decreased

specificity.[25] The high negative predictive value is valuable with patients who have a negative scan showing superior progression-free and overall survival.[26] A randomized controlled trial (PET-NECK trial) of 564 patients showed that 18F-FDG PET/CT surveillance after primary chemoradiation therapy in HNSCC patients with N2 or N3 disease was associated with a reduction in neck dissections, which results in fewer surgical complications and lower treatment cost (approximately US$2190). There was no significant difference in the results based on the HPV status of the tumors.[27]

Qualitative Treatment Response Assessment Criteria

In the recent past, there have been multiple proposed qualitative treatment response assessment criteria in HNC patients. These include the Neck Imaging Reporting and Data System (NI-RADS), Hopkins, Porceddu, and Deauville criteria.[28,29] All these criteria use a proposed scoring system or categorization based on the qualitative assessment of the metabolic activity at the site of the primary tumor or cervical lymph nodes and some criteria comparing this uptake to reference blood pool and liver metabolic activity to suggest the presence or absence of recurrent disease. An example of one of these treatment response criteria (Hopkins criteria) is presented in Table 1. This scoring system categorizes scores of 1, 2, and 3 as negative and scores of 4 and 5 as positive for residual disease. The authors reported a sensitivity, specificity, positive predictive value, negative predictive value, and diagnostic accuracy of 68%, 92%, 71%, 91%, and 87%, respectively. The high negative predictive value favors using such criteria for treatment response assessment to prevent unnecessary invasive evaluations. These categories were also able to predict survival in these patients.[30] Since introducing these criteria, there have been many validation studies and studies comparing the different criteria. In a prospective multicenter study (the ECLYPS study), Hopkins criteria for treatment response assessment in locally advanced HNSCC patients after primary chemoradiation indicated high negative predictive value (92%), specificity (91%), and accuracy (86%). The authors observed a time-dependent decrease in recurrent disease detection, with optimal performance approximately 12 weeks after completion of treatment.[31] A similar high negative predictive value for this criteria was seen in other clinical trials (NRG-HN002).[32] A recent study comparing the above-mentioned different qualitative assessment criteria concluded that all 4 treatment response

Table 1
Five-point qualitative posttreatment assessment scoring system (Hopkins criteria)

Score	^{18}F-FDG Uptake	Response Category
1	Less than IJV blood pool	Complete metabolic response
2	Focal uptake greater than IJV but less than liver	Likely complete metabolic response
3	Diffuse uptake greater than IJV or liver	Likely inflammation
4	Focal uptake greater than liver	Likely residual tumor
5	Focal and intense uptake	Residual tumor

Abbreviation: IJV, internal jugular vein.
Adapted from Marcus C, Ciarallo A, Tahari AK, et al. Head and Neck PET/CT: Therapy Response Interpretation Criteria (Hopkins Criteria)–Interreader Reliability, Accuracy, and Survival Outcomes. J Nucl Med [Internet]. 2014;55:1411–1416.

assessment criteria had similar diagnostic performance in detecting recurrent disease in a large (n = 562) study of HNSCC patients treated with chemoradiation or radiation therapy alone in the site of primary tumor and nodal disease. A significant difference in progression-free and overall survival was associated with all 4 criteria (P<.0001). The highest number of overall indeterminate scores was associated with NI-RADS, while the least was associated with Hopkins criteria, likely related to the more subjective nature of the NI-RADS criteria. Marginal improvement in negative predictive value was observed with Deauville and Porceddu criteria while keeping the number of indeterminate scores low[33] (**Fig. 3**).

OCCULT PRIMARY DETECTION

Metastatic cancer identified in cervical lymph nodes without a clinically evident primary head and neck tumor is a diagnostic dilemma requiring a streamlined evidence-based algorithm for optimal diagnosis and management of these patients. The workup of these patients often includes a comprehensive clinical evaluation, imaging, pan-endoscopy, tonsillectomy, etc, which improves the detection rate with improvement in the

prognosis of these patients.[34] The most common location of the unknown primary tumors is in the oropharynx, especially in the palatine tonsil, followed by the base of the tongue, nasopharynx, and hypopharynx. Identification of the occult primary tumor results in improved outcomes in these patients.[35] Applying ^{18}F-FDG PET/CT has the added advantage of detecting occult primary tumors with high diagnostic accuracy (89%). However, some studies report lower sensitivity likely due to inflammatory radiotracer uptake similar to that of common conditions like tonsillitis. Overall, studies report that ^{18}F-FDG PET/CT can detect primary tumors in approximately 40% of patients.[35–37] Using a simplified qualitative Likert scale of metabolic activity, sensitivity was 94% and specificity was 73% in detecting the primary tumor at a per-patient level. No significant difference was identified in comparison with diffusion-weighted MR imaging (DWI). The authors also found a significant difference in quantitative assessment (SUVmax) in detected primary tumor compared with unknown primary tumors (11.56 vs 6.43; P = .002). In quantitative assessment, ^{18}F-FDG PET/CT was superior to DWI.[38] Given that the most common location of these occult

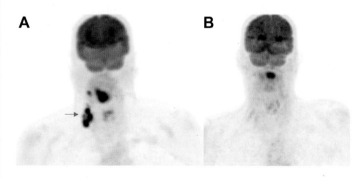

A   B

Fig. 3. Coronal MIP (*A*) of a staging ^{18}F-FDG PET/CT of a 70-year-old man with a newly diagnosed HPV-associated T2N1M0 squamous cell carcinoma of the right base of tongue demonstrates a hypermetabolic right tongue base mass (*yellow arrow*) and metastatic right cervical lymphadenopathy (*blue arrow*). Coronal MIP (*B*) of a re-staging ^{18}F-FDG PET/CT performed approximately 12 weeks after completion of concurrent chemoradiation demonstrates resolution of the previously noted areas of abnormal ^{18}F-FDG uptake, consistent with complete metabolic response (Hopkins score 1).

head and neck tumors is the palatine tonsil, careful evaluation of tonsillar metabolic activity is important. An SUVmax cutoff ratio of 1.5 between the bilateral tonsils resulted in 100% sensitivity and specificity in detecting cancers. The mean SUVmax of cancers of the tonsils was significantly higher than for the contralateral normal side and control patients (9.4 vs 2.5 vs 3.0; $P<.0001$).[39]

PET/CT also appears to assist in decreasing false-positive diagnoses. The most encountered locations of a second primary malignancy include esophagus, stomach, thyroid, lung, colon, and breast. A second primary malignancy diagnosis is associated with poor overall survival (HR = 3.07; P = .002) and progression-free survival (HR = 2.3; P = .016)[40] (Fig. 4).

SECOND PRIMARY MALIGNANCY DETECTION

In a prospective study of 248 patients with HNC, a second primary malignancy was detected in approximately 7% of patients.[40] A meta-analysis of 12 studies demonstrated a pooled sensitivity of 88% and pooled specificity of 95% for detection of distant metastases and second primary malignancies by ^{18}F-FDG PET/CT.[41] Physiologic metabolic activity in organs like the esophagus decreases the ability of ^{18}F-FDG PET/CT to detect a second primary malignancy, and hence, close attention while evaluating sites with normal background physiologic metabolic activity is crucial. Compared with a conventional workup, ^{18}F-FDG

DISEASE RECURRENCE DETECTION

Timely disease recurrence detection is of utmost priority in these patients and can have a significant impact on patient outcome and survival. The value of ^{18}F-FDG PET/CT in evaluating treatment response early during patient follow-up has been discussed above. Following treatment with primary radiation therapy, the positive (100%) and negative (100%) predictive values for detecting recurrent disease are high, especially 1 year after treatment. The corresponding values are slightly lower but still good 6 months after treatment (71%-100% and 93%-100%, respectively).[42] Compared with routine imaging, [18]F-

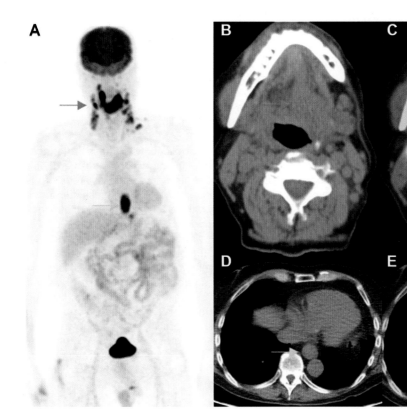

Fig. 4. Coronal MIP (A), axial CT (B, D), axial fused ^{18}F-FDG PET/CT (C, E) images of a 66-year-old male demonstrating hypermetabolic large left tongue base mass extending into the right base of the tongue with bilateral metastatic cervical lymphadenopathy (*blue arrows*), consistent with a p16 negative squamous cell carcinoma. He also had a synchronous second primary malignant mass of the distal thoracic esophagus (*yellow arrows*) with adjacent metastatic lymphadenopathy.

FDG PET/CT had diagnostic performance in identifying primary tumor recurrence similar to that of MR imaging and had superior performance in detecting nodal disease recurrence. Combining ^{18}F-FDG PET/CT and MR imaging offered the best overall locoregional disease recurrence detection rates.[43,44] In evaluating disease recurrence, among quantitative PET parameters, metabolic tumor volume (MTV) appears to provide the most prognostic information about disease progression and postradiation locoregional disease control.[45] ^{18}F-FDG PET/CT also appears to predict disease recurrence or progression in pretreatment evaluation, which can be valuable in treatment planning for these patients. A systematic review has shown that quantitative metabolic parameters—MTV and total lesion glycolysis (TLG)—could predict disease progression after primary surgical treatment.[46] In patients with suspected recurrent disease, ^{18}F-FDG PET/CT can detect distant disease in up to 30% of patients, with the most common site of distant disease being the lungs, followed by bone. In patients without extensive recurrent disease or distant metastases, those who had salvage surgical management had better survival than those who did not (22 months vs 6 months), showing that accurate detection of disease recurrence and appropriate management can improve outcome in these patients[47] (Fig. 5).

PROGNOSIS PREDICTION

It is well known that ^{18}F-FDG uptake in tumors and detection of metastatic disease can predict patient outcome and provide valuable information to appropriately tailor treatment for these patients to improve prognosis. Compared with conventional imaging techniques, ^{18}F-FDG PET/CT staging categorization of local, locally advanced, locoregional, and distant metastatic disease has been significantly associated with prognosis, especially disease-specific survival in patients with recurrent HNSCC.[48] Quantitative PET parameters have long been evaluated for prognosis prediction in many cancers including HNC. For example, MTV and TLG of the primary tumor and metastatic lymph nodes have been found to predict survival outcomes.[49] These parameters have also been shown to predict progressive disease in patients who underwent primary surgical management. This valuable information can help identify patients who may need additional treatment strategies to improve outcomes. These volumetric parameters have also been found to have outcome predictions superior to the most clinically estimated SUVmax in many studies.[46] In patients

with recurrent disease, a high SUVmax of the recurrent tumor (>8.7) has been shown to be a prognostic indicator of overall survival in patients with HNSCC.[50] Following primary surgical management, persistent FDG uptake was associated with unfavorable overall and disease-specific survival.[51] Tumor radiomics has been of special interest in PET/CT imaging of cancers recently. Tumor heterogeneity and texture analysis are some of the most studied entities. Studies have shown that texture analysis can predict treatment response in HNC patients undergoing primary chemoradiation.[52] Tumors that are less heterogeneous and have localized disease as indicated by focal increased FDG uptake, compared with more extensive and heterogeneous disease, are associated with better prognosis.[53,54]

ALTERNATIVE PET RADIOTRACERS IN HEAD AND NECK CANCERS

^{18}F-FDG PET/CT has been routinely incorporated in the indicated clinical evaluation of HNC patients as described above. Multiple other investigational PET radiotracers have not yet been used in the routine clinical evaluation of HNC patients. These radiotracers reflect different tumor characteristics than glucose uptake and metabolism evaluated with ^{18}F-FDG. Some of these include tumor hypoxia, amino acid metabolism, and tumor proliferation. The most studied are tumor hypoxia-specific radiotracers, especially ^{18}F-fluoromisonidazole, followed by ^{18}F-fluoroazomycinarabinoside, ^{18}F-flortanidazole, etc.[55–57] One of the most useful applications of these radiotracers is in treatment planning. Hypoxic cells are resistant to radiation and correlated to areas of disease recurrence.[58] Identifying these tumor foci noninvasively can help in optimally configuring radiation treatment delivery to these tumors, thereby improving treatment response and leading to better tumor control.[59,60] Following treatment, reoxygenation of these tumor cells shows decreased radiotracer uptake and can be useful in treatment response assessment.[61,62] High uptake of radiotracers is associated with poor prognosis and can help clinicians change treatment approaches to improve outcomes in these patients.[63,64] The advantage of amino acid transport-related radiotracer uptake in PET agents such as ^{11}C-methionine, radiolabeled tyrosine, and ^{11}C-choline appears to be uptake in tumor with minimal to no uptake in inflammatory cells and normal brain tissue, which can be extremely useful in differentiating disease recurrence from treatment-related inflammation and in certain HNCs such as nasopharyngeal or

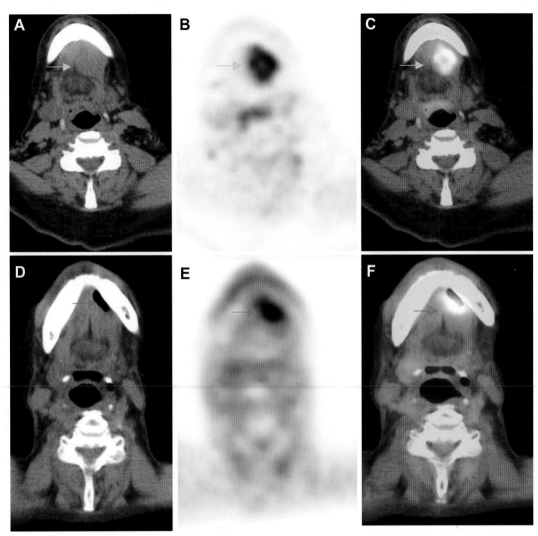

Fig. 5. Axial CT (*A*), axial PET (*B*), axial fused PET/CT (*C*) of a 77-year-old man who underwent a staging ¹⁸F-FDG PET/CT demonstrating a left floor of mouth mass (*yellow arrows*), consistent with a T3N0 HPV-associated squamous cell carcinoma (SUVmax 11.3). He underwent primary chemoradiation therapy. Axial CT (*D*), axial PET (*E*), axial fused PET/CT (*F*) of a follow-up ¹⁸F-FDG PET/CT performed approximately 1 year after initial treatment demonstrated an ulcerated hypermetabolic lesion (*blue arrows*) in the left floor of the mouth (SUVmax 6.1), which was biopsy-proven to be recurrent disease.

paranasal sinus tumors that may demonstrate intracranial extension, which can be challenging to evaluate on ¹⁸F-FDG PET/CT.[65–67] Radiotracers reflecting tumor proliferation, such as ¹⁸F-fluorothymidine, correlate with ¹⁸F-FDG uptake. Although these agents have not been found superior to ¹⁸F-FDG, they can be useful in special clinical situations such as monitoring treatment response following chemotherapeutic anti-VEGF monoclonal antibody agents (bevacizumab), predicting early treatment response preceding changes in ¹⁸F-FDG uptake, and planning optimal radiation treatment focusing on areas of high tumor proliferation.[68–71]

PET/MR IMAGING IN HEAD AND NECK CANCER

The recent introduction of hybrid positron emission tomography-magnetic resonance imaging (PET/MR imaging) combines the unique features of MR imaging, including higher soft tissue contrast, emerging pulse sequences (eg, diffusion-weighted imaging, dynamic contrast-enhanced MR), and multiplanar image acquisition, with the quantifiable functional and molecular information provided by PET.[72] Data on the clinical utility of hybrid ¹⁸F-FDG PET/MR imaging in oncology patients are rapidly emerging. In recent

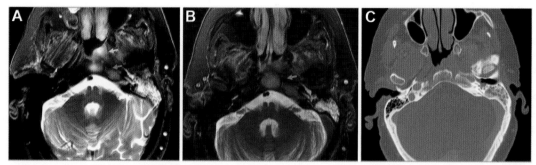

Fig. 6. Axial fused ¹⁸F-FDG PET/MR (*A*), axial T2-weighted MR (*B*), and axial CT (*C*) of a patient with nasopharyngeal cancer (*yellow arrow*) demonstrating MR signal change with associated increased metabolic activity (*blue arrows*) in the clivus and left petrous apex, concerning for tumor involvement. No osseous change is noted in the corresponding CT image.

years, a growing number of studies have evaluated the utility of hybrid ¹⁸F-FDG PET/MR imaging in patients with HNC and its potential added value in cancer staging and treatment planning.

A meta-analysis of 10 studies comprising 421 HNSCC patients showed that ¹⁸F-FDG PET/MR imaging has high sensitivity (91%) and moderate specificity (63%) in the diagnosis of HNCs.[73] The most promising application of ¹⁸F-FDG PET/MR imaging is in the staging workup of HNC.[74] Hybrid ¹⁸F-FDG PET/MR imaging has superior diagnostic accuracy in T-category staging[72,75–77] and at least comparable diagnostic accuracy for nodal (N) and metastatic (M) staging of HNC[74,77,78] compared with FDG-PET/CT or MR imaging. ¹⁸F-FDG PET/MR imaging has been more accurate in defining the tumor infiltration boundary (T4b status), depicting intracranial invasion, perineural infiltration, prevertebral or retropharyngeal invasion, muscular involvement (eg, mandibular/medial pterygoid muscle invasion), and bone/skull base invasion (eg, clivus)[75,79] (**Fig. 6**). Thus, contrast-enhanced PET/MR imaging can serve as a reliable modality for defining local resectability of HNC with excellent and comparable performance to contrast-enhanced PET/CT.[80] According to the eighth edition of the *AJCC Cancer Staging Manual* (2018), ¹⁸F-FDG PET/MR imaging has the potential to replace the combination of contrast-enhanced MR imaging and ¹⁸F-FDG PET/CT in TNM staging of oral cavity or oropharyngeal cancers.[72] A potential challenge of hybrid ¹⁸F-FDG PET/MR imaging is in evaluating lung metastases, mostly due to the impact of susceptibility and motion artifact on image quality. However, this can be overcome in the near future by implementing new MR imaging techniques such as high-resolution Dixon, breath-hold, or ultrashort echo-time sequences.

Preliminary data also suggest that hybrid ¹⁸F-FDG PET/MR imaging can improve accuracy of gross tumor volume (GTV) delineation in primary tumor and lymph nodes during radiation treatment

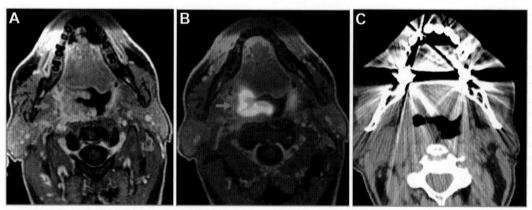

Fig. 7. Axial T1-weighted contrast-enhanced MR (*A*), axial fused ¹⁸F-FDG PET/MR (*B*), and axial CT (*C*) demonstrate superior soft tissue characterization of the extent of tumor in this patient with oropharyngeal squamous cell carcinoma (*blue arrows*). The delineation of the tumor on the corresponding CT image is extremely limited secondary to artifact from dental amalgam.

planning, due to higher soft tissue contrast[81] (Fig. 7). However, further studies on a larger patient population need to validate this result and establish a standardized technique for GTV delineation using PET/MR imaging.

Besides staging, multiparametric hybrid ^{18}F-FDG PET/MR imaging can improve therapeutic response assessment and predict clinical outcome/treatment failure in HNC patients following chemotherapy, radiotherapy, or surgery.[82–84] A recent study on 72 patients suggested that combined PET/MR imaging metabolo-volumetric parameters corrected by tumor cellularity (eg, MTV/ADC and TLG/ADC) are independent prognostic factors for predicting treatment failure in surgically resected HNC.[83] Another study suggested that a combination of pretreatment SUVmax and ADC can improve risk stratification of HNC patients; high SUVmax and ADC are associated with poor clinical outcomes.[85]

Despite the many potential advantages of hybrid ^{18}F-FDG PET/MR imaging, clinical adoption of this imaging technique is challenging based on scanner availability, reimbursement issues, lack of standardized technique/protocols, longer scan time, and limited radiological expertise in interpreting images from PET/MR imaging. In addition, there are still insufficient data on the comparative effectiveness and cost-utility of ^{18}F-FDG PET/MR imaging in HNC patients, and it is unclear whether routine use of PET/MR imaging can significantly improve patient outcomes and survival compared with PET/CT or MR imaging alone. These issues deserve further investigation.

SUMMARY

^{18}F-FDG PET/CT has been clinically useful in the evaluation, treatment, and follow-up of HNC patients for decades, with a significant impact on the management and outcome of these patients. PET/CT information can add value or be superior to routine anatomic imaging in special situations. Recent advances in treatment planning and response assessment have shown improve outcomes in these patients. Alternative PET tracers have not found routine clinical applications yet but can add important information like radioresistant tumor hypoxia that can contribute to optimal treatment planning. The introduction of clinical ^{18}F-FDG PET/MR imaging has provided the advantage of combining the superior soft tissue resolution of MR imaging with the metabolic information provided by ^{18}F-FDG PET.

CLINICS CARE POINTS

- In the staging of head and neck cancer, ^{18}F-FDG PET/CT is especially useful in detecting nodal and distant metastatic disease and should be considered prior to any surgical intervention.
- ^{18}F-FDG PET/CT may have limitations in the evaluation of small tumors. Soft-tissue extent delineation, evaluation of depth of invasion, perineural spread or marrow involvement.
- ^{18}F-FDG PET/CT guided radiation planning can provide additional information resulting in changes in treatment planning in up to 10% of the patients.
- ^{18}F-FDG PET/CT is useful for treatment response assessment and should be performed 3-6 months after treatment completion to reduce the rates of false positive results.
- ^{18}F-FDG PET/CT can provide prognostic information such as disease free survival, progression free survival, overall survival which can be valuable for treatment planning.
- ^{18}F-FDG PET/MR can be especially useful in the staging work-up providing superior accuracy in T-category staging with the superior soft tissue contrast.

REFERENCES

1. National Cancer Institute. Nation Cancer Institute: surveillance, epidemiology, and end results program [Internet]. Cancer Stat Facts. 2020. Available at: https://seer.cancer.gov/statfacts/. Accessed November 12, 2020.
2. Chegini S, Mitsimponas K, Shakib K. A review of recent advances in histopathological assessment of head and neck squamous cell carcinoma. J Oral Pathol Med 2020;49:9–13. Available at: https://onlinelibrary.wiley.com/doi/abs/10.1111/jop.12943.
3. Glastonbury CM. Head and neck squamous cell cancer: approach to staging and surveillance. 2020. p. 215–22. Available at: http://link.springer.com/10.1007/978-3-030-38490-6_17.
4. Glastonbury CM. Critical changes in the staging of head and neck cancer. Radiol Imaging Cancer 2020;2:e190022. Available at: http://pubs.rsna.org/doi/10.1148/rycan.2019190022.
5. Lee J, Emmett L, Tang R, et al. Prospective evaluation of the impact of <scp>human papilloma vi-

rus</scp> status and small node size on the diagnostic accuracy of <scp>18F</scp> -fluorodeoxyglucose <scp>positron emission tomography/computed tomography</scp> for primary head and neck squa. ANZ J Surg 2020;90:1396–401. Available at: https://onlinelibrary.wiley.com/doi/abs/10.1111/ans.16093.

6. Huang Y-H, Yeh C-H, Cheng N-M, et al. Cystic nodal metastasis in patients with oropharyngeal squamous cell carcinoma receiving chemoradiotherapy: relationship with human papillomavirus status and failure patterns. PLoS One 2017;12:e0180779. Available at: https://dx.plos.org/10.1371/journal.pone.0180779.

7. NCCN Clinical Practice Guidelines in Oncology (NCCN Guideline): Head and Neck Cancers. National Comprehensive Cancer Network. Version 1. 2020. Available at: www.nccn.org. Accessed November 12, 2020.

8. Ceylan Y, Ömür Ö, Hatipoğlu F. Contribution of 18F-FDG PET/CT to staging of head and neck malignancies. Mol Imaging Radionucl Ther 2018;27:19–24. Available at: http://cms.galenos.com.tr/Uploads/Article_16635/MIRT-27-1-En.pdf.

9. Chaput A, Robin P, Podeur F, et al. Diagnostic performance of 18 fluorodesoxyglucose positron emission/computed tomography and magnetic resonance imaging in detecting T1-T2 head and neck squamous cell carcinoma. Laryngoscope 2018;128:378–85. Available at: http://doi.wiley.com/10.1002/lary.26729.

10. Hong HR, Jin S, Koo HJ, et al. Clinical values of 18 F-FDG PET/CT in oral cavity cancer with dental artifacts on CT or MRI. J Surg Oncol 2014;110:696–701. Available at: http://doi.wiley.com/10.1002/jso.23691.

11. Lowe VJ, Duan F, Subramaniam RM, et al. Multicenter trial of [18 F]fluorodeoxyglucose positron emission tomography/computed tomography staging of head and neck cancer and negative predictive value and surgical impact in the N0 neck: results from ACRIN 6685. J Clin Oncol 2019;37:1704–12. Available at: http://ascopubs.org/doi/10.1200/JCO.18.01182.

12. Hollenbeak CS, Lowe VJ, Stack BC. The cost-effectiveness of fluorodeoxyglucose 18-F positron emission tomography in the N0 neck. Cancer 2001;92:2341–8. Available at: https://onlinelibrary.wiley.com/doi/10.1002/1097-0142(20011101)92:9%3C2341::AID-CNCR1581%3E3.0.CO;2-8.

13. Yongkui L, Jian L, Wanghan, et al. 18FDG-PET/CT for the detection of regional nodal metastasis in patients with primary head and neck cancer before treatment: a meta-analysis. Surg Oncol 2013;22:e11–6. Available at: https://linkinghub.elsevier.com/retrieve/pii/S0960740413000200.

14. Arora A, Husain N, Bansal A, et al. Development of a new outcome prediction model in early-stage squamous cell carcinoma of the oral cavity based on histopathologic parameters with multivariate analysis. Am J Surg Pathol 2017;41:950–60. Available at: http://journals.lww.com/00000478-201707000-00010.

15. Duprez F, Berwouts D, De Neve W, et al. Distant metastases in head and neck cancer. Head Neck 2017;39:1733–43. Available at: http://doi.wiley.com/10.1002/hed.24687.

16. Liu JC, Bhayani M, Kuchta K, et al. Patterns of distant metastasis in head and neck cancer at presentation: implications for initial evaluation. Oral Oncol 2019;88:131–6. Available at: https://linkinghub.elsevier.com/retrieve/pii/S1368837518304329.

17. Xu G, Li J, Zuo X, et al. Comparison of whole body positron emission tomography (PET)/PET-computed tomography and conventional anatomic imaging for detecting distant malignancies in patients with head and neck cancer: a meta-analysis. Laryngoscope 2012;122:1974–8. Available at: http://doi.wiley.com/10.1002/lary.23409.

18. Mazzola R, Alongi P, Ricchetti F, et al. 18F-Fluorodeoxyglucose-PET/CT in locally advanced head and neck cancer can influence the stage migration and nodal radiation treatment volumes. Radiol Med 2017;122:952–9. Available at: http://link.springer.com/10.1007/s11547-017-0804-0.

19. Pedraza S, Ruiz-Alonso A, Hernández-Martínez AC, et al. 18F-FDG PET/TC para la estadificación y la delineación del volumen de radioterapia en el cáncer de cabeza y cuello. Rev Esp Med Nucl Imagen Mol (Engl Ed) 2019;38:154–9. Available at: https://linkinghub.elsevier.com/retrieve/pii/S2253654X18300520.

20. van den Bosch S, Doornaert PAH, Dijkema T, et al. 18F-FDG-PET/CT-based treatment planning for definitive (chemo)radiotherapy in patients with head and neck squamous cell carcinoma improves regional control and survival. Radiother Oncol 2020;142:107–14. Available at: https://linkinghub.elsevier.com/retrieve/pii/S016781401933018X.

21. Berwouts D, Olteanu LAM, Speleers B, et al. Intensity modulated arc therapy implementation in a three phase adaptive 18F-FDG-PET voxel intensity-based planning strategy for head-and-neck cancer. Radiat Oncol 2016;11:52. Available at: http://ro-journal.biomedcentral.com/articles/10.1186/s13014-016-0629-3.

22. Morgan R, Chin B, Lanning R. Feasibility of rapid integrated radiation therapy planning with follow-up FDG PET/CT to improve overall treatment assessment in head and neck cancer. Am J Nucl Med Mol Imaging 2019;15:24–9. Available at: https://pubmed.ncbi.nlm.nih.gov/30911435/.

23. van den Bosch S, Dijkema T, Kunze-Busch MC, et al. Uniform FDG-PET guided GRAdient Dose prEscription

to reduce late Radiation Toxicity (UPGRADE-RT): study protocol for a randomized clinical trial with dose reduction to the elective neck in head and neck squamous cell carcinoma. BMC Cancer 2017;17:208. Available at: http://bmccancer.biomedcentral.com/articles/10. 1186/s12885-017-3195-7.

24. Sivarajah S, Isaac A, Cooper T, et al. Association of Fludeoxyglucose F 18–labeled positron emission tomography and computed tomography with the detection of oropharyngeal cancer recurrence. JAMA Otolaryngol Neck Surg 2018;144:1037. Available at: http://archotol.jamanetwork.com/article.aspx?doi=10.1001/jamaoto.2018.2143.

25. Helsen N, Van den Wyngaert T, Carp L, et al. FDG-PET/CT for treatment response assessment in head and neck squamous cell carcinoma: a systematic review and meta-analysis of diagnostic performance. Eur J Nucl Med Mol Imaging 2018;45: 1063–71. Available at: http://link.springer.com/10. 1007/s00259-018-3978-3.

26. Ghosh-Laskar S, Mummudi N, Rangarajan V, et al. Prognostic value of response assessment fluorodeoxyglucose positron emission tomography-computed tomography scan in radically treated squamous cell carcinoma of head and neck: long-term results of a prospective study. J Cancer Res Ther 2019;15:596. Available at: http://www.cancerjournal.net/text.asp?2019/15/3/596/244466.

27. Mehanna H, Wong W-L, McConkey CC, et al. PET-CT surveillance versus neck dissection in advanced head and neck cancer. N Engl J Med 2016;374: 1444–54. Available at: http://www.nejm.org/doi/10. 1056/NEJMoa1514493.

28. Hsu D, Chokshi FH, Hudgins PA, et al. Predictive value of first posttreatment imaging using standardized reporting in head and neck cancer. Otolaryngol Neck Surg 2019;161:978–85. Available at: http://journals.sagepub.com/doi/10.1177/0194599819865235.

29. Strauss SB, Aiken AH, Lantos JE, et al. Best practices for post-treatment surveillance imaging in head and neck cancer: application of the neck imaging reporting and data system (NI-RADS). Am J Roentgenol 2020;216(6):1438–51.

30. Marcus C, Ciarallo A, Tahari AK, et al. Head and neck PET/CT: therapy response interpretation criteria (Hopkins Criteria)–Interreader reliability, accuracy, and survival outcomes. J Nucl Med 2014;55: 1411–6. Available at: http://jnm.snmjournals.org/cgi/doi/10.2967/jnumed.113.136796.

31. Van den Wyngaert T, Helsen N, Carp L, et al. Fluorodeoxyglucose-positron emission tomography/computed tomography after concurrent chemoradiotherapy in locally advanced head-and-neck squamous cell cancer: the ECLYPS study. J Clin Oncol 2017;35:3458–64. Available at: https://ascopubs.org/doi/10.1200/JCO.2017.73.5845.

32. Subramaniam RM, Demora L, Yao M, et al. 18 FDG PET/CT prediction of treatment outcomes in patients with p16-positive, non-smoking associated, locoregionally advanced oropharyngeal cancer (LA-OPC) receiving deintensified therapy: results from NRG-HN002. J Clin Oncol 2020;38:6563. Available at: https://ascopubs.org/doi/10.1200/JCO.2020.38.15_suppl.6563.

33. Zhong J, Sundersingh M, Dyker K, et al. Post-treatment FDG PET-CT in head and neck carcinoma: comparative analysis of 4 qualitative interpretative criteria in a large patient cohort. Sci Rep 2020;10: 4086. Available at: http://www.nature.com/articles/s41598-020-60739-3.

34. Golusinski P, Di Maio P, Pehlivan B, et al. Evidence for the approach to the diagnostic evaluation of squamous cell carcinoma occult primary tumors of the head and neck. Oral Oncol 2019;88:145–52. Available at: https://linkinghub.elsevier.com/retrieve/pii/S1368837518304299.

35. Cheol Park G, Roh J-L, Cho K-J, et al. 18 F-FDG PET/CT vs . human papillomavirus, p16 and Epstein-Barr virus detection in cervical metastatic lymph nodes for identifying primary tumors. Int J Cancer 2017;140:1405–12. Available at: http://doi.wiley.com/10.1002/ijc.30550.

36. Chen Y-H, Yang X-M, Li S-S, et al. Value of fused positron emission tomography CT in detecting primaries in patients with primary unknown cervical lymph node metastasis. J Med Imaging Radiat Oncol 2012;56:66–74. Available at: http://doi.wiley.com/10.1111/j.1754-9485.2011.02331.x.

37. Wong WL, Sonoda LI, Gharpurhy A, et al. 18F-fluorodeoxyglucose Positron emission tomography/computed tomography in the assessment of occult primary head and neck cancers — An audit and review of published studies. Clin Oncol 2012;24: 190–5. Available at: https://linkinghub.elsevier.com/retrieve/pii/S0936655511009022.

38. Noij DP, Martens RM, Zwezerijnen B, et al. Diagnostic value of diffusion-weighted imaging and 18F-FDG-PET/CT for the detection of unknown primary head and neck cancer in patients presenting with cervical metastasis. Eur J Radiol 2018;107: 20–5. Available at: https://linkinghub.elsevier.com/retrieve/pii/S0720048X18302778.

39. Davison JM, Ozonoff A, Imsande HM, et al. Squamous cell carcinoma of the palatine tonsils: FDG standardized uptake value ratio as a biomarker to differentiate tonsillar carcinoma from physiologic uptake. Radiology 2010;255:578–85. Available at: http://pubs.rsna.org/doi/10.1148/radiol.10091479.

40. Ryu IS, Roh J-L, Kim JS, et al. Impact of 18F-FDG PET/CT staging on management and prognostic stratification in head and neck squamous cell carcinoma: a prospective observational study. Eur J Cancer 2016; 63:88–96. Available at: http://linkinghub.elsevier.com/retrieve/pii/S0959804916321244.

41. Xu G-Z, Guan D-J, He Z-Y. 18FDG-PET/CT for detecting distant metastases and second primary cancers in patients with head and neck cancer. A meta-analysis. Oral Oncol 2011;47:560–5. Available at: https://linkinghub.elsevier.com/retrieve/pii/S1368837511001618.

42. Risør LM, Loft A, Berthelsen AK, et al. FDG-PET/CT in the surveillance of head and neck cancer following radiotherapy. Eur Arch Otorhinolaryngol 2020;277:539–47. Available at: http://link.springer.com/10.1007/s00405-019-05684-2.

43. Kim ES, Yoon DY, Moon JY, et al. Detection of locoregional recurrence in malignant head and neck tumors: a comparison of CT, MRI, and FDG PET-CT. Acta Radiol 2019;60:186–95. Available at: http://journals.sagepub.com/doi/10.1177/0284185118776504.

44. Breik O, Kumar A, Birchall J, et al. Follow up imaging of oral, oropharyngeal and hypopharyngeal cancer patients: comparison of PET-CT and MRI post treatment. J Craniomaxillofac Surg 2020;48:672–9. Available at: https://linkinghub.elsevier.com/retrieve/pii/S1010518220301268.

45. Velez MA, Veruttipong D, Wang P-C, et al. FDG-PET metabolic tumor parameters for the reirradiation of recurrent head and neck cancer. Laryngoscope 2018;128:2345–50. Available at: http://doi.wiley.com/10.1002/lary.27173.

46. Creff G, Devillers A, Depeursinge A, et al. Evaluation of the prognostic value of FDG PET/CT parameters for patients with surgically treated head and neck cancer. JAMA Otolaryngol Neck Surg 2020;146:471. Available at: https://jamanetwork.com/journals/jamaotolaryngology/fullarticle/2763433.

47. Nøhr A, Gram SB, Charabi B, et al. PET/CT prior to salvage surgery in recurrent head and neck squamous cell carcinoma. Eur Arch Otorhinolaryngol 2019;276:2895–902. Available at: http://link.springer.com/10.1007/s00405-019-05550-1.

48. Rohde M, Nielsen AL, Pareek M, et al. PET/CT versus standard imaging for prediction of survival in patients with recurrent head and neck squamous cell carcinoma. J Nucl Med 2019;60:592–9. Available at: http://jnm.snmjournals.org/lookup/doi/10.2967/jnumed.118.217976.

49. Castelli J, Depeursinge A, Devillers A, et al. PET-based prognostic survival model after radiotherapy for head and neck cancer. Eur J Nucl Med Mol Imaging 2019;46:638–49. Available at: http://link.springer.com/10.1007/s00259-018-4134-9.

50. Ha SC, Roh J-L, Kim JS, et al. Clinical utility of 18 F-FDG PET/CT for patients with recurrent head and neck squamous cell carcinoma. Acta Otolaryngol 2019;139:810–5. Available at: https://www.tandfonline.com/doi/full/10.1080/00016489.2019.1632483.

51. Jung AR, Roh J-L, Kim JS, et al. Post-treatment 18F-FDG PET/CT for predicting survival and recurrence in patients with advanced-stage head and neck cancer undergoing curative surgery. Oral Oncol 2020;107:104750. Available at: https://linkinghub.elsevier.com/retrieve/pii/S136883752030186X.

52. Feliciani G, Fioroni F, Grassi E, et al. Radiomic profiling of head and neck cancer: 18 F-FDG PET texture analysis as predictor of patient survival. Contrast Media Mol Imaging 2018;2018:1–8. Available at: https://www.hindawi.com/journals/cmmi/2018/3574310/.

53. Bogowicz M, Riesterer O, Stark LS, et al. Comparison of PET and CT radiomics for prediction of local tumor control in head and neck squamous cell carcinoma. Acta Oncol (Madr) 2017;56:1531–6. Available at: https://www.tandfonline.com/doi/full/10.1080/0284186X.2017.1346382.

54. Choi J, Gim J-A, Oh C, et al. Association of metabolic and genetic heterogeneity in head and neck squamous cell carcinoma with prognostic implications: integration of FDG PET and genomic analysis. EJNMMI Res 2019;9:97. Available at: https://ejnmmires.springeropen.com/articles/10.1186/s13550-019-0563-0.

55. Sato J, Kitagawa Y, Watanabe S, et al. 18 F-Fluoromisonidazole positron emission tomography (FMISO-PET) may reflect hypoxia and cell proliferation activity in oral squamous cell carcinoma. Oral Surg Oral Med Oral Pathol Oral Radiol 2017;124:261–70. Available at: https://linkinghub.elsevier.com/retrieve/pii/S221244031730826X.

56. Wack LJ, Mönnich D, van Elmpt W, et al. Comparison of [18F]-FMISO, [18F]-FAZA and [18F]-HX4 for PET imaging of hypoxia – a simulation study. Acta Oncol (Madr) 2015;54:1370–7. Available at: http://www.tandfonline.com/doi/full/10.3109/0284186X.2015.1067721.

57. Chen L, Zhang Z, Kolb HC, et al. 18F-HX4 hypoxia imaging with PET/CT in head and neck cancer. Nucl Med Commun 2012;33:1096–102. Available at: http://content.wkhealth.com/linkback/openurl?sid=WKPTLP:landingpage&an=00006231-201210000-00015.

58. Boeke S, Thorwarth D, Mönnich D, et al. Geometric analysis of loco-regional recurrences in relation to pre-treatment hypoxia in patients with head and neck cancer. Acta Oncol (Madr) 2017;56:1571–6. Available at: https://www.tandfonline.com/doi/full/10.1080/0284186X.2017.1372626.

59. Lin Z, Mechalakos J, Nehmeh S, et al. The influence of changes in tumor hypoxia on dose-painting treatment plans based on 18F-FMISO positron emission tomography. Int J Radiat Oncol 2008;70:1219–28. Available at: https://linkinghub.elsevier.com/retrieve/pii/S0360301607043684.

60. Chang JH, Wada M, Anderson NJ, et al. Hypoxia-targeted radiotherapy dose painting for head and neck cancer using 18 F-FMISO PET: a biological modeling study. Acta Oncol (Madr) 2013;52:1723–9. Available at: http://www.tandfonline.com/doi/full/10.3109/0284186X.2012.759273.

61. Koh W-J, Rasey JS, Evans ML, et al. Imaging of hypoxia in human tumors with [F-18]fluoromisonidazole. Int J Radiat Oncol 1992;22: 199–212. Available at: https://linkinghub.elsevier.com/retrieve/pii/0360301692910014.

62. Yeh S-H, Liu R-S, Wu L-C, et al. Fluorine-18 fluoromisonidazole tumour to muscle retention ratio for the detection of hypoxia in nasopharyngeal carcinoma. Eur J Nucl Med 1996;23:1378–83. Available at: http://link.springer.com/10.1007/BF01367595.

63. Kikuchi M, Yamane T, Shinohara S, et al. 18F-fluoromisonidazole positron emission tomography before treatment is a predictor of radiotherapy outcome and survival prognosis in patients with head and neck squamous cell carcinoma. Ann Nucl Med 2011;25:625–33. Available at: http://link.springer.com/10.1007/s12149-011-0508-9.

64. Sato J, Kitagawa Y, Watanabe S, et al. Hypoxic volume evaluated by 18 F-fluoromisonidazole positron emission tomography (FMISO-PET) may be a prognostic factor in patients with oral squamous cell carcinoma: preliminary analyses. Int J Oral Maxillofac Surg 2018; 47:553–60. Available at: https://linkinghub.elsevier.com/retrieve/pii/S090150271731617X.

65. Lindholm P, Leskinen S, Lapela M. Carbon-11-methionine uptake in squamous cell head and neck cancer. J Nucl Med 1998;39:1393–7.

66. de Boer JR, van der Laan BF, Pruim J, et al. Carbon-11 tyrosine PET for visualization and protein synthesis rate assessment of laryngeal and hypopharyngeal carcinomas. Eur J Nucl Med Mol Imaging 2002;29: 1182–7. Available at: http://link.springer.com/10.1007/s00259-002-0863-9.

67. Khan N, Oriuchi N, Ninomiya H, et al. Positron emission tomographic imaging with11C-choline in differential diagnosis of head and neck tumors: comparison with18F-FDG PET. Ann Nucl Med 2004;18: 409–17. Available at: http://link.springer.com/10.1007/BF02984484.

68. Nyflot MJ, Kruser TJ, Traynor AM, et al. Phase 1 trial of bevacizumab with concurrent chemoradiation therapy for squamous cell carcinoma of the head and neck with exploratory functional imaging of tumor hypoxia, proliferation, and perfusion. Int J Radiat Oncol 2015;91: 942–51. Available at: https://linkinghub.elsevier.com/retrieve/pii/S0360301614044381.

69. Hoshikawa H, Mori T, Kishino T, et al. Changes in 18F-fluorothymidine and 18F-fluorodeoxyglucose positron emission tomography imaging in patients with head and neck cancer treated with chemoradiotherapy. Ann Nucl Med 2013;27:363–70. Available at: http://link.springer.com/10.1007/s12149-013-0694-8.

70. Kishino T, Hoshikawa H, Nishiyama Y, et al. Usefulness of 3'-Deoxy-3'-18F-Fluorothymidine PET for predicting early response to chemoradiotherapy in head and neck cancer. J Nucl Med 2012;53:1521–7.

Available at: http://jnm.snmjournals.org/cgi/doi/10.2967/jnumed.111.099200.

71. Baxa J, Ferda J, Ferdova E, et al. Hybrid imaging PET/CT with application of 18 F-Fluorothymidine in patients with head and neck carcinoma undergoing radiotherapy. Anticancer Res 2018;38:4153–7. Available at: http://ar.iiarjournals.org/lookup/doi/10.21873/anticanres.12708.

72. Tsujikawa T, Narita N, Kanno M, et al. Role of PET/MRI in oral cavity and oropharyngeal cancers based on the 8th edition of the AJCC cancer staging system: a pictorial essay. Ann Nucl Med 2018;32: 239–49. Available at: http://link.springer.com/10.1007/s12149-018-1244-1.

73. Xiao Y, Chen Y, Shi Y, et al. The value of fluorine-18 fluorodeoxyglucose PET/MRI in the diagnosis of head and neck carcinoma. Nucl Med Commun 2015;36:312–8. Available at: http://content.wkhealth.com/linkback/openurl?sid=WKPTLP:landingpage&an=00006231-201504000-00002.

74. Sekine T, de Galiza Barbosa F, Kuhn FP, et al. PET+MR versus PET/CT in the initial staging of head and neck cancer, using a trimodality PET/CT+MR system. Clin Imaging 2017;42:232–9. Available at: https://linkinghub.elsevier.com/retrieve/pii/S0899707117300037.

75. Chan S-C, Yeh C-H, Yen T-C, et al. Clinical utility of simultaneous whole-body 18F-FDG PET/MRI as a single-step imaging modality in the staging of primary nasopharyngeal carcinoma. Eur J Nucl Med Mol Imaging 2018;45:1297–308. Available at: http://link.springer.com/10.1007/s00259-018-3986-3.

76. Samolyk-Kogaczewska N, Sierko E, Dziemianczyk-Pakiela D, et al. Usefulness of Hybrid PET/MRI in Clinical Evaluation of Head and Neck Cancer Patients. Cancers (Basel) 2020;12:511. Available at: https://www.mdpi.com/2072-6694/12/2/511.

77. Schaarschmidt BM, Heusch P, Buchbender C, et al. Locoregional tumour evaluation of squamous cell carcinoma in the head and neck area: a comparison between MRI, PET/CT and integrated PET/MRI. Eur J Nucl Med Mol Imaging 2016;43:92–102. Available at: http://link.springer.com/10.1007/s00259-015-3145-z.

78. Platzek I, Beuthien-Baumann B, Schneider M, et al. FDG PET/MR for lymph node staging in head and neck cancer. Eur J Radiol 2014;83:1163–8. Available at: https://linkinghub.elsevier.com/retrieve/pii/S0720048X14001612.

79. Hayashi K, Kikuchi M, Imai Y, et al. Clinical value of fused PET/MRI for surgical planning in patients with oral/oropharyngeal carcinoma. Laryngoscope 2020; 130:367–74. Available at: https://onlinelibrary.wiley.com/doi/abs/10.1002/lary.27911.

80. Sekine T, Barbosa F de G, Delso G, et al. Local resectability assessment of head and neck cancer: positron emission tomography/MRI versus positron emission tomography/CT. Head Neck 2017;39:

1550–8. Available at: http://doi.wiley.com/10.1002/hed.24783.

81. Samołyk-Kogaczewska N, Sierko E, Zuzda K, et al. PET/MRI-guided GTV delineation during radiotherapy planning in patients with squamous cell carcinoma of the tongue. Strahlenther Onkol 2019; 195:780–91. Available at: http://link.springer.com/10.1007/s00066-019-01480-3.

82. Romeo V, Iorio B, Mesolella M, et al. Simultaneous PET/MRI in assessing the response to chemo/radiotherapy in head and neck carcinoma: initial experience. Med Oncol 2018;35:112. Available at: http://link.springer.com/10.1007/s12032-018-1170-z.

83. Kim Y, Cheon GJ, Kang SY, et al. Prognostic value of simultaneous 18F-FDG PET/MRI using a combination of metabolo-volumetric parameters and apparent diffusion coefficient in treated head and neck cancer. EJNMMI Res 2018;8:2. Available at: https://ejnmmires.springeropen.com/articles/10.1186/s13550-018-0357-9.

84. Becker M, Varoquaux AD, Combescure C, et al. Local recurrence of squamous cell carcinoma of the head and neck after radio(chemo)therapy: diagnostic performance of FDG-PET/MRI with diffusion-weighted sequences. Eur Radiol 2018;28:651–63. Available at: http://link.springer.com/10.1007/s00330-017-4999-1.

85. Preda L, Conte G, Bonello L, et al. Combining standardized uptake value of FDG-PET and apparent diffusion coefficient of DW-MRI improves risk stratification in head and neck squamous cell carcinoma. Eur Radiol 2016;26:4432–41. Available at: http://link.springer.com/10.1007/s00330-016-4284-8.

PET Imaging of Neuroendocrine Tumors

Samuel J. Galgano, MD[a,b,*], Benjamin Wei, MD[b,c], J. Bart Rose, MD[b,d]

KEYWORDS

- Neuroendocrine tumors • SSTR-PET • DOTATATE • Carcinoid
- Peptide receptor radionuclide therapy

KEY POINTS

- SSTR-PET has significantly improved staging of NETs compared to historical radiotracers.
- Knowledge of NET pathology is essential for selection of appropriate PET radiotracer.
- PET imaging with both SSTR-PET tracers and FDG may play a significant role in guiding treatment decisions for patients with moderately or poorly differentiated NETs.

INTRODUCTION

Neuroendocrine tumors (NETs) consist of a wide array of lesions arising from multiple organs throughout the body with an estimated 12,000 people diagnosed in the United States each year and approximately 170,000 people alive with a known diagnosis of NET.[1] These tumors arise from cells in both the endocrine and nervous systems and can demonstrate varying levels of hormone secretion, which may elicit symptoms that prompt their discovery. Most commonly, NETs arise from the bowel, pancreas, and lung but can be found in multiple additional organs. Typically, these are first discovered through a combination of anatomic imaging with either computed tomography (CT) or MR imaging and endoscopy with or without endoscopic ultrasound (EUS). Once diagnosed, accurate staging and tumor grading is needed to determine the optimal treatment algorithm for these patients, as they can range from slow-growing and indolent to highly aggressive with a propensity to metastasize.

Traditionally, molecular imaging has played a large role in the noninvasive diagnosis of NETs through the use of [111In]pentetreotide scintigraphy with planar gamma camera imaging and single positron emission computed tomography (SPECT), as this radiotracer targets somatostatin receptors (SSTRs) that are overexpressed on NETs in varying degrees. In 2016, the United States Food and Drug Administration (FDA) approved [68Ga]DOTATATE as a PET radiotracer for PET imaging of NETs, with improved performance of this agent over planar and SPECT somatostatin receptor scintigraphy.[2,3] In addition, in 2018, the United States FDA approved a targeted systemic therapy ([177Lu]DOTATATE) to somatostatin-receptor-expressing gastroenteropancreatic NETs, using a theranostic approach where patients are first imaged with [68Ga]DOTATATE to noninvasively determine SSTR expression and subsequently treat with a therapeutic radioisotope targeting the exact same receptor used in PET imaging. These advances have led to substantial increases in PET imaging utilization for NETs, and thus, knowledge of strengths and weaknesses of PET imaging of NETs is essential to both the general radiologist and subspecialty

[a] Department of Radiology, University of Alabama at Birmingham, Birmingham, AL, USA; [b] O'Neal Comprehensive Cancer Center, University of Alabama at Birmingham, Birmingham, AL, USA; [c] Division of Cardiothoracic Surgery, Department of Surgery, University of Alabama at Birmingham, 703 19th St South, Zeigler Research Building 707, Birmingham, AL 35249, USA; [d] Division of Surgical Oncology, Department of Surgery, University of Alabama at Birmingham, 1808 7th Avenue South, Boshell Diabetes Building 605, Birmingham, AL 35249, USA

* Corresponding author. Department of Radiology, University of Alabama at Birmingham, 619 19th Street South, JT N325, Birmingham, AL 35249.

E-mail address: samuelgalgano@uabmc.edu

Radiol Clin N Am 59 (2021) 789–799
https://doi.org/10.1016/j.rcl.2021.05.006

radiologist. The focus of this article is current and future applications of PET in several of the most common NETs, current PET radiotracers available for NET imaging, and pathologic considerations in molecular imaging of NETs.

TUMOR GRADING AND IMPACT OF TUMOR PATHOLOGY ON PET IMAGING

As stated previously, NETs are a heterogeneous group of tumors with varying degrees of aggressiveness and differentiation. In 2017, the World Health Organization (WHO) revised the pathologic classification of pancreatic NETs (PNETs) which was further adapted to NETs of other origin in 2019.[4] NETs, or neuroendocrine neoplasms (NENs), are classified on the basis of differentiation, tumor grade, mitotic rate, and Ki-67 index. NENs are then categorized into NETs grades 1 to 3, neuroendocrine carcinoma (small-cell and large-cell variants), and mixed neuroendocrine–non-neuroendocrine neoplasms (MiNENs) with pathologic criteria outlined in **Table 1**. Most MiNENs are mixed adenoneuroendorine carcinomas, with pathologic features of both tumors, and can occur at any primary site that both neuroendocrine and adenocarcinoma can arise.[5] Many NETs that are initially diagnosed on EUS may be diagnosed by fine-needle aspiration, which may limit pathologic classification or cause inaccurate tumor grading.[6] Thus, EUS-guided fine-needle core biopsies are preferable, providing important additional information to the cytologic evaluation and improving diagnostic sensitivity.[7] Accurate pathologic characterization of NETs is an essential topic for guiding molecular imaging, as tumor grade can have a significant impact on choice of radiotracers. Well-differentiated NETs are more likely to maintain expression of SSTRs and are best imaged with PET SSTR ligands while poorly differentiated NECs are more likely to not express SSTRs but instead are best imaged with 2-deoxy-2-[^{18}F]fluoro-D-glucose (FDG) PET because of their high mitotic count and increased glucose utilization.[8] Thus, a collaborative multidisciplinary approach between several departments should be taken to optimize diagnosis, imaging, and management of patients with NETs.

PET RADIOTRACERS, BIODISTRIBUTION, AND IMAGING PROTOCOLS

Historically, molecular imaging has long played a role in the imaging of NETs. The earliest imaging agent, [^{111}In]pentetreotide, targeted SSTRs at the surface of the cell, mainly subtypes SSTR2 and SSTR5.[9] These SSTRs (predominantly SSTR2) are overexpressed on the surface of NET cells and are preferentially imagined through this mechanism. [^{111}In]Pentetreotide imaging involved a combination of planar, SPECT, and SPECT/CT imaging to accurately diagnose and localize NETs. Building on this same principle, several PET radiotracers have been developed for improving imaging of NETs (**Table 2**) because of their improved spatial resolution and signal-to-noise ratio when compared with SPECT imaging agents. Notably, all DOTA-peptide radiotracers demonstrate a higher affinity for SSTR2 than [^{111}In]pentetreotide, which improved detection and accurate characterization of lesions.[10] Knowledge of normal radiotracer biodistribution is important to avoid interpretation errors. For [^{68}Ga]DOTATATE and similar SSTR ligands, the spleen demonstrates

---

Table 1
WHO 2019 classification of neuroendocrine neoplasms

Terminology	Differentiation	Grade	Mitotic rate (mitoses/2 mm²)	Ki-67 Index
Neuroendocrine tumor				
Grade 1 (G1)	Well	Low	<2	<3%
Grade 2 (G2)	Well	Intermediate	2–20	3%–20%
Grade 3 (G3)	Well	High	>20	>20%
Neuroendocrine carcinoma				
Small cell	Poor	High	>20	>20%
Large cell	Poor	High	>20	>20%
MiNEN	Variable (usually poor)	Variable	Variable	Variable

Abbreviations: MiNEN, mixed neuroendocrine–non-neuroendocrine neoplasms; WHO, World Health Organization.

Table 2
Radiotracers in development or clinical use for NET imaging

Name	SSTR affinity	Half-life	Production	Approval status
[68Ga]DOTATATE	SSTR2	68 min	Ga/Ge generator	Yes (2016)
[68Ga]DOTATOC	SSTR2, SSTR5	68 min	Ga/Ge generator	Yes (2019)
[68Ga]DOTANOC	SSTR2, SSTR5>SSTR3	68 min	Ga/Ge generator	No
[64Cu]DOTATATE	SSTR2	12.7 h	Cyclotron	Yes (2020)

Abbreviations: NET, neuroendocrine tumors; SSTR, somatostatin receptor.

the highest level of radiotracer activity, followed by the adrenal glands, pituitary, kidneys, and liver (Fig. 1). Less activity is noted in the salivary and thyroid glands with variable amounts of activity noted in the bowel.

Currently, SSTR-PET/CT and PET/MR imaging are used for several clinical scenarios including localization of NET of unknown primary, staging of patients with known NET, follow-up for patients with NET to evaluate response to treatment and/or progression, and for noninvasive determination of SSTR expression and potential treatment with peptide receptor radionuclide therapy (PRRT). Unlike [18F]FDG-PET/CT, there is no need for patients to fast before SSTR-PET/CT, as blood sugar levels do not alter tracer distribution. Many patients with known diagnoses of NETs are frequently on long-acting somatostatin analogs to treat their symptoms, and there is a theoretic potential for these nonradiolabelled analogs to interfere with and decrease sensitivity of SSTR-PET. Thus, some advocate for timing the SSTR-PET scan just before the next scheduled injection. However, a recent prospective study found that lanreotide had a minimal effect on DOTATATE uptake in tumors and should not influence timing of the PET scan.[11] Adult patients are typically administered an intravenous dose of DOTATATE between 2.7 and 5.4 mCi (100–200 MBq), and the typical uptake period is approximately 60 minutes.[12] Patients are encouraged to void before scanning to minimize radiation dose to the urinary bladder and decrease activity in the pelvis. Once on the PET scanner, patients are scanned typically from skull base to mid-thigh using 3- to 5-minute PET bed positions.

GASTROENTEROPANCREATIC NEUROENDOCRINE TUMORS

Gastroenteropancreatic neuroendocrine tumors (GEP-NETs) are the most common type of NET and account for approximately 70% of NETs, with an estimated incidence of 3.56 per 100,000 and accounting for 2% of all primary gastrointestinal and pancreatic neoplasms.[1,13] Most GEP-NETs occur sporadically, but these tumors are associated with multiple genetic syndromes, including multiple endocrine neoplasia type 1 (MEN-1), neurofibromatosis type 1, Von Hippel-Lindau disease, and tuberous sclerosis. The gastrointestinal tract is the most common site of NET origin, accounting for 67% of cases.[14] Once thought to be a rare tumor, PNETs are being

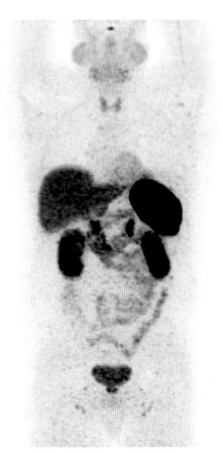

Fig. 1. Maximum-intensity projection PET image of the normal biodistribution of [68Ga]DOTATATE.

diagnosed more frequently in the past several decades, likely due to an increase in medical imaging, as many of these tumors (70%–90%) are hormonally nonfunctional and are discovered incidentally.[15] Owing to the lack of symptoms, a significant number of GEP-NETs are diagnosed late and are at an advanced stage at presentation. Functional NETs tend to present earlier, and symptoms can differ depending on tumor type, with insulinomas and gastrinomas being most common.[16] Carcinoid syndrome is classically associated with small bowel NETs but occurs in the minority of patients with nonmetastatic small bowel NETs (6%–30%) and the presence significantly increasing in the setting of hepatic metastases (95% of cases).[17] While the initial diagnosis of GEP-NET often is made on conventional imaging with CT and MR imaging, molecular imaging has long played a role in the accurate diagnosis and staging of these patients with [68Ga]DOTATATE PET/CT offering significant improvement over [111In]pentetreotide scintigraphy.

Several studies and meta-analyses have directly compared the performance of [68Ga]DOTATATE PET/CT and [111In]pentetreotide scintigraphy. An early study evaluating the use of [68Ga]DOTATATE PET/CT in patients with known NETs (predominantly GEP-NETs) found that [68Ga]DOTATATE PET/CT identified significantly more lesions than [111In]pentetreotide scintigraphy and changed management of 36/51 patients (70.6%).[18] In a study by Deppen and colleagues, [68Ga]DOTATATE PET/CT performed equally or superior to [111In]pentetreotide scintigraphy in all patients (n = 78) with a sensitivity and specificity of 96% and 93%, respectively, for [68Ga]DOTATATE PET/CT compared with 72% and 93%, respectively, for [111In]pentetreotide scintigraphy.[3] In addition, this study found that [68Ga]DOTATATE PET/CT correctly identified 3 patients for potential PRRT that were inaccurately classified by [111In] pentetreotide.[3] This same study also examined safety of the [68Ga]DOTATATE radiotracer and found no instances of a trial-related event requiring treatment.[3] A separate prospective study evaluating the use of [68Ga]DOTATATE PET/CT, [111In] pentetreotide SPECT/CT, multiphasic CT, and/or MR imaging for detection of unknown primary and metastatic GEP-NETs found that [68Ga]DOTATATE PET/CT detected 95.1% of lesions, compared with anatomic imaging detecting 45.3%, and [111In]pentetreotide SPECT/CT detecting 30.9% of lesions.[19] A 2016 meta-analysis of the literature estimated a sensitivity of 90.9% and specificity of 90.6% for [68Ga]DOTATATE PET/CT for the diagnosis and staging of NETs (Fig. 2).[2] As a result of this superior

performance, both the North American Neuroendocrine Tumor Society (NANETS) and National Comprehensive Cancer Network (NCCN) include [68Ga]DOTATATE PET/CT as a recommendation for staging patients with newly diagnosed GEP-NET (Fig. 3).[20,21]

GEP-NETs (particularly PNETs) are a heterogeneous group of tumors with varying degrees of differentiation and proliferation. As outlined previously, the WHO 2019 classification subdivides PNETs into three grades (G1-3) for well-differentiated lesions based on the Ki-67 index and characterizes poorly differentiated tumors separately.[4] As a result, these tumors demonstrate varying degrees of SSTR expression on the cell surface, which impacts their imaging with molecular radiotracers. For low-grade well-differentiated NETs (G1 tumors), SSTR expression is maintained, and these lesions are best imaged with PET SSTR ligands. However, as the proliferative index increases in G2 and G3 tumors, the need for non–SSTR-based PET imaging increases. For these more aggressive lesions, consideration should be given to imaging with [18F]FDG PET/CT, as the increased cellular glucose metabolism often results in a disease that is FDG-avid that may no longer express SSTRs and be DOTATATE negative. Prior research comparing [18F]FDG PET/CT to [111In]pentetreotide scintigraphy found that tumor differentiation was important in guiding molecular imaging, with [111In]pentetreotide scintigraphy more sensitive for detection of well-differentiated NETs and [18F]FDG PET/CT more sensitive for detection of poorly differentiated NETs.[22] Additional studies comparing the impact of [18F]FDG PET/CT and [68Ga]DOTATATE PET/CT have found that [18F]FDG PET/CT has no clinical impact on G1 NETs and moderate impact on G2 NETs, while [18F]FDG PET/CT played a significant role in poorly differentiated NETs.[23] In the study by Panagiotidis and colleagues, the maximum standardized uptake value (SUV_{max}) on [68Ga]DOTATATE PET/CT was higher for G1 tumors and lower for G3 tumors.[23] Thus, this research emphasizes the need for a multidisciplinary approach with knowledge of NET pathology to guide appropriate imaging for NETs.

Surgical resection of GEP-NETs can be complex and often involves multiple sites of disease. Resection of primary tumors and oligometastatic disease has been shown to confer both a palliative and survival benefit.[24,25] Accurate staging is therefore paramount to preoperative planning, especially when 13% of NETs were historically diagnosed with an unknown primary site.[26] As mentioned previously, [68Ga]DOTATATE PET/CT has shown improvement over prior imaging

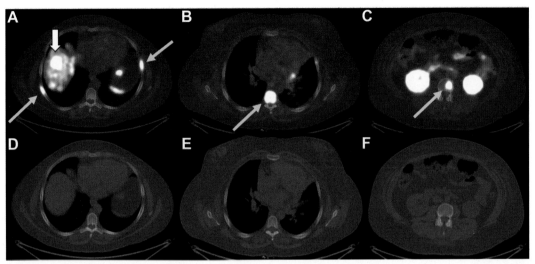

Fig. 2. Fused [68Ga]DOTATATE-PET/CT (*A–C*) and CT (*D–F*) images of a patient with metastatic gastroenteropancreatic neuroendocrine tumor to the liver (*white arrow*) and multiple bones (*green arrows*). Osseous metastases are not visible on CT images even in retrospect.

modalities by identifying a previously unknown primary site 60% of the time.[27] In a meta-analysis of 14 studies that included 1561 patients, this improved detection rate changed management 44% of the time with 77% of these changes involving a switch in treatment modality.[28] Furthermore, when considering noncurative cytoreduction of hepatic metastases, knowing the receptor status of tumors may help in planning resection as early evidence suggests debulking may improve response to subsequent PRRT.[29] If the receptor status is heterogeneous, then the surgeon may focus on noncurative resection of less DOTATATE-PET avid lesions and leave disease that is potentially targetable.

THORACIC NEUROENDOCRINE TUMORS

Lung carcinoid tumors account for approximately 1% to 2% of all lung cancers, with approximately 2000 to 4500 newly diagnosed cases in the United States each year.[30] Thymic carcinoid tumors (also referred to as NETs of the thymus) are rare tumors, accounting for only 2% to 5% of thymic tumors and 0.4% of all carcinoid tumors, with an estimated incidence of 0.2 per million in the United States.[31,32] Carcinoid tumors of the lung are most commonly well-differentiated NETs with indolent behavior that may be detected incidentally or present with symptoms of cough, hemoptysis, or pneumonia.[33] Most lung carcinoid tumors are spontaneous, whereas thymic NETs are associated with the genetic syndrome MEN-1. Unlike lung carcinoid tumors, thymic carcinoid tumors can range from asymptomatic and indolent

to highly aggressive and symptomatic, either due to local mass effect and invasion of the tumor or due to hormonal secretion of adrenocorticotropic hormone by the tumor.[33,34] Unlike GEP-NETs, carcinoid syndrome is an uncommon clinical presentation for thoracic NETs. In addition, owing to the more aggressive behavior of thymic NETs, up to 30% of patients present with advanced-stage disease which is much higher than lung carcinoid tumors.

Lung carcinoid tumors express SSTRs similarly to GEP-NETs and have historically been evaluated with molecular imaging using [111In]pentetreotide, [18F]FDG, and most recently [68Ga]DOTATATE. Often, before a histologic confirmation of the diagnosis, many lung carcinoid tumors are detected incidentally as a solitary pulmonary nodule and undergo PET imaging with [18F]FDG to evaluate for potential lung cancer. Unlike primary lung cancers, lung carcinoids tend to be more well-circumscribed and round on CT, as opposed to the spiculations seen with primary lung cancers. Although many well-differentiated lung carcinoids will not demonstrate increased FDG uptake, a more aggressive subset of these represent atypical carcinoids and may demonstrate significant FDG uptake similar to other lung malignancies.[35–37] Similar to GEP-NETs, thoracic NETs that demonstrate significant FDG uptake are associated with a more aggressive histology, clinical course, and decreased survival (**Fig. 4**).[38] More recently, [68Ga]DOTATATE has replaced [111In]pentetreotide for imaging well-differentiated (typical) lung carcinoid tumors.[2] However, [18F] FDG outperforms [68Ga]DOTATATE for atypical

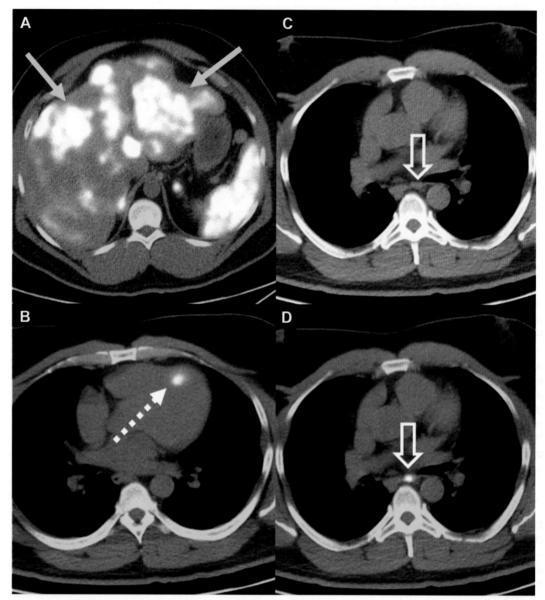

Fig. 3. Fused [^{68}Ga]DOTATATE-PET/CT (*A, B, D*) and CT (*C*) images of a patient with known hepatic metastatic disease (*green arrows*) undergoing evaluation for liver-directed therapy demonstrate unexpected metastases in the myocardium (*dotted arrow*) and subcentimeter paraesophageal lymph node (*open arrow*).

lung carcinoid tumors.[35] Thus, in the absence of a histologic diagnosis, both [^{18}F]FDG and [^{68}Ga] DOTATATE are useful in evaluation of a potential lung carcinoid and provide comprehensive and often complementary staging information.

PET/CT findings are less likely to influence the preoperative and surgical management of carcinoid tumors, than noncarcinoid lung cancers. This is due to the fact that neoadjuvant treatment is generally much less effective for carcinoid lung tumors and that the prognosis after surgical resection for stage II and III carcinoid tumors

(locoregional disease) tends to be more favorable than noncarcinoid lung cancers.[39,40] Tissue biopsy with some type of invasive modality (such as endobronchial ultrasound-fine needle aspiration or mediastinoscopy) would be considered mandatory for patients with hypermetabolic and/or enlarged mediastinal lymph nodes on [^{18}F]FDG-PET/CT scan for noncarcinoid lung cancer, while many would consider conventional imaging alone sufficient for mediastinal staging of carcinoid tumors. Good surgical candidates may be considered for resection even if they have evidence of

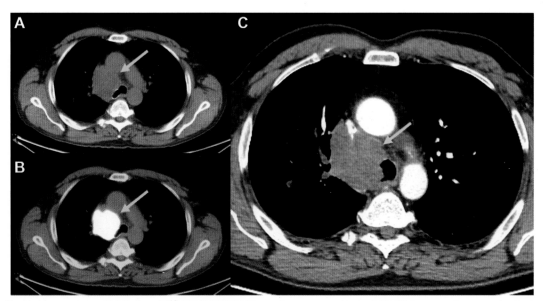

Fig. 4. Noncontrast CT (*A*), fused [^{18}F]FDG-PET/CT (*B*), and contrast-enhanced CT (*C*) images of a central mass in the right lung (*green arrows*) with invasion into trachea and bronchus, biopsy-proven to represent an atypical carcinoid tumor.

hilar or mediastinal disease on PET/CT scan. In addition, many carcinoid tumors are not FDG avid on PET/CT, and this absence of activity does not necessarily influence the decision about resection in patients with a known diagnosis. PET/CT scan can, however, help identify stage IV patients, who would not generally be considered candidates for lung resection.[41]

OTHER NEUROENDOCRINE TUMORS

Many other NETs are able to be imaged with SSTR PET, including pheochromocytomas, paragangliomas, NETs of the genitourinary tract, medullary thyroid cancer (MTC), and Merkel cell carcinoma (MCC). Pheochromocytomas and paragangliomas are rare NETs with an estimated 500 to 1600 cases diagnosed each year in the United States.[20] These lesions may be nonsecretory or secrete catecholamines, and when secretory, they will present with severe hypertension and other symptoms related to excess catecholamine release. These tumors may arise from either the sympathetic or parasympathetic paraganglia in the head and neck, adrenal gland, or along the abdominopelvic sympathetic chain. Molecular imaging has offered noninvasive definitive diagnosis of paragangliomas and pheochromocytomas. For secretory pheochromocytomas, [^{123}I] or [^{131}I]meta-iodobenzylguanidine (MIBG) is a molecular imaging analog of norepinephrine that targets the presynaptic norepinephrine transporter.[42] This mechanism results in accumulation of radiotracer in patients with secretory lesions. For nonsecretory lesions, SSTR-PET/CT can be used to image owing to overexpression of SSTRs at the cell surface of both pheochromocytomas and paragangliomas. Early studies comparing molecular imaging modalities report that [^{68}Ga]DOTATATE-PET/CT performs similarly in evaluation and identification of the primary lesion but superior to [^{131}I]MIBG and [^{18}F]FDG-PET/CT scan in identification and localization of metastases.[43–45] [^{18}F]FDG-PET/CT may also play a role for malignant paragangliomas that may not express SSTRs at the cell surface to the degree of nonmalignant paragangliomas.

MCC is a rare cutaneous neoplasm with an aggressive behavior and poor prognosis. Traditionally, the management of MCC has been guided through [^{18}F]FDG-PET/CT, as it is recommended by the NCCN as either initial imaging or after initial wide local excision and positive sentinel lymph node biopsy.[46] However, MCC is derived from neuroendocrine cells and demonstrates SSTRs at the cell surface. An early study evaluating the use of SSTR-PET for MCC demonstrated a high patient-based sensitivity for detection of metastatic disease and changed management in 13% of patients.[47] An additional case report of a patient with metastatic MCC that underwent dual radiotracer PET with both [^{68}Ga]DOTATATE and [^{18}F]FDG found that [^{68}Ga]DOTATATE revealed a more extensive tumor burden than [^{18}F]FDG.[48] Thus, as further research is conducted, [^{68}Ga]DOTATATE may become increasingly used for comprehensive staging of patients with MCC.

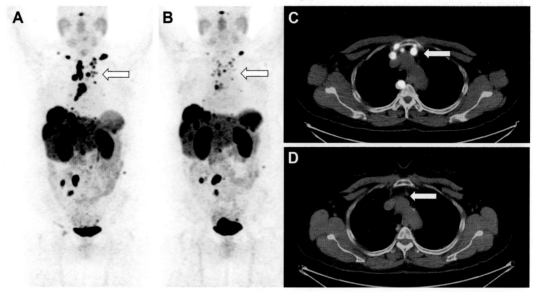

Fig. 5. Maximum-intensity projection (*A, B*) and fused PET/CT (*C, D*) images from [⁶⁸Ga]DOTATATE-PET/CT demonstrating significant improvement in thoracic nodal metastatic disease (*white arrows*) after four cycles of [¹⁷⁷Lu] DOTATATE therapy.

MTC is a rare subtype of thyroid cancer that arises from parafollicular C cells in the thyroid gland and is associated with the genetic syndrome multiple endocrine neoplasia types 2A and 2B. The parafollicular C cells are of neural crest origin, and these tumors result in hypersecretion of calcitonin, leading to decreased serum calcium levels. Given their neural crest origin, these cells express SSTRs and have the potential to be imaged with SSTR-PET. Several studies comparing multiple molecular imaging modalities have found that [⁶⁸Ga]DOTA-TATE outperforms [¹⁸F]FDG and [¹¹¹In]pentetreotide in patients with MTC, but other studies find that no single radiotracer can fully map and detect the entire metastatic disease burden.[49-51] Further research is needed to establish the role of SSTR-PET in the diagnosis and management of patients with MTC and to evaluate a potential theranostic approach for patients with metastatic MTC.

ROLE OF PET IMAGING IN PRRT

After obtaining FDA approval of [¹⁷⁷Lu]DOTATATE in 2018, SSTR-PET with [⁶⁸Ga]DOTATATE has become a cornerstone for diagnosis, management, and treatment of patients with metastatic GEP-NETs. Using the theranostic approach, SSTR-PET is used for diagnostic PET imaging, and then a therapeutic radionuclide ([¹⁷⁷Lu], a beta-emitter) is substituted into the DOTATATE compound to deliver targeted therapeutic radiation to all sites of disease identified on SSTR-PET. Eligibility for PRRT relies entirely on the NET histology and results of SSTR-PET, and the

current NCCN and NANETS guidelines recommend the use of SSTR PET in the initial staging of all patients with NETs.[21,52] In addition, PRRT eligibility also requires progression of disease in the setting of lanreotide, and many NETs are slow growing, making documentation of progression on conventional imaging challenging. SSTR-PET allows for detection of small-volume metastatic disease before it becomes evident on conventional imaging, and restaging of patients with metastatic GEP-NET is frequently performed through a combination of conventional imaging and SSTR-PET (**Fig. 5**). Beyond GEP-NETs, many of the other NETs described previously have been evaluated in the setting of clinical trials involving PRRT, all of which demonstrate safety and feasibility for the new and emerging indications.[53-56] As a result, SSTR-PET has become an essential molecular imaging modality in the management of patients with NET and will continue to play a major role as approved indications for PRRT are expanded beyond GEP-NETs.

SUMMARY

NETs are a heterogeneous group of tumors arising from all parts of the body, with varying pathologies, prognosis, and treatment options. SSTR expression is a key pathologic feature of NETs that allows for targeted imaging of these tumors, with SSTR-PET now replacing [¹¹¹In]pentetreotide and serving a complementary role to [¹⁸F]FDG PET. In addition, the theranostic approach used in GEP-NETs is being evaluated in other NETs and may result in even greater utilization of SSTR-PET in the future.

CLINICS CARE POINTS

- SSTR-PET has significantly improved molecular imaging of NETs when compared to [111In]pentetreotide scintigraphy.
- Knowledge of NET pathology is essential to select the most appropriate PET radiotracer, with some requiring both SSTR-PET and FDG.
- SSTR-PET is paramount in establishing eligibility for PRRT.

DISCLOSURE

The authors have nothing to disclose.

REFERENCES

1. Dasari A, Shen C, Halperin D, et al. Trends in the incidence, prevalence, and survival outcomes in patients with neuroendocrine tumors in the United States. JAMA Oncol 2017;3(10):1335–42.
2. Deppen SA, Blume J, Bobbey AJ, et al. 68Ga-DOTATATE compared with 111In-DTPA-octreotide and conventional imaging for pulmonary and gastroenteropancreatic neuroendocrine tumors: a systematic review and meta-analysis. J Nucl Med 2016;57(6):872–8.
3. Deppen SA, Liu E, Blume JD, et al. Safety and efficacy of 68Ga-DOTATATE PET/CT for diagnosis, staging, and treatment management of neuroendocrine tumors. J Nucl Med 2016;57(5):708–14.
4. Rindi G, Klimstra DS, Abedi-Ardekani B, et al. A common classification framework for neuroendocrine neoplasms: an International Agency for Research on Cancer (IARC) and World Health Organization (WHO) expert consensus proposal. Mod Pathol 2018;31(12):1770–86.
5. Nagtegaal ID, Odze RD, Klimstra D, et al. The 2019 WHO classification of tumours of the digestive system. Histopathology 2020;76(2):182–8.
6. Laskiewicz L, Jamshed S, Gong Y, et al. The diagnostic value of FNA biopsy in grading pancreatic neuroendocrine tumors. Cancer Cytopathol 2018;126(3):170–8.
7. Eusebi LH, Thorburn D, Toumpanakis C, et al. Endoscopic ultrasound-guided fine-needle aspiration vs fine-needle biopsy for the diagnosis of pancreatic neuroendocrine tumors. Endosc Int Open 2019;7(11):E1393–9.
8. Kaemmerer D, Peter L, Lupp A, et al. Molecular imaging with 68Ga-SSTR PET/CT and correlation to immunohistochemistry of somatostatin receptors in neuroendocrine tumours. Eur J Nucl Med Mol Imaging 2011;38(9):1659–68.
9. Balon HR, Brown TL, Goldsmith SJ, et al. The SNM practice guideline for somatostatin receptor scintigraphy 2.0. J Nucl Med Technol 2011;39(4):317–24.
10. Reubi JC, Schar JC, Waser B, et al. Affinity profiles for human somatostatin receptor subtypes SST1-SST5 of somatostatin radiotracers selected for scintigraphic and radiotherapeutic use. Eur J Nucl Med 2000;27(3):273–82.
11. Aalbersberg EA, de Wit-van der Veen BJ, Versleijen MWJ, et al. Influence of lanreotide on uptake of (68)Ga-DOTATATE in patients with neuroendocrine tumours: a prospective intra-patient evaluation. Eur J Nucl Med Mol Imaging 2019;46(3):696–703.
12. Bozkurt MF, Virgolini I, Balogova S, et al. Guideline for PET/CT imaging of neuroendocrine neoplasms with (68)Ga-DOTA-conjugated somatostatin receptor targeting peptides and (18)F-DOPA. Eur J Nucl Med Mol Imaging 2017;44(9):1588–601.
13. Walczyk J, Sowa-Staszczak A. Diagnostic imaging of gastrointestinal neuroendocrine neoplasms with a focus on ultrasound. J Ultrason 2019;19(78):228–35.
14. Chang S, Choi D, Lee SJ, et al. Neuroendocrine neoplasms of the gastrointestinal tract: classification, pathologic basis, and imaging features. Radiographics 2007;27(6):1667–79.
15. McKenna LR, Edil BH. Update on pancreatic neuroendocrine tumors. Gland Surg 2014;3(4):258–75.
16. Tan EH, Tan CH. Imaging of gastroenteropancreatic neuroendocrine tumors. World J Clin Oncol 2011;2(1):28–43.
17. Modlin IM, Oberg K, Chung DC, et al. Gastroenteropancreatic neuroendocrine tumours. Lancet Oncol 2008;9(1):61–72.
18. Srirajaskanthan R, Kayani I, Quigley AM, et al. The role of 68Ga-DOTATATE PET in patients with neuroendocrine tumors and negative or equivocal findings on 111In-DTPA-octreotide scintigraphy. J Nucl Med 2010;51(6):875–82.
19. Sadowski SM, Neychev V, Millo C, et al. Prospective study of 68Ga-DOTATATE positron emission tomography/computed tomography for detecting gastro-entero-pancreatic neuroendocrine tumors and unknown primary sites. J Clin Oncol 2016;34(6):588–96.
20. Chen H, Sippel RS, O'Dorisio MS, et al. The North American Neuroendocrine Tumor Society consensus guideline for the diagnosis and management of neuroendocrine tumors: pheochromocytoma, paraganglioma, and medullary thyroid cancer. Pancreas 2010;39(6):775–83.
21. National Comprehensive Cancer Network. Neuroendocrine and Adrenal Tumors (Version 2.2020). Available at: https://www.nccn.org/professionals/

physician_gls/pdf/neuroendocrine.pdf. [Accessed 5 October 2020].

22. Squires MH 3rd, Volkan Adsay N, Schuster DM, et al. Octreoscan versus FDG-PET for neuroendocrine tumor staging: a biological approach. Ann Surg Oncol 2015;22(7):2295–301.

23. Panagiotidis E, Alshammari A, Michopoulou S, et al. Comparison of the impact of 68Ga-DOTATATE and 18F-FDG PET/CT on clinical management in patients with neuroendocrine tumors. J Nucl Med 2017;58(1):91–6.

24. Chambers AJ, Pasieka JL, Dixon E, et al. The palliative benefit of aggressive surgical intervention for both hepatic and mesenteric metastases from neuroendocrine tumors. Surgery 2008;144(4):645–51. discussion 651-3.

25. Graff-Baker AN, Sauer DA, Pommier SJ, et al. Expanded criteria for carcinoid liver debulking: maintaining survival and increasing the number of eligible patients. Surgery 2014;156(6):1369–76. discussion 1376-7.

26. Yao JC, Hassan M, Phan A, et al. One hundred years after "carcinoid": epidemiology of and prognostic factors for neuroendocrine tumors in 35,825 cases in the United States. J Clin Oncol 2008;26(18):3063–72.

27. Naswa N, Sharma P, Kumar A, et al. 68Ga-DOTANOC PET/CT in patients with carcinoma of unknown primary of neuroendocrine origin. Clin Nucl Med 2012;37(3):245–51.

28. Barrio M, Czernin J, Fanti S, et al. The impact of somatostatin receptor-directed PET/CT on the management of patients with neuroendocrine tumor: a systematic review and meta-analysis. J Nucl Med 2017;58(5):756–61.

29. Bertani E, Fazio N, Radice D, et al. Resection of the primary tumor followed by peptide receptor radionuclide therapy as upfront strategy for the treatment of G1-G2 pancreatic neuroendocrine tumors with unresectable liver metastases. Ann Surg Oncol 2016;23(Suppl 5):981–9.

30. Hilal T. Current understanding and approach to well differentiated lung neuroendocrine tumors: an update on classification and management. Ther Adv Med Oncol 2017;9(3):189–99.

31. Chaer R, Massad MG, Evans A, et al. Primary neuroendocrine tumors of the thymus. Ann Thorac Surg 2002;74(5):1733–40.

32. Gaur P, Leary C, Yao JC. Thymic neuroendocrine tumors: a SEER database analysis of 160 patients. Ann Surg 2010;251(6):1117–21.

33. Rosado de Christenson ML, Abbott GF, Kirejczyk WM, et al. Thoracic carcinoids: radiologic-pathologic correlation. Radiographics 1999;19(3):707–36.

34. Walts AE, Frye J, Engman DM, et al. Carcinoid tumors of the thymus and Cushing's syndrome: clinicopathologic features and current best evidence regarding the cell of origin of these unusual neoplasms. Ann Diagn Pathol 2019;38:71–9.

35. Jindal T, Kumar A, Venkitaraman B, et al. Evaluation of the role of [18F]FDG-PET/CT and [68Ga] DOTATOC-PET/CT in differentiating typical and atypical pulmonary carcinoids. Cancer Imaging 2011;11:70–5.

36. Moore W, Freiberg E, Bishawi M, et al. FDG-PET imaging in patients with pulmonary carcinoid tumor. Clin Nucl Med 2013;38(7):501–5.

37. Erasmus JJ, McAdams HP, Patz EF Jr, et al. Evaluation of primary pulmonary carcinoid tumors using FDG PET. AJR Am J Roentgenol 1998;170(5):1369–73.

38. Chan DL, Bernard E, Schembri G, et al. High metabolic tumour volume on FDG PET predicts poor survival from neuroendocrine neoplasms. Neuroendocrinology 2020;110(11–12):950–8.

39. Ramirez RA, Beyer DT, Diebold AE, et al. Prognostic factors in typical and atypical pulmonary carcinoids. Ochsner J 2017;17(4):335–40.

40. Gosain R, Mukherjee S, Yendamuri SS, et al. Management of typical and atypical pulmonary carcinoids based on different established guidelines. Cancers 2018;10(12):510.

41. Singh S, Bergsland EK, Card CM, et al. Commonwealth Neuroendocrine Tumour Research Collaboration and the North American Neuroendocrine Tumor Society Guidelines for the Diagnosis and Management of Patients With Lung Neuroendocrine Tumors: An International Collaborative Endorsement and Update of the 2015 European Neuroendocrine Tumor Society Expert Consensus Guidelines. J Thorac Oncol 2020;15(10):1577–98.

42. Vallabhajosula S, Nikolopoulou A. Radioiodinated metaiodobenzylguanidine (MIBG): radiochemistry, biology, and pharmacology. Semin Nucl Med 2011;41(5):324–33.

43. Tan TH, Hussein Z, Saad FF, et al. Diagnostic performance of (68)Ga-DOTATATE PET/CT, (18)F-FDG PET/CT and (131)I-MIBG scintigraphy in mapping metastatic pheochromocytoma and paraganglioma. Nucl Med Mol Imaging 2015;49(2):143–51.

44. Jing H, Li F, Wang L, et al. Comparison of the 68Ga-DOTATATA PET/CT, FDG PET/CT, and MIBG SPECT/CT in the evaluation of suspected primary pheochromocytomas and paragangliomas. Clin Nucl Med 2017;42(7):525–9.

45. Han S, Suh CH, Woo S, et al. Performance of (68) Ga-DOTA-conjugated somatostatin receptor-targeting peptide PET in detection of pheochromocytoma and paraganglioma: a systematic review and metaanalysis. J Nucl Med 2019;60(3):369–76.

46. Network NCC. Merkel Cell Carcinoma (Version 1.2020). Available at: https://www.nccn.org/professionals/physician_gls/pdf/mcc.pdf. [Accessed 18 December 2020].

47. Buder K, Lapa C, Kreissl MC, et al. Somatostatin receptor expression in Merkel cell carcinoma as target for molecular imaging. BMC Cancer 2014; 14:268.

48. Epstude M, Tornquist K, Riklin C, et al. Comparison of (18)F-FDG PET/CT and (68)Ga-DOTATATE PET/CT imaging in metastasized Merkel cell carcinoma. Clin Nucl Med 2013;38(4):283–4.

49. Yamaga LYI, Cunha ML, Campos Neto GC, et al. (68)Ga-DOTATATE PET/CT in recurrent medullary thyroid carcinoma: a lesion-by-lesion comparison with (111)In-octreotide SPECT/CT and conventional imaging. Eur J Nucl Med Mol Imaging 2017;44(10): 1695–701.

50. Ozkan ZG, Kuyumcu S, Uzum AK, et al. Comparison of ^{68}Ga-DOTATATE PET-CT, ^{18}F-FDG PET-CT and 99mTc-(V)DMSA scintigraphy in the detection of recurrent or metastatic medullary thyroid carcinoma. Nucl Med Commun 2015;36(3): 242–50.

51. Conry BG, Papathanasiou ND, Prakash V, et al. Comparison of (68)Ga-DOTATATE and (18)F-fluorodeoxyglucose PET/CT in the detection of recurrent medullary thyroid carcinoma. Eur J Nucl Mcd Mol Imaging 2010;37(1):49–57.

52. Halfdanarson TR, Strosberg JR, Tang L, et al. The North American Neuroendocrine Tumor Society Consensus Guidelines for surveillance and medical management of pancreatic neuroendocrine tumors. Pancreas 2020;49(7):863–81.

53. Mirvis E, Toumpanakis C, Mandair D, et al. Efficacy and tolerability of peptide receptor radionuclide therapy (PRRT) in advanced metastatic bronchial neuroendocrine tumours (NETs). Lung Cancer 2020;150:70–5.

54. Jaiswal SK, Sarathi V, Memon SS, et al. 177Lu-DOTATATE therapy in metastatic/inoperable pheochromocytoma-paraganglioma. Endocr Connect 2020; 9(9):864–73.

55. Basu S, Ranade R. Favorable response of metastatic merkel cell carcinoma to targeted 177Lu-DOTATATE therapy: will PRRT evolve to become an important approach in receptor-positive cases? J Nucl Med Technol 2016;44(2):85–7.

56. Satapathy S, Mittal BR, Sood A, et al. Efficacy and safety of concomitant 177Lu-DOTATATE and low-dose capecitabine in advanced medullary thyroid carcinoma: a single-centre experience. Nucl Med Commun 2020;41(7):629–35.

PET Imaging for Prostate Cancer

Bital Savir-Baruch, MD[a],*, Rudolf A. Werner, MD[b], Steven P. Rowe, MD, PhD[c], David M. Schuster, MD[d]

KEYWORDS

- Fluciclovine • Prostate-specific membrane antigen • PET imaging • Prostate cancer
- Biochemical recurrence • Theranostics

KEY POINTS

- ^{18}F-fluciclovine and prostate-specific membrane antigen (PSMA) PET/CT have demonstrated high positive predictive value in detecting extraprostatic malignancy in patients with biochemical recurrence with diagnostic performance exceeding that of conventional imaging.
- Although ^{18}F-fluciclovine is not FDA approved for use in initial staging, both ^{18}F-fluciclovine and PSMA PET/CT may help identify patients with occult metastasis who may not benefit from curative surgery in primary prostate cancer.
- Early data indicate that the use of ^{18}F-fluciclovine and PSMA PET improves patient outcomes.
- ^{18}F-fluciclovine excels in local disease detection because of limited urinary excretion, whereas PSMA has superior performance in extraprostatic disease detection.
- PSMA PET can serve as a means of selection for treatment with PSMA radioligand therapy.

INTRODUCTION

The role of PET imaging with ^{11}C-choline and ^{18}F-fluciclovine in evaluating patients with prostate cancer (PCa) has become more important over the years and has been incorporated into the NCCN guidelines. A new generation of PET radiotracers targeting the prostate-specific membrane antigen (PSMA) is widely used outside the United States to evaluate patients with primary PCa and PCa recurrence.

CHOLINE PET

Choline is a component of phosphatidylcholine incorporated into the cell membrane. The enzyme choline kinase is upregulated in many cancers, including PCa.[1] In September 2012, ^{11}C-choline was FDA approved for PET imaging of patients with suspected PCa recurrence. Choline radiotracers have been mostly replaced by PSMA PET worldwide and are not widely available in the United States compared with the FDA-approved synthetic amino acid PET radiotracer ^{18}F-fluciclovine.

^{18}F-FLUCICLOVINE PET
Pathophysiology and Biodistribution

[18]F-fluciclovine is a fluorinated synthetic amino acid PET tracer approved by the FDA for imaging of patients with suspected PCa recurrence after prior treatment. In PCa cells, amino acid transport is significantly upregulated.[2] ^{18}F-fluciclovine physiologic activity is most intense in the pancreas and liver.[3] Variable mild to moderate physiologic uptake is seen in salivary glands, pituitary, adrenals, muscle, esophagus, bowel, and bone marrow;

[a] Division of Nuclear Medicine, Department of Radiology, Loyola University Medical Center, 2160 South 1st Avenue, Maywood, IL 60153, USA; [b] Department of Nuclear Medicine, University Hospital Würzburg, Oberdürrbacherstr. 6, Würzburg 97080, Germany; [c] Division of Nuclear Medicine and Molecular Imaging, The Russell H. Morgan Department of Radiology and Radiological Science, Johns Hopkins University School of Medicine, 601 North Caroline Street Room 3233, Baltimore, MD 21287, USA; [d] Division of Nuclear Medicine and Molecular Imaging, Department of Radiology and Imaging Sciences, Emory University, 1364 Clifton Road NE, Atlanta, GA 30322, USA
* Corresponding author.
E-mail address: bsavirbaruch@luc.edu

Radiol Clin N Am 59 (2021) 801–811
https://doi.org/10.1016/j.rcl.2021.05.008
0033-8389/21/© 2021 Elsevier Inc. All rights reserved.

[18]F-fluciclovine has greater heterogeneity than seen with ^{18}F-fluorodeoxyglucose (FDG). Mild uptake is noted within the blood pool and brain parenchyma. ^{18}F-fluciclovine is only minimally excreted by the kidneys with little to no resulting bladder activity, though a minority of patients may exhibit an early excretion pattern.[3]

Normal Variants/Pitfalls

[18]F-fluciclovine is not prostate specific, as other benign and malignant neoplasia have upregulated amino acid metabolism and may have increased ^{18}F-fluciclovine uptake, such as lung, breast, and gynecologic cancers as well as meningioma and osteoid osteoma.[4,5] It is not uncommon to have mild to moderate symmetric ^{18}F-fluciclovine benign activity in inguinal, distal external iliac, and axillary nodes. Periurethral tissue may have mild to moderate activity, and therefore, sagittal images can help differentiate physiologic uptake from recurrence at the vesicourethral anastomosis. The early appearance of bladder or ureteral activity may mimic tumor or abnormal lymph nodes, respectively.[6]

Degenerative uptake is less intense and less commonly described than with FDG PET. Though amino acid imaging demonstrates less inflammatory uptake than FDG, amino acid transport also occurs in benign inflammation, and therefore fluciclovine uptake not specific to malignancy can occur.[3] For bone lesions, uptake is typically more intense with lytic or mixed sclerotic lesions. Indolent, dense sclerotic lesions may have little or no ^{18}F-fluciclovine uptake. Occasional ^{18}F-fluciclovine uptake seen in isolated red marrow in the pelvis or proximal femurs may stimulate metastasis. In these cases, bone-specific MR imaging, skeletal scintigraphy with agents such as sodium ^{18}F-fluoride or ^{99m}Tc-methylene diphosphate, or biopsy may be required.[7]

Patient Preparation and Imaging Protocol

Patient preparation and imaging protocol for ^{18}F-fluciclovine PET have been described in detail.[7,8] In brief, the patient is advised to fast (except for medications) for 4 hours and avoid excessive physical activity starting 24 hours before the scan. If possible, patients should refrain from voiding 15 to 30 minutes before the study to mitigate early urine tracer excretion.

PET images should start at 4 minutes (3–5 min) postinjection of 10 mCi (370 MBq) ^{18}F-fluciclovine as an IV bolus. As the dynamic tracer washout is relatively fast, it is important not to delay the start of the PET images. The CT can be acquired within the 4-minute interval between ^{18}F-fluciclovine

injection and PET acquisition. CT images with IV contrast should be performed after the PET, as the IV contrast may act as a diuretic and increase early urinary excretion.

Image Interpretation

[18]F-fluciclovine image interpretation is based on the uptake compared with defined background regions such as bone marrow and blood pool.[7,9] Typical PCa recurrence patterns should be kept in mind when interpreting ^{18}F-fluciclovine PET.[7,10] Overall, any lesion with increased uptake equal to or higher than bone marrow (level of normal L3 vertebrae) should be considered suspicious for malignancy. Lesions smaller than 1 cm may demonstrate lower activity due to partial volume artifact, and therefore the threshold for positivity is lower. Hence, subcentimeter structures should be considered suspicious when uptake is significantly above the adjacent visualized blood pool uptake and approaches the bone marrow uptake.[7,9] For bone lesions, focal activity should be clearly seen on the maximum intensity projection (MIP) image.

Primary Disease and Staging

Neither characterization of the primary lesion nor initial staging are FDA-approved indications for ^{18}F-fluciclovine. While primary malignant lesions have higher uptake versus normal prostate tissue, there is a significant overlap in uptake between PCa and nonmalignant processes such as benign prostatic hypertrophy.[11,12] Multiple studies have demonstrated a correlation between Gleason grade and ^{18}F-fluciclovine uptake.[11–15] Approximately 28% of patients are undergraded on biopsy compared with prostatectomy.[16] The possibility of using ^{18}F-fluciclovine to help direct biopsy to more aggressive occult lesions, especially with the addition of multiparametric PET/MR to refine characterization, is intriguing.

A multicenter Phase 2 trial for initial staging of primary PCa with ^{18}F-fluciclovine PET/CT in 28 patients reported sensitivity and specificity of 66.7% and 86.4%, respectively, for extraprostatic nodal disease.[17] Another study of 28 patients with high-risk PCa in patients who underwent ^{18}F-fluciclovine PET/MR imaging before surgery reported patient-based and region-based sensitivity of 40% and 30%, respectively, with 100% specificity for the detection of regional lymph node metastases with a higher PPV of PET versus MR imaging alone.[18]

A prospective study using ^{18}F-fluciclovine PET for preoperative staging in patients with intermediate-risk to high-risk primary PCa of 57 patients who subsequently underwent robotic radical prostatectomy with extended pelvic lymph node dissection reported a sensitivity and specificity for malignant nodal detection of 55.3% and 84.8% per patient, respectively, and 54.8% and 96.4% per region, respectively.[19] The sensitivity was significantly higher than conventional imaging both on a patient-based (55.3% vs 33.3%, P<.01) and region-based (54.8% vs 19.4%, P<.01) analysis with similar high specificity. Metastasis detection correlates to the size of metastatic deposits within lymph nodes and overall metastatic burden.[18,19] Hence, ^{18}F-fluciclovine PET can be useful to guide lymph node dissection because of its high specificity and to help identify patients with occult metastasis who may not benefit from curative surgery.

Recurrence/Restaging

[18]F-fluciclovine PET/CT demonstrated promising initial results in detecting malignancy in patients with biochemical recurrence (BCR).[20] In a prospective clinical trial in which there was a 96.1% level of histologic proof, the detection rate was related to the prostate-specific antigen (PSA) level: 37.5% at a PSA of less than 1 ng/mL, 77.8% at 1 to 2 ng/mL, 91.7% at >2 to 5 ng/mL, and 83.3% at greater than 5 ng/mL, which was significantly better than CT.[21] The sensitivity and specificity in the treated prostate or prostate bed were 90.2% and 40.0%, respectively; sensitivity and specificity for extraprostatic disease were 55.0% and 96.7%, respectively. Confounding uptake due to inflammation or prostatic hypertrophy was likely responsible for the lower specificity in the treated prostate.[22] A subsequent study using ^{18}F-fluciclovine-guided transrectal ultrasound-guided biopsies reported that using a higher threshold of intensity minimizes false-positive results in the treated prostate.[23] A multisite study of 596 patients reported a sensitivity of 88.1%, specificity of 32.6%, and PPV of 71.8% for local recurrence.[24] Thus, histologic confirmation of findings in the treated prostate is recommended, yet there is high specificity for extraprostatic disease detection mirrored by the multisite study that reported a PPV of 92.3%.[24]

In the prospective multicenter intention-to-treat LOCATE trial enrolling 213 patients with BCR, detection rate varied with PSA level: 31%, 79%, and 81% with a PSA (ng/mL) of 0 to 0.5, greater than 1.0, and greater than 2.0, respectively. A postscan change in management occurred in 59% of patients.[25] The FALCON prospective trial enrolled 104 patients and reported a 64% change in management with detection rates of 29.5% and

93% in PSAs of less than and greater than 2.0 ng/mL, respectively.[26] Interestingly, there was a 28.9% patient-level detection rate with PSA less than 0.5 ng/ml. A retrospective report of 152 patients from clinically performed ^{18}F-fluciclovine PET/CT demonstrated positivity rates of 58%, 87%, 100%, and 92% for PSA (ng/mL) levels of less than 1, 1 to 2, 2 to 5, and greater than 5, respectively.[27]

A final analysis of patients from a randomized prospective trial of 165 patients (NCT01666808) in a postprostatectomy setting with BCR reported a 35.4% change in therapy approach in patients who underwent standard of care imaging (abdominopelvic CT or MR imaging) followed by ^{18}F-fluciclovine PET/CT.[28] Upon examining outcomes from salvage radiotherapy planning with standard imaging only versus those whose planning was based on the additional ^{18}F-fluciclovine PET/CT, a significant improvement in failure-free survival at 3 years (75.5% vs 63.0; P = .003) and 4 years (75.5% vs 51.2%; P<.001) was reported. A second similar randomized clinical trial (NCT03762759) will compare ^{18}F-fluciclovine and ^{68}Ga-PSMA in patients with BCR postprostatectomy.

The detection of recurrent disease at low PSA levels has assumed importance as salvage radiotherapy is being offered at increasingly lower PSA levels. The reported detection rate of ^{18}F-fluciclovine at low PSA levels has varied widely. In the randomized salvage therapy outcomes trial above, there was a 72% detection rate with PSA less than 1 ng/mL while Wang and coworkers reported a 33% detection rate at this level.[29,30] Others have reported values in between 46.4% and 58% for PSA< or ≤1 ng/mL.[27,31] These differences in detection rates are likely related to specifics of trial populations, such as aggressiveness of disease.

Therapy Response Assessment with ^{18}F-Fluciclovine PET

Preliminary studies suggested that ^{18}F-fluciclovine could be used to assess response to therapy.[32,33] A small prospective study of patients with primary PCa undergoing androgen-deprivation therapy (ADT) reported a significant decrease in standardized uptake values (ie, SUVmax) of detected local and metastatic lesions on a subsequent PET/MR imaging scan.[33] A second small retrospective study in patients with BCR found a correlation between PSA and the number of lesions to findings on post-therapy PET/CT scans.[32] However, this needs to be further evaluated in larger prospective clinical trials.

PROSTATE-SPECIFIC MEMBRANE ANTIGEN-TARGETED PET

Introduction to Prostate-Specific Membrane Antigen-Targeted PET

PSMA radiotracers are widely used throughout the world for PCa imaging and therapy. PSMA is a type II transmembrane glycoprotein with folate hydrolase activity and an extracellular domain that includes the enzyme active site.[34] Expression of PSMA is seen in approximately 95% of PCa tumors.[35] At the histologic level, aggressive and advanced PCa shows increased levels of PSMA expression.[36] The accessibility of the active site to high-affinity ligands, combined with rapid internalization of PSMA from the cell surface, allows for high-contrast imaging.[37]

Early in the clinical adoption of PSMA PET agents, ^{68}Ga-labeled radiotracers proliferated because of several factors including facile synthesis and the ability to make such compounds without access to a cyclotron. ^{68}Ga-PSMA-HBED-CC, later more commonly known as ^{68}Ga-PSMA-11 or simply ^{68}Ga-PSMA, became the dominant agent in the field.[38] However, parallel to the development of ^{68}Ga-labeled radiotracers, PSMA-targeted agents labeled with fluorine-18 were also being explored, initially ^{18}F-DCFBC[39] and other first-generation compounds, and later more widely used radiotracers such as ^{18}F-DCFPyL,[40] ^{18}F-PSMA-1007, and ^{18}F-rhPSMA-7.[41,42]

Patient Preparation and Imaging Protocol

Patient preparation and imaging protocol for PSMA-directed imaging PET were previously described.[43,44] Patients do not fast and are encouraged to be well hydrated. Voiding before imaging may decrease the frequency of halo artifacts. The dose range from 1.8 to 2.2 MBq (0.05–0.06 mCi) per kilogram for ^{68}Ga-labeled PSMA radiotracers,[43] and 200 to 370 MBq (5–10 mCi) for the ^{18}F-labeled counterparts.[44] After bolus injection, an uptake time of 1 h is recommended, although delayed acquisition or the use of furosemide may improve lesion detection.[45] Field of view includes the base of the skull to midthigh with 3 to 4 min per bed position and images.[43]

Normal Variants/Pitfalls

For most PSMA radiotracers, biodistribution includes the lacrimal glands, salivary glands, liver, spleen, kidneys, small bowel, ganglia, and urinary tract due to renal excretion.[43] There are some variations among radiotracers. ^{18}F-DCFPyL has higher hepatic uptake than ^{68}Ga-PSMA-11, whereas ^{68}Ga-PSMA-11 has increased accumulation in the kidneys.[46] ^{18}F-PSMA-1007 has less renal excretion, which can increase the lesion detection rate for small pelvic lymph node lesions or local recurrence.[41] With increasing clinical availability of PSMA-directed imaging, the number of reported pitfalls is steadily increasing (Fig. 1). Multiple benign pathologies with increased PSMA expression can be misinterpreted as malignant, for example, sympathetic ganglia,[47] benign tumors (meningioma, schwannoma), soft tissue lesions (desmoid tumors, myxoma), or lung lesions (sarcoidosis, tuberculosis, or anthracosilicosis). Nonprostatic malignant tumors, however, may also have substantial PSMA expression; these include medullary thyroid carcinoma, renal cell carcinoma, breast cancer, and lung cancer.[48]

Interpretative Criteria

Multiple standardized frameworks for image interpretation have been introduced for PSMA PET. For instance, Eiber and coworkers recently introduced the "PROMISE" system, which is based on a molecular imaging TNM classification ("miTNM," version 1.0). Using the "miPSMA expression score," different uptake levels are considered relative to normal uptake in the blood pool, liver, and parotid glands. The local tumor is classified, which refers to extent and organ confinement ranging from "miT0" to "miT4". In addition, a sextant segmentation of the prostate is used for intraprostatic tumor extension. Pelvic lymph node lesions are categorized (from "miN0" to "miN1b"). Last, the extrapelvic nodes ("miM1a") and distant metastases ("miM1b" referring to bone or "miM1c" to other organ involvement) are also evaluated.[49] In a prospective trial applying PROMISE to ^{68}Ga-PSMA-11 PET/CT in 635 men afflicted with PCa, interreader reproducibility was substantial, with a Fleiss κ of 0.65 to 0.78.[50] Also providing reliable standards in PSMA PET/CT interpretation, the PSMA Reporting and Data System (RADS) framework has been recently introduced. In brief, a 5-point scale is applied to a maximum of 5 target lesions, with increasing numbers indicating a higher likelihood of malignancy. PSMA-RADS ranges from 1 = no evidence of disease and definitively benign to 5 = high certainty that prostate carcinoma is present and refers to the site of disease and the intensity of radiotracer uptake. Depending on the derived RADS score, PSMA-RADS also triggers further clinical workup—for example, by recommending biopsy or follow-up imaging. Taken together, this framework should increase the level of reader confidence, should facilitate communication with other specialists, and may guide the reader in determining

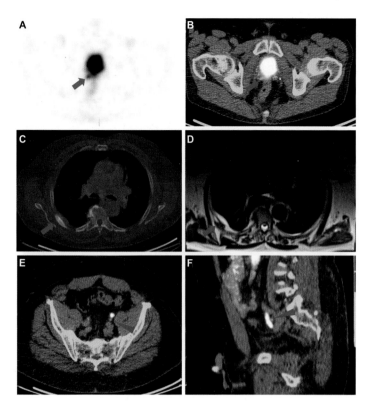

Fig. 1. (A) (PET axial) (B) (axial fused PET-CT) 51-year-old man postprostatectomy with positive margin (Gleason 3 + 4 = 7). PSA at time of [11]Ga-PSMA PET was 0.23 ng/mL. Uptake in right lateral surgical margin (arrows) obscured by intense bladder activity. Patient underwent EBRT to prostate bed with ADT with subsequent PSA less than 0.01 ng/ml. (C) (PET/CT fused axial) 65-year-old man postprostatectomy presented with PSA of 0.03 ng/mL. [11]Ga-PSMA images demonstrate abnormal uptake in the right fifth rib with sclerosis and new soft tissue thickening (arrow). The patient denies trauma. An MR image (D axial T2 HASTE) showed a characteristic healing fracture (arrows). (E) PET/CT fused axial and (F) sagittal images demonstrate abnormal uptake in a left external iliac lymph node measuring 0.6 × 0.5 cm behind and obscured by intense left ureteral activity (arrowheads).

whether radioligand therapy for PCa should be recommended.[51] In a prospective setting enrolling 50 ^{18}F-DCFPyL PET/CTs, the interobserver agreement rate using PSMA-RADS was excellent.[52]

Prostate-Specific Membrane Antigen-Targeted PET in Primary Prostate Cancer and Initial Staging

Identification of primary PCa is ongoing research with PSMA PET. An early study with the first-generation agent ^{18}F-DCFBC noted that PET had an improved specificity for high-grade disease than MR imaging, although with a lower sensitivity.[53] Other studies have been more promising. Eiber and colleagues found that ^{68}Ga-PSMA-11 PET had a significantly higher area under the receiver-operating-characteristic curve (AUC, 0.83) than multiparametric MR imaging (0.73).[54] The combination of both modalities led to the highest AUC (0.88).[54] Similarly, Hicks and colleagues found that ^{68}Ga-PSMA-11 PET/MR imaging sensitivity was superior to multiparametric MR imaging at the anatomic-region level.[55] These findings suggest that PSMA PET may be appropriate to incorporate into biopsy planning.[56]

PSMA PET is a useful staging modality for patients at risk of occult locoregional nodal involvement or distant metastatic disease. In single-center retrospective[57] and prospective studies in men with intermediate-risk or high-risk PCa,[58] PSMA PET has demonstrated moderate sensitivity and very high specificity for identifying pelvic lymph node involvement. The first published study on this topic reported a relatively low patient-level sensitivity of 33.3%,[57] which is in line with larger multicenter trials, such as OSPREY (sensitivity 30.6%–41.9% among three readers)[59] or a study with ^{68}Ga-PSMA-11 that reported sensitivity of 40%.[60] The apparently low sensitivity of PSMA PET in multicenter trials suggests that there may be heterogeneity between centers and that care will need to be taken in translating PSMA PET beyond large tertiary care medical centers with specific expertise.

PSMA PET can predict biochemical persistence (BCP) after radical prostatectomy with lymph node dissection. Van Leeuwen and colleagues found that BCP was noted in 50% of men in whom lymph node involvement was seen on PSMA PET and confirmed histologically, whereas only 16.7% BCP was noted in men with lymph node involvement histologically but not identified on PSMA PET.[61]

The recently published proPSMA trial found that PSMA PET outperformed conventional imaging for the systemic staging of men with high-risk PCa.[62] Therefore, despite limitations in sensitivity, PSMA PET may become a clinical standard for staging patients being considered for curative-intent local therapy.

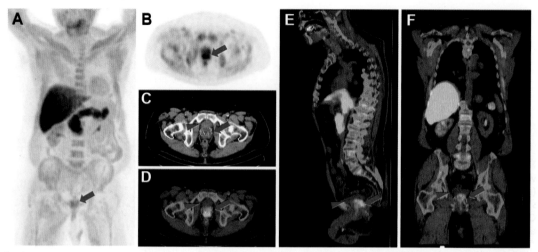

Fig. 2. A 72-year-old-man with biochemical recurrence of PCa with PSA 4 ng/mL after prior brachytherapy (initial PSA of 11 ng/mL). ^{18}F-fluciclovine PET/CT images (A) MIP, (B) axial PET, (C) axial CT, (D) axial PET/CT, (E) sagittal PET/CT (F), and coronal PET/CT images demonstrate increased tracer uptake within the prostate extending to the seminal vesicles (arrows). A prostate biopsy confirmed the presence of recurrent disease. Compared with ^{68}Ga-PSMA-11 or ^{18}F-PSMA- DCFPyL PET tracers, ^{18}F-fluciclovine urine washout to the bladder is usually mild (arrowheads), improving the evaluation of local recurrence.

Prostate-Specific Membrane Antigen-Targeted PET for Recurrence, Restaging, and Metastatic Disease

The most widely studied aspect of PSMA PET imaging is detection efficiency in recurrent disease, as identifying the site of recurrence influences the approach to salvage therapy.[63] Early studies on PSMA PET in the recurrence population varied in the reported detection efficiencies, which may have been due in part to the retrospective nature of many of the studies and differences in the degree of inclusion of patients with visible lesions on conventional imaging.[37] However, the limitations from early studies have begun to be addressed by improved study designs. For example, Fendler and colleagues reported in a two-center prospective trial that sites of PCa were localized in 75% of men with recurrent disease and that the PPV of PSMA PET findings was 0.84 on a per-patient basis with histologic validation.[50] Another recent prospective study that specifically excluded patients with evidence of disease on conventional imaging found a detection rate of 67.7%.[64] Although detection efficiency generally tracks with serum PSA level,[37] the rates of lesion localization are still moderate at low PSAs, and there are no current recommendations to exclude patients from imaging based on PSA level.

Phillips and colleagues reported the results of the ORIOLE trial, in which patients were randomized to either stereotactic ablative body radiation (SABR) or observation for oligometastatic disease identified on conventional imaging. SABR improved progression-free survival, particularly in a post hoc analysis that showed that inclusion of all PSMA-positive sites of disease in the treatment plan was beneficial.[65] We can expect that the high sensitivity of PSMA PET will popularize metastasis-directed therapy in oligometastatic patients.

Therapy Response Assessment with Prostate-Specific Membrane Antigen-Targeted PET

There is a complex interplay between androgen signaling and PSMA expression, making interpretation of response assessment difficult. Hope and coworkers demonstrated that short-term ADT led to a flare phenomenon with increased uptake in known lesions and the appearance of new lesions.[66] Longer-term ADT generally leads to decreased conspicuity of lesions.[67] The initiation of second-generation anti-androgen therapy can also confuse patterns of changes in uptake on PSMA PET.[68] Due to the apparent complexity of response assessment with PSMA PET, interest has arisen in developing response criteria.[69] However, prospective data are needed to evaluate systemic therapy effects on PSMA expression.

Prostate-Specific Membrane Antigen Ligands Versus ^{18}F-Fluciclovine

[18]F-fluciclovine is a metabolic radiotracer, whereas PSMA is targeted to receptors. Thus, each radiotracer reflects a different aspect of PCa biology. Intrapatient comparisons of ^{18}F-fluciclovine and ^{68}Ga-PSMA-11 reported superior performance for [68]GA-PSMA-11 in detecting

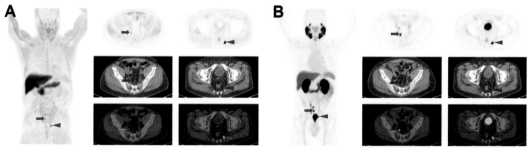

Fig. 3. A 74-year-old man with biochemical recurrence of PCa after radical prostatectomy. (A) ^{18}F-fluciclovine PET whole-body MIP image showing multiple radiotracer-avid pelvic lymph nodes as well as axial PET (*top row*), CT (*middle row*), and PET/CT (*bottom row*) images. (B) PSMA-targeted ^{18}F-DCFPyL PET whole-body MIP image showing multiple radiotracer-avid pelvic lymph nodes as well as axial PET (*top row*), CT (*middle row*), and PET/ CT (*bottom row*) images. Although some lesions are more conspicuous with the PSMA agent (*red arrows*), it also has high urinary excretion that obscures lesions in some images, such as on the MIP (*red arrowheads*). This patient was imaged on the CONDOR clinical trial protocol (NCT03739684).

metastatic lymph nodes and skeletal disease, particularly for patients with PSAs less than 2 ng/ mL.[70,71] For detecting local recurrence, ^{18}F-fluci- clovine is reported to be superior to ^{68}Ga-PSMA- 11 because of much lower urinary excretion, which could interfere with the detection of recurrence adjacent to the bladder (**Figs. 2** and **3**).

[18]F-fluciclovine is FDA approved for the detection of recurrent PCa and is widely commercially avail- able.[68] Ga-PSMA-11 is now FDA approved for pa- tients with suspected PCa metastasis who are potentially curable by surgery or radiation therapy (primary PCa) and for patients with suspected PCa recurrence based on elevated PSA. The approval is specific to the University of California, Los Angeles, and the University of California, San Francisco. More recently, 18F-DCFPyL PET was approved by the FDA for commercial use in the

United States for patients with prostate cancer. Other PSMA radiotracers, including fluorinated var- iants, are expected to gain FDA approval in the near future. With time, it is expected that PSMA-based radiotracers will assume a dominant role, though fluciclovine may be of value in the definition of local recurrence and with PSMA-negative or equivocal lesions. As noted above, flare has been reported with PSMA radiotracers post initiation of ADT. More study is needed to determine which radio- tracer may be useful in posttherapy monitoring and under which circumstances.

For patients with a more extensive disease burden, PSMA PET can serve as a means of selec- tion for treatment with PSMA radioligand therapy (PRLT), **Fig. 4**. PRLT appears to be effective with limited toxicities[72] and is expected to move toward regulatory approval in the future.

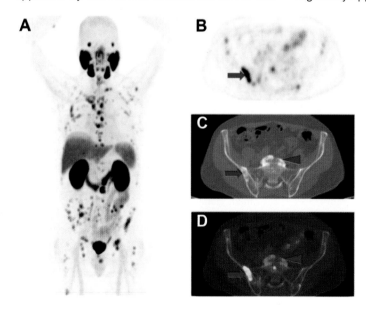

Fig. 4. An 86-year-old man with extensive bone metastatic PCa. (A) MIP, (B) axial PET, (C) axial CT, and (D) axial PET/CT images from a PSMA-targeted ^{18}F-DCFPyL scan showing extensive abnormal uptake in the visualized skeleton. Note the intense uptake in sclerotic lesions consistent with bone metastases (*red arrows*), whereas there is no uptake in degenerative sclerosis (*red arrowheads*).

CLINICS CARE POINTS

- 18F-fluciclovine and PSMA PET/CT are highly useful in detecting prostate cancer recurrence and metastases.

- Low urinary activity is an advantage for 18F-fluciclovine in detecting local recurrence, while high affinity and low background are advantages for PSMA in detecting extra-prostatic disease.

- 18F-fluciclovine PET is FDA approved for patients with biochemical recurrence, yet early data also suggest the benefit of evaluating for occult metastases in patients with higher-risk primary prostate cancer.

- The FDA recently approved the clinical use of 68Ga-PSMA-11 and 18F-DCFPyL for patients with primary and recurrent prostate cancer. It is expected that those PSMA-based radiotracers will become more predominant, with 18F-fluciclovine reserved for niche situations such as PSMA negative disease.

- PSMA PET radiotracers can be used for selecting patients for PSMA radioligand therapy (PRLT).

DISCLOSURE

B. Savir-Baruch: Grand sponsor and Consultant: Blue earth diagnostics, Lecturer: PET/NET and Blue earth diagnostics. R.A. Werner: Nothing to disclose. S.P. Rowe: Consultant, salary support, research funding from Progenics Pharmaceuticals, Inc.; Co-founder, consultant, equity in Precision Molecular, Inc.; Co-founder, consultant, equity in Plenary.ai, Inc. D.M. Schuster: Consultant: Syncona; AIM Specialty Health; Global Medical Solutions Taiwan; Progenics Pharmaceuticals, Inc. Participates through the Emory Office of Sponsored Projects in sponsored grants including those funded or partially funded by Blue Earth Diagnostics, Ltd; Nihon MediPhysics Co, Ltd.; Telix Pharmaceuticals (US) Inc.; Advanced Accelerator Applications; FUJIFILM Pharmaceuticals U.S.A., Inc; Amgen Inc.

REFERENCES

1. Zheng QH, Gardner TA, Raikwar S, et al. [11C] Choline as a PET biomarker for assessment of prostate cancer tumor models. Bioorg Med Chem 2004; 12(11):2887–93.
2. Fuchs BC, Bode BP. Amino acid transporters ASCT2 and LAT1 in cancer: partners in crime? Semin Cancer Biol 2005;15(4):254–66.
3. Schuster DM, Nanni C, Fanti S, et al. Anti-1-amino-3-18F-fluorocyclobutane-1-carboxylic acid: physiologic uptake patterns, incidental findings, and variants that may simulate disease. J Nucl Med 2014;55:1986–92.
4. Savir-Baruch B, Zanoni L, Schuster DM. Imaging of Prostate Cancer Using Fluciclovine. Urol Clin North Am 2018;45(3):489–502.
5. Tade F, Buehner T, Potkol R, et al. Feasibility of Fluciclovine PET-CT Imaging of Endometrial, Cervical, and Ovarian Cancers: Preliminary Findings. J Nucl Med 2019;60(supplement 1):558.
6. Lovrec P, Schuster DM, Wagner RH, et al. Characterizing and Mitigating Bladder Radioactivity on (18)F-Fluciclovine PET/CT. J Nucl Med Technol 2020; 48(1):24–9.
7. Savir-Baruch B, Banks KP, McConathy JE, et al. ACR-ACNM Practice Parameter for the Performance of Fluorine-18 Fluciclovine-PET/CT for Recurrent Prostate Cancer. Clin Nucl Med 2018;43(12):909–17.
8. Tade FI, Sajdak RA, Gabriel M, et al. Best practices for 18F-Fluciclovine PET/CT imaging of recurrent prostate cancer: a guide for technologists. J Nucl Med Technol 2019;47(4):282–7.
9. Nanni C, Zanoni L, Bach-Gansmo T, et al. [(18)F]Fluciclovine PET/CT: joint EANM and SNMMI procedure guideline for prostate cancer imaging-version 1.0. Eur J Nucl Med Mol Imaging 2020;47(3):579–91.
10. Barbosa FG, Queiroz MA, Nunes RF, et al. Revisiting prostate cancer recurrence with PSMA PET: atlas of typical and atypical patterns of spread. Radiographics 2019;39(1):186–212.
11. Schuster DM, Taleghani PA, Nieh PT, et al. Characterization of primary prostate carcinoma by anti-1-amino-2-[(18)F]-fluorocyclobutane-1-carboxylic acid (anti-3-[(18)F] FACBC) uptake. Am J Nucl Med Mol Imaging 2013;3(1):85–96.
12. Turkbey B, Mena E, Shih J, et al. Localized prostate cancer detection with 18F FACBC PET/CT: comparison with MR imaging and histopathologic analysis. Radiology 2014;270(3):849–56.
13. Elschot M, Selnæs KM, Sandsmark E, et al. A PET/MRI study towards finding the optimal [(18)F]Fluciclovine PET protocol for detection and characterisation of primary prostate cancer. Eur J Nucl Med Mol Imaging 2017;44(4):695–703.
14. Jambor I, Kuisma A, Kähkönen E, et al. Prospective evaluation of (18)F-FACBC PET/CT and PET/MRI versus multiparametric MRI in intermediate-to high-risk prostate cancer patients (FLUCIPRO trial). Eur J Nucl Med Mol Imaging 2018;45(3):355–64.
15. Kendall JJAA, Abiodun-Ojo OA, Alemozaffar M, et al. Fluciclovine detection of primary prostate cancer at the sextant level and correlation of SUVmax with Gleason grades. Oral Presentation presented at RSNA; 2020. Virtual.

16. Chun FK, Briganti A, Shariat SF, et al. Significant upgrading affects a third of men diagnosed with prostate cancer: predictive nomogram and internal validation. BJU Int 2006;98(2):329–34.

17. Suzuki H, Jinnouchi S, Kaji Y, et al. Diagnostic performance of 18F-fluciclovine PET/CT for regional lymph node metastases in patients with primary prostate cancer: a multicenter phase II clinical trial. Jpn J Clin Oncol 2019;49(9):803–11.

18. Selnaes KM, Kruger-Stokke B, Elschot M, et al. (18)F-Fluciclovine PET/MRI for preoperative lymph node staging in high-risk prostate cancer patients. Eur Radiol 2018;28(8):3151–9.

19. Alemozaffar M, Akintayo AA, Abiodun-Ojo OA, et al. [(18)F]Fluciclovine positron emission tomography/Computerized tomography for preoperative staging in patients with intermediate to high risk primary prostate cancer. J Urol 2020;204(4):734–40.

20. Schuster DM, Votaw JR, Nieh PT, et al. Initial experience with the radiotracer anti-1-amino-3-18F-fluorocyclobutane-1-carboxylic acid with PET/CT in prostate carcinoma. J Nucl Med 2007;48(1):56–63.

21. Odewole OA, Tade FI, Nieh PT, et al. Recurrent prostate cancer detection with anti-3-[(18)F]FACBC PET/CT: comparison with CT. Eur J Nucl Med Mol Imaging 2016;43(10):1773–83.

22. Schuster DM, Nieh PT, Jani AB, et al. Anti-3-[(18)F]FACBC positron emission tomography-computerized tomography and (111)In-capromab pendetide single photon emission computerized tomography-computerized tomography for recurrent prostate carcinoma: results of a prospective clinical trial. J Urol 2014;191(5):1446–53.

23. Abiodun-Ojo OA, Akintayo AA, Akin-Akintayo OO, et al. 18F-Fluciclovine parameters on targeted prostate biopsy associated with true positivity in recurrent prostate cancer. J Nucl Med 2019;60(11):1531–6.

24. Bach-Gansmo T, Nanni C, Nieh PT, et al. Multisite experience of the safety, detection rate and diagnostic performance of Fluciclovine ((18)F) positron emission tomography/Computerized tomography imaging in the staging of biochemically recurrent prostate cancer. J Urol 2017;197(3 Pt 1):676–83.

25. Andriole GL, Kostakoglu L, Chau A, et al. The impact of positron emission tomography with 18F-Fluciclovine on the treatment of biochemical recurrence of prostate cancer: results from the LOCATE trial. J Urol 2019;201(2):322–31.

26. Scarsbrook AF, Bottomley D, Teoh EJ, et al. Effect of (18)F-Fluciclovine positron emission tomography on the management of patients with recurrence of prostate cancer: results from the FALCON trial. Int J Radiat Oncol Biol Phys 2020;107(2):316–24.

27. Savir-Baruch B, Lovrec P, Solanki AA, et al. Fluorine-18-Labeled Fluciclovine PET/CT in clinical practice: factors affecting the rate of detection of recurrent prostate cancer. AJR Am J Roentgenol 2019; 213(4):851–8.

28. Jani AB, Schreibmann E, Goyal S, et al. Initial report of a randomized trial comparing conventional- vs conventional plus fluciclovine (18F) PET/CT imaging-guided post-prostatectomy radiotherapy for prostate cancer. Int J Radiat Oncol Biol Phys 2020;108(5):P1397.

29. Akin-Akintayo OO, Jani AB, Odewole O, et al. Change in salvage radiotherapy management based on guidance with FACBC (Fluciclovine) PET/CT in postprostatectomy recurrent prostate cancer. Clin Nucl Med 2017;42(1):e22–8.

30. Wang Y, Chow DZ, Ebert E, et al. Utility of (18)F-Fluciclovine PET/CT for detecting prostate cancer recurrence in patients with low (< 1 ng/mL) or very low (< 0.3 ng/mL) prostate-specific antigen levels. AJR Am J Roentgenol 2020;215(4):997–1001.

31. England JR, Paluch J, Ballas LK, et al. 18F-Fluciclovine PET/CT detection of recurrent prostate carcinoma in patients with serum PSA </= 1 ng/mL after definitive primary treatment. Clin Nucl Med 2019;44(3):e128–32.

32. Kim YPLP, Wagner RH, Gabriel MS, et al. Potential use of fluciclovine PET/CT as follow-up modality in patients with biochemically recurrent prostate cancer. Chicago: RSNA; 2019. Monday, Dec. 2 8:55AM - 9:05AM, 2019.

33. Galgano SJ, McDonald AM, Rais-Bahrami S, et al. Utility of ^{18}F-Fluciclovine PET/MRI for staging newly diagnosed high-risk prostate cancer and evaluating response to initial androgen deprivation therapy: a prospective single-arm pilot study. AJR Am J Roentgenol 2020. [Epub ahead of print].

34. Barinka C, Rojas C, Slusher B, et al. Glutamate carboxypeptidase II in diagnosis and treatment of neurologic disorders and prostate cancer. Curr Med Chem 2012;19(6):856–70.

35. Wright GL Jr, Haley C, Beckett ML, et al. Expression of prostate-specific membrane antigen in normal, benign, and malignant prostate tissues. Urol Oncol 1995;1(1):18–28.

36. Perner S, Hofer MD, Kim R, et al. Prostate-specific membrane antigen expression as a predictor of prostate cancer progression. Hum Pathol 2007; 38(5):696–701.

37. Rowe SP, Gorin MA, Pomper MG. Imaging of prostate-specific membrane antigen with small-molecule PET radiotracers: from the bench to advanced clinical applications. Annu Rev Med 2019;70:461–77.

38. Perera M, Papa N, Christidis D, et al. Sensitivity, specificity, and predictors of positive (68)Ga-prostate-specific membrane antigen positron emission tomography in advanced prostate cancer: a systematic review and meta-analysis. Eur Urol 2016;70(6):926–37.

39. Cho SY, Gage KL, Mease RC, et al. Biodistribution, tumor detection, and radiation dosimetry of 18F-DCFBC, a low-molecular-weight inhibitor of prostate-specific membrane antigen, in patients with metastatic prostate cancer. J Nucl Med 2012; 53(12):1883–91.

40. Szabo Z, Mena E, Rowe SP, et al. Initial Evaluation of [(18)F]DCFPyL for Prostate-Specific Membrane Antigen (PSMA)-targeted PET imaging of prostate cancer. Mol Imaging Biol 2015;17(4):565–74.

41. Giesel FL, Hadaschik B, Cardinale J, et al. F-18 labelled PSMA-1007: biodistribution, radiation dosimetry and histopathological validation of tumor lesions in prostate cancer patients. Eur J Nucl Med Mol Imaging 2017;44(4):678–88.

42. Oh SW, Wurzer A, Teoh EJ, et al. Quantitative and qualitative analyses of biodistribution and PET image quality of a novel radiohybrid PSMA, (18)F-rhPSMA-7, in patients with prostate cancer. J Nucl Med 2020;61(5):702–9.

43. Fendler WP, Eiber M, Beheshti M, et al. 68)Ga-PSMA PET/CT: Joint EANM and SNMMI procedure guideline for prostate cancer imaging: version 1.0. Eur J Nucl Med Mol Imaging 2017;44(6):1014–24.

44. Werner RA, Derlin T, Lapa C, et al. 18F-Labeled, PSMA-targeted radiotracers: leveraging the advantages of radiofluorination for prostate cancer molecular imaging. Theranostics 2020;10(1):1–16.

45. Schmuck S, Nordlohne S, von Klot CA, et al. Comparison of standard and delayed imaging to improve the detection rate of [(68)Ga]PSMA I&T PET/CT in patients with biochemical recurrence or prostate-specific antigen persistence after primary therapy for prostate cancer. Eur J Nucl Med Mol Imaging 2017;44(6):960–8.

46. Ferreira G, Iravani A, Hofman MS, et al. Intra-individual comparison of (68)Ga-PSMA-11 and (18)F-DCFPyL normal-organ biodistribution. Cancer Imaging 2019; 19(1):23.

47. Werner RA, Sheikhbahaei S, Jones KM, et al. Patterns of uptake of prostate-specific membrane antigen (PSMA)-targeted (18)F-DCFPyL in peripheral ganglia. Ann Nucl Med 2017;31(9):696–702.

48. Sheikhbahaei S, Werner RA, Solnes LB, et al. Prostate-Specific Membrane Antigen (PSMA)-targeted PET imaging of prostate cancer: an update on important pitfalls. Semin Nucl Med 2019;49(4):255–70.

49. Eiber M, Herrmann K, Calais J, et al. Prostate Cancer Molecular Imaging Standardized Evaluation (PROMISE): proposed miTNM classification for the interpretation of PSMA-Ligand PET/CT. J Nucl Med 2018;59(3):469–78.

50. Fendler WP, Calais J, Eiber M, et al. Assessment of 68Ga-PSMA-11 PET accuracy in localizing recurrent prostate cancer: a prospective single-arm clinical trial. JAMA Oncol 2019;5(6):856–63.

51. Rowe SP, Pienta KJ, Pomper MG, et al. Proposal for a structured reporting system for prostate-specific membrane antigen-targeted PET imaging: PSMA-RADS Version 1.0. J Nucl Med 2018;59(3):479–85.

52. Werner RA, Bundschuh RA, Bundschuh L, et al. Interobserver agreement for the standardized reporting system PSMA-RADS 1.0 on (18)F-DCFPyL PET/CT imaging. J Nucl Med 2018;59(12):1857–64.

53. Rowe SP, Gage KL, Faraj SF, et al. 1)(8)F-DCFBC PET/CT for PSMA-based detection and characterization of primary prostate cancer. J Nucl Med 2015;56(7):1003–10.

54. Eiber M, Weirich G, Holzapfel K, et al. Simultaneous (68)Ga-PSMA HBED-CC PET/MRI improves the localization of primary prostate cancer. Eur Urol 2016;70(5):829–36.

55. Hicks RM, Simko JP, Westphalen AC, et al. Diagnostic accuracy of (68)Ga-PSMA-11 PET/MRI compared with multiparametric MRI in the detection of prostate cancer. Radiology 2018;289(3):730–7.

56. Azadi J, Nguyen ML, Leroy A, et al. The emerging role of imaging in prostate cancer secondary screening: multiparametric magnetic resonance imaging and the incipient incorporation of molecular imaging. Br J Radiol 2018;91(1090):20170960.

57. Budaus L, Leyh-Bannurah SR, Salomon G, et al. Initial experience of (68)Ga-PSMA PET/CT imaging in high-risk prostate cancer patients prior to radical prostatectomy. Eur Urol 2016;69(3):393–6.

58. Gorin MA, Rowe SP, Patel HD, et al. Prostate Specific Membrane Antigen Targeted (18)F-DCFPyL Positron Emission Tomography/Computerized Tomography for the Preoperative Staging of High Risk Prostate Cancer: Results of a Prospective, Phase II, Single Center Study. J Urol 2018;199(1): 126–32.

59. Rowe S, Gorin M, Pienta K, et al. Results from the OSPREY trial: A PrOspective Phase 2/3 Multi-Center Study of 18F-DCFPyL PET/CT Imaging in Patients with PRostate Cancer - Examination of Diagnostic AccuracY. J Nucl Med 2019;60(supplement 1):586.

60. Robertson GS, Johnson PR, Bolia A, et al. Long-term results of unilateral neck exploration for preoperatively localized nonfamilial parathyroid adenomas. Am J Surg 1996;172(4):311–4.

61. van Leeuwen PJ, Donswijk M, Nandurkar R, et al. Gallium-68-prostate-specific membrane antigen ((68)Ga-PSMA) positron emission tomography (PET)/ computed tomography (CT) predicts complete biochemical response from radical prostatectomy and lymph node dissection in intermediate- and high-risk prostate cancer. BJU Int 2019;124(1):62–8.

62. Hofman MS, Lawrentschuk N, Francis RJ, et al. Prostate-specific membrane antigen PET-CT in patients with high-risk prostate cancer before curative-intent surgery or radiotherapy (proPSMA):

a prospective, randomised, multicentre study. Lancet 2020;395(10231):1208–16.

63. Rowe SP, Macura KJ, Mena E, et al. PSMA-Based [(18)F]DCFPyL PET/CT is superior to conventional imaging for lesion detection in patients with metastatic prostate cancer. Mol Imaging Biol 2016;18(3): 411–9.

64. Rowe SP, Campbell SP, Mana-Ay M, et al. Prospective Evaluation of PSMA-Targeted (18)F-DCFPyL PET/CT in Men with biochemical failure after radical prostatectomy for prostate cancer. J Nucl Med 2020; 61(1):58–61.

65. Phillips R, Shi WY, Deek M, et al. Outcomes of observation vs stereotactic ablative radiation for oligometastatic prostate cancer: The ORIOLE Phase 2 Randomized Clinical Trial. JAMA Oncol 2020;6(5): 650–9.

66. Hope TA, Truillet C, Ehman EC, et al. 68Ga-PSMA-11 PET Imaging of response to androgen receptor inhibition: first human experience. J Nucl Med 2017; 58(1):81–4.

67. Afshar-Oromieh A, Debus N, Uhrig M, et al. Impact of long-term androgen deprivation therapy on PSMA ligand PET/CT in patients with castration-sensitive prostate cancer. Eur J Nucl Med Mol Imaging 2018;45(12):2045–54.

68. Aggarwal R, Wei X, Kim W, et al. Heterogeneous flare in prostate-specific membrane antigen positron emission tomography tracer uptake with initiation of androgen pathway blockade in metastatic prostate cancer. Eur Urol Oncol 2018;1(1):78–82.

69. Fanti S, Hadaschik B, Herrmann K. Proposal for systemic-therapy response-assessment criteria at the time of PSMA PET/CT imaging: The PSMA PET progression criteria. J Nucl Med 2020;61(5):678–82.

70. Calais J, Ceci F, Eiber M, et al. 18F-fluciclovine PET-CT and (68)Ga-PSMA-11 PET-CT in patients with early biochemical recurrence after prostatectomy: a prospective, single-centre, single-arm, comparative imaging trial. Lancet Oncol 2019;20(9):1286–94.

71. Pernthaler B, Kulnik R, Gstettner C, et al. A prospective head-to-head comparison of 18F-Fluciclovine With 68Ga-PSMA-11 in biochemical recurrence of prostate cancer in PET/CT. Clin Nucl Med 2019;44(10):e566–73.

72. Hofman MS, Violet J, Hicks RJ, et al. [(177)Lu]-PSMA-617 radionuclide treatment in patients with metastatic castration-resistant prostate cancer (LuPSMA trial): a single-centre, single-arm, phase 2 study. Lancet Oncol 2018;19(6):825–33.

PET Imaging for Gynecologic Malignancies

Saul N. Friedman, MD, PhD[a], Malak Itani, MD[b], Farrokh Dehdashti, MD[c],*

KEYWORDS

• PET • Endometrial cancer • Ovarian cancer • Cervical cancer • Vaginal cancer • Vulvar cancer

KEY POINTS

• 2-Deoxy-2-[^{18}F]fluoro-D-glucose (FDG) PET generally has high sensitivity for advanced disease but limited specificity, making it a useful tool for late-stage disease and detecting malignant recurrence, but limiting its role for diagnosis.
• FDG uptake has been correlated with tumor aggressiveness, and can help with treatment planning, particularly of radiation treatment fields.
• Vaginal and vulvar cancers are less common than endometrial, ovarian, and cervical cancers, and investigations on the role of PET are less conclusive and require further studies.
• Many new and emerging PET tracers are promising for evaluating and mapping different receptors, cell proliferation rates, and even hypoxia, helping to direct treatment, but most still require additional testing before they are ready for standard clinical use.

INTRODUCTION

Approximately 94,000 new cases of gynecologic cancer are diagnosed in the United States each year. Gynecologic cancers are typically separated into 5 groups based on anatomy, listed here from most to least common: endometrium/uterine body, ovary, cervix, vagina, and vulva.[1] Incidence rates are summarized in **Table 1**. These cancers have diverse clinical presentations and prognoses, and their treatment typically includes a combination of radical surgery, chemotherapy, and/or radiotherapy based on the stage of disease.

The stage of disease at diagnosis is predictive of prognosis and is crucial for selection of the best mode of therapy. Gynecologic cancers are typically staged using the International Federation of Gynecology and Obstetrics (FIGO) criteria. Imaging plays an important role in pretreatment evaluation of patients with gynecologic malignancies as well as in the follow-up for response assessment to therapy and detection of disease recurrence. Imaging of the female pelvis can be achieved using a combination of ultrasonography (US), computed tomography (CT), magnetic resonance (MR) imaging, and PET/CT using 2-deoxy-2-[^{18}F]fluoro-D-glucose (FDG) and other emerging radiopharmaceuticals. PET/CT is known to be more accurate than CT or MR imaging alone for staging and can help direct management.[2]

This article discusses the use of FDG-PET/CT and PET/MR for clinical evaluation of the most common types of gynecologic cancers: endometrial, ovarian, cervical, vaginal, and vulvar cancers.

PET RADIOPHARMACEUTICALS AND IMAGING PROTOCOLS

Anatomic evaluation of gynecologic malignancies is typically performed with a combination of CT and MR imaging.[2–4] PET is commonly coupled with concurrent CT for attenuation correction and

[a] Division of Nuclear Medicine, Edward Mallinckrodt Institute of Radiology, Washington University School of Medicine, 510 South Kingshighway Boulevard, St Louis, MO 63110, USA; [b] Section of Abdominal Imaging, Edward Mallinckrodt Institute of Radiology, Washington University School of Medicine, 510 South Kingshighway Boulevard, St Louis, MO 63110, USA; [c] Division of Nuclear Medicine, Edward Mallinckrodt Institute of Radiology, Alvin J. Siteman Cancer Center, Washington University School of Medicine, 510 South Kingshighway Boulevard, St Louis, MO 63110, USA
* Corresponding author.
E-mail address: dehdashtif@wustl.edu

Radiol Clin N Am 59 (2021) 813–833
https://doi.org/10.1016/j.rcl.2021.05.011

Table 1
Incidence of primary gynecologic cancers based on the Centers for Disease Control and Prevention US data from 2012 to 2016[1]

Cancer Location	Incident Cases per 100,000
Uterine body	26.82
Ovary	11.18
Cervix	7.60
Vulvar	2.62
Vaginal	0.66

anatomic localization, which is often of lower resolution than dedicated CT studies and is often performed without contrast. PET/MR imaging is a more recent innovation, but access remains limited to larger institutions and it is not in widespread use. To allow a more in-depth PET review, anatomic evaluation is not the focus of this article. The focus is on FDG because of its widespread clinical use and accepted role in evaluation in malignant diseases. However, it also briefly reviews clinically approved non-FDG radiopharmaceuticals, including somatostatin-receptor and steroid-receptor imaging agents, as well as radiopharmaceuticals that are currently used in research settings that have clinical potential, including human epidermal growth factor receptors (EGFR), DNA-precursor use, and cell hypoxia imaging tracers. The PET tracers discussed here are summarized in **Table 2** along with key procedural parameters.

Glucose Metabolism

FDG ([18]F: half-life $T_{1/2} = 109.7$ minutes), a glucose analogue, is the most common tracer used for clinical evaluation of patients with gynecologic malignancies. The biological basis for the use of FDG in oncology is the Warburg effect, which describes an increase in glycolysis under aerobic conditions and is characteristic of the malignant state. FDG is taken up by the cell using glucose transporters and phosphorylated by hexokinase to FDG–6 phosphate (FDG-6P). FDG-6P is not a good substrate for further metabolism and is trapped within the cell, because glucose 6-phosphatase is markedly downregulated in cancer cells.

Patient preparation for FDG-PET imaging of gynecologic tumors typically follows the Society of Nuclear Medicine and Molecular Imaging guidelines, which includes fasting for at least 4 hours and fasting blood glucose level less than or equal to 200 mg/dL. Typical doses are within 10 to 20 mCi (370–740 MBq). Urinary tract preparation that involves placement of a Foley catheter, intravenous administration of fluids, and furosemide may be performed for evaluation of gynecologic cancers for evaluating lesions close to the bladder. Imaging typically begins 60 minutes after administration of FDG. Standard imaging from the skull base to the thighs typically takes approximately 20 minutes, but depends on patient size and scanner technology. Anatomic imaging protocols differ between institutions and scanners. Although CT oral contrast is used in many centers, the use of intravenous contrast is controversial and limited to some centers. CT images are typically acquired before PET acquisition.

For PET/MR imaging, routine pelvic MR protocols are acquired with and without intravenous contrast, use of antiperistaltic medications, and intravaginal contrast. Acquired sequences differ between institutions, but typically include T1-weighted and T2-weighted sequences, diffusion-weighted imaging, and postcontrast imaging, which enables better evaluation of structures and possible tumor invasion. The use of dynamic contrast-enhanced imaging allows the evaluation of tissue perfusion and oxygenation.[5,6] Although PET/CT enables direct calculation of attenuation correction from the CT data, MR imaging relies on determining tumor composition and associated look-up tables. A common technique relies on Dixon sequences to delineate up to 4 materials within a given pixel, typically background/air, soft tissue, fat, and lung. Limitations include the inability to always properly delineate organs, particularly the lungs, and the inability to accurately identify cortical bone because of insufficient signal, both of which affect the attenuation correction and resulting standardized uptake value (SUV) accuracy.[7,8]

PET analysis is both qualitative and quantitative. Qualitative analysis compares potential malignant uptake with physiologic uptake, including hepatic uptake, blood pool activity, and adjacent organ parenchymal activity. Quantitative uptake most commonly relies on the maximum SUV (SUV_{max}) because of ease of measurement, but SUV mean and peak, as well as metabolic tumor volume (MTV) and total lesion glycolysis (TLG), are becoming more accepted.

Estrogen Receptors

There are 2 types of estrogen receptors (ERs): ERα and ERβ.[9] 16α-^{18}F-fluoro-17β-estradiol (FES) is an estrogen analogue that was recently approved by US Food and Drug Administration (FDA) for imaging advanced breast cancer and provides imaging

Table 2
PET tracers for evaluation of gynecologic cancers

PET Tracer	Half-Life $(T_{1/2})$	Typical Dose	Uptake Time	Fasting State
^{18}F-FDG	109.7 min	370–740 MBq (10–20 mCi)	60 min	At least 4 h
^{68}Ga-DOTATOC ^{68}Ga-DOTATATE ^{68}Ga-DOTANOC	68 min	132–222 MBq (4–6 mCi); should not be <100 MBq (2.7 mCi)	60 min	Not required
[64]Cu-DOTATATE	12.7 h	148 MBq (4 mCi)	45–90 min	Not required
^{18}F-FES	109.7 min	222 MBq (6 mCi); range 111–222 MBq (3–6 mCi)	60 min; range 20–80 min	Not required
[89]Zr-labeled lumretuzumab	3.27 d	37 MBq (1 mCi)	2, 4, and 7 d	Not required
^{18}F-FLT	109.7 min	2.6 MBq/kg (0.07 mCi/kg); maximum dose 185 MBq (5 mCi)	60–70 min	Not required
^{18}F-FMISO	109.7 min	3.7 MBq/kg (0.1 mCi/kg); maximum 260 MBq (7 mCi)	$\geq$2 h	Not required
[60]Cu-ATSM ^{64}Cu-ATSM	23.7 min 12.7 h	481–740 MBq (13–20 mCi) 925 MBq (25 mCi)	60-min dynamic imaging and/or static imaging at 30 min	Not required

^{18}F-FDG, ^{68}Ga-DOTA-peptides, and ^{64}Cu-DOTATATE are commonly used in clinical practice, whereas the remaining tracers are mostly investigational.

Abbreviations: ATSM, diacetyl-bis(N4-ethylthiosemicarbazone); DOTATOC, 1, 4, 7, 10-tetraazacyclododecane- N, N′, N″, N‴-tetraacetic acid-D-Phe 1-Tyr 3-octreotide; DOTATATE, 1, 4, 7, 10-tetraazacyclododecane- N, N′, N″, N‴-tetraacetic acid-D-Phe 1, Tyr 3-octreotate; DOTANOC, 1, 4, 7, 10-tetraazacyclododecane- N, N′, N″, N‴-tetraacetic acid-Nal3-octreotide; FES, 16α-^{18}F-fluoro-17β-estradiol; FLT, 3′-deoxy-3′-[^{18}F]fluorothymidine; FMISO, 1-(2′nitro-1′-imidazolyl)-3-fluoro-2-propranol.

of ERs through selective binding of the ERα isoform.[10,11] However, its use in other cancers, including gynecologic cancers, is limited to research settings under investigational new drug applications. FES is the most investigated steroid-receptor tracer. Typical dose is 6 mCi (222 MBq) with a typical range of 3 to 6 mCi (111–222 MBq). Recommended imaging is 80 minutes (range of 20–80 minutes), but typically investigators use 60 minutes after administration before starting imaging.[10] Fasting is not required.

Cell Proliferation

3′-Deoxy-3′-[^{18}F]fluorothymidine (FLT)[12,13] is a pyrimidine analogue of thymidine, a DNA precursor intended to evaluate cell proliferation rate, but is more a measure of S-phase fraction. Its uptake is via passive diffusion and facilitated transport by type 1 equilibrate nucleoside transporters (ENT1).[14] Although FLT is a specific marker for cell proliferation and a better marker for evaluation of response to therapy than FDG, physiologic uptake of FLT in the bone marrow caused by increased cell proliferation, in the liver secondary to hepatic glucuronidation, and in the urinary tract

as part of the renal clearance of the tracer represent the main limitations of the method.[15] Investigators have used a dose of 0.07 mCi/kg (2.6 MBq/kg), maximum dose of 5 mCi (185 MBq), infused intravenously over 2 minutes, with PET images acquired 60 to 70 minutes after injection for imaging of cervical cancer.[16,17] Patient fasting was not an explicit requirement of the protocol.

Hypoxia

Tumor hypoxia inhibits radiation therapy by decreasing the availability of oxygen free radicals that cause tumor DNA damage and cell death. Tumor hypoxia also likely limits the efficacy of chemotherapy. Polarographic oxygen sensors are the gold standard of evaluating hypoxia but are limited by the invasive technique and inherent sampling limitations. PET offers a noninvasive means to reliably evaluate the entire tumor and multiple tumor sites at the same time. The PET agents for assessing hypoxia are in 2 groups.[18] The first is fluorine-labeled nitroimidazoles such as 1-(2′nitro-1′-imidazolyl)-3-fluoro-2-propranol (FMISO)[19]; [^{18}F]fluoroazomycin arabinoside (FAZA), a second-generation 2-nitroimidazole; and [^{18}F]fluoroerythronitroimidazole

(FETNIM), which is more hydrophilic than FMISO. The second group is copper-labeled diacetyl-bis(N4-ethylthiosemicarbazone) (Cu-ATSM) analogues (^{60}Cu, $T_{1/2}$ = 23.7 minutes; ^{61}Cu, $T_{1/2}$ = 3.32 hours; ^{62}Cu, $T_{1/2}$ = 9.7 minutes; and ^{64}Cu, $T_{1/2}$ = 12.7 hours), which have neutral lipophilic molecules with high cell membrane permeability, and are reduced and trapped in hypoxic cells.

A standard dose of FMISO is 0.1 mCi/kg (3.7 MBq/kg) up to a maximum of 7 mCi (260 MBq).[19] A combination of low tumor uptake, slow accumulation in hypoxic tissues, and slow clearance from normoxic tissue caused by the lipophilic nature of the tracer necessitates long wait periods, of 2 hours or more, between injection and imaging.[20]

For ^{60}Cu-ATSM, a typical dose of 13 to 20 mCi (481–740 MBq) and for ^{64}Cu-ATSM, a typical dose of 25 mCi (925 MBq) injected intravenously, followed by 60 minutes of dynamic imaging[21,22] or static imaging at 30 minutes after injections, have been reported.[23]

ENDOMETRIAL CANCER

Approximately 75% to 80% of patients with endometrial cancer are postmenopausal. This disease typically presents with abnormal bleeding resulting in early-stage diagnosis in 75% of patients.[24] The risk factors include abdominal obesity, multiparity, late menopause, smoking, unopposed estrogen therapy, tamoxifen, Lynch syndrome, and diabetes; hormone replacement therapy, although a risk factor, is no longer typically prescribed.[25] There are 2 histologic subtypes: type 1 are well differentiated estrogen-associated endometrioid adenocarcinomas accounting for 75% to 80% and expressing high levels of ERs. Type 2 are aggressive, undifferentiated, estrogen-independent cancers that typically develop in atrophic endometrium and include adenosquamous, serous papillary, clear cell, and undifferentiated types.[25] FIGO staging of endometrial cancer, which was revised in 2009 and is summarized in Table 3,[26] does not include an imaging component. However, MR imaging is highly sensitive and specific for revealing important prognostic factors and thus, when available, is recommended as an adjunct to clinical examination.[27,28]

FIGO staging does include involvement of locoregional and distant nodal metastases, which PET can aid in detecting. Nodal metastatic pattern is predominately pelvic, following anterior pelvic, lateral pelvic, hypogastric, and presacral routes, but can then spread to para-aortic lymph nodes[29]; this reflects stage III disease, with para-aortic involvement being more advanced IIIC2 (see Table 3). Fig. 1 shows an example of recurrent endometrial cancer. More distant nodal spread to abdominal and/or inguinal lymph nodes reflects stage IV disease.[27] Fig. 2 shows recurrent endometrial adenocarcinoma with distant metastasis.

FDG-PET

FDG-PET has a limited role in initial staging. Chang and colleagues[30] reported a pooled sensitivity for the detection of pelvic and/or para-aortic metastasis of only 63% based on their meta-analysis, which is insufficient to replace lymphadenectomy. A more recent meta-analysis showed the overall pooled sensitivity, specificity, and area under the curve (AUC) of FDG-PET/CT for detection of lymph node metastases to be 72% (95% confidence interval [CI], 63%–80%), 94% (CI, 93%–96%), and 94% (CI, 85%–99%), respectively, with an overall diagnostic accuracy (Q* index) of 88%.[31] Most patients with advanced disease also benefit from surgical debulking, and thus the results of FDG-PET are unlikely to deter surgery. However, FDG-PET can play a role in identification of distant metastases and treatment planning, particularly for radiation therapy.[24] Furthermore, greater uterine tumor SUV_{max} has been correlated with greater tumor aggressiveness. In particular, Kitajima and colleagues[32] discovered that patients with SUV_{max} 12.7 or greater had a significantly lower disease-free survival rate (P = .00042). FDG-PET also has high sensitivity for detection of both local and distant recurrence, ranging from 85.7% to 100%,[33,34] and may therefore be useful for post-therapy surveillance and detection of recurrent disease. In a recent meta-analysis, FDG-PET/CT had an overall pooled sensitivity, specificity, and AUC for detection of endometrial cancer recurrence of 95% (CI, 91%–98%), 91% (CI, 86%–94%), and 97% (CI, 95%–98%), respectively, with overall diagnostic accuracy (Q* index) of 93%.[31] The National Comprehensive Cancer Network (NCCN) suggests considering FDG-PET/CT if metastasis is suspected at initial staging and for evaluation of suspected recurrence.

2-Deoxy-2-[^{18}F]fluoro-D-glucose PET/ Magnetic Resonance

Data on PET/MR are not as extensive as for PET/CT because of its recent clinical adoption. However, in gynecologic as well as nongynecologic malignancies, several investigators[35–37] have already noted that PET/MR is superior to PET/CT in diagnosing brain and liver metastases, as well as removing the diagnostic uncertainty of some abdominal findings; nonetheless, PET/CT remains superior for diagnosing lung metastases. No statistically significant advantage of PET/MR compared

Table 3
Summary of the revised International Federation of Gynecology and Obstetrics staging of endometrial cancer with adaptation of magnetic resonance findings[27]

Stage I	Carcinoma confined to the uterus
IA	<50% invasion of the myometrium MR: abnormal signal intensity in endometrial cavity or confined to inner half of myometrium
IB	≥50% invasion of the myometrium MR: extends into the outer half of myometrium
Stage II	Cervical stromal invasion without extension beyond the uterus MR: disruption or focal thinning of cervical stroma
Stage III	Carcinoma spread locally
IIIA	Serosal or adnexal invasion MR: disruption or irregular uterine contour caused by tumor; ovarian nodular tumor
IIIB	Vaginal or parametrial involvement MR: direct tumor extension of upper vagina or/and parametrial tissues
IIIC	Metastasis to pelvic or para-aortic lymph nodes
IIIC1	Metastasis to pelvic lymph node MR: lymph nodes >8 mm in short axis
IIIC2	Metastasis to para-aortic lymph node MR: lymph nodes >10 mm in short axis
Stage IV	Extension to the pelvic wall, lower one-third of the vagina, or hydronephrosis or nonfunctioning kidney
IVA	Bladder or bowel mucosal invasion MR: disruption of bladder or bowel muscular wall with mucosal invasion; not bullous edema
IVB	Distant metastases, including abdominal, or involvement of inguinal lymph nodes MR: tumor deposits at distal sites including peritoneal metastasis, bladder, bone liver metastasis, and distal lymph node metastases

with PET/CT has been ascertained, but data remain limited. Tsuyoshi and colleagues[38] found that non-enhanced PET/MR has similar accuracy to contrast-enhanced CT and that greater SUV/apparent diffusion coefficient (ADC) ratio correlated with high-risk cancers.[39] One of the important advantages of PET/MR, which contributed to the addition of MR, is the evaluation of myometrial invasion because of its high soft tissue resolution.[40] Integrated PET/MR proved significantly more accurate than PET/CT. Bian and colleagues[40] reported an overall detection accuracy of myometrial invasion for PET/CT and integrated PET/MR of 45.9% and 81.8%, respectively (P<.001). The depth of myometrial invasion is an important prognostic factor because it strongly correlates with the risk of lymph node metastasis and prognosis in patients with endometrial cancer.[41] **Fig. 3** shows an example of FDG-PET/MR and the superiority of MR in evaluation of endometrial cancer.

16α-^{18}F-fluoro-17β-estradiol PET

Endometrial cancer is traditionally divided into estrogen dependent (type 1) and estrogen independent (type 2).[42] The presence of ERα and progesterone receptor in endometrial carcinoma correlates positively with clinical response rate and improved survival, and thus is a potential predictive and prognostic biomarker.[43] Tsujikawa and colleagues[44,45] showed that increasing ratios of FDG/FES uptake can be used as a predictor of not only malignant versus benign tumors but also of malignant aggressiveness and stage. They determined an optimal cutoff ratio of 2.0 resulting in 73% sensitivity, 100% specificity, and 86% accuracy for differentiating malignant from benign lesions, outperforming the 77% accuracy for MR imaging, and noted that a cutoff ratio of 0.5 differentiated carcinoma from hyperplasia with 100% accuracy.[44,45] Results suggest that endometrial carcinoma has a

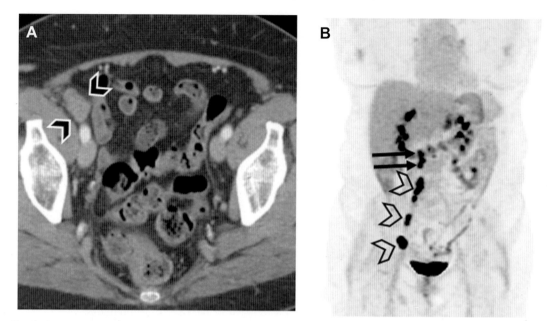

Fig. 1. Restaging FDG-PET/CT of a 72-year-old woman with recurrent endometrial malignant mixed müllerian tumor (carcinosarcoma) after hysterectomy, salpingo-oophorectomy, and adjuvant chemotherapy. (A) Axial contrast-enhanced CT image shows a large multilobulated right external iliac lymph node (*arrowheads*). (B) Maximum intensity projection (MIP) image show markedly hypermetabolic lymphadenopathy along the right external and common iliac chains (*arrowheads*), as well as in the retroperitoneum (*arrows*).

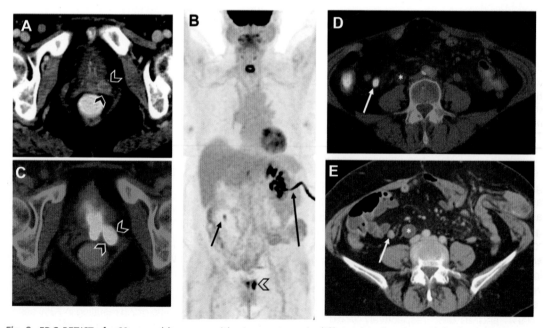

Fig. 2. FDG-PET/CT of a 69-year-old woman with recurrent poorly differentiated endometrial adenocarcinoma in the vaginal wall, presenting 13 years after original cancer resection. (A) Axial contrast-enhanced CT image shows an enhancing nodule along the left vaginal wall (*arrowheads*) without additional sites of metastasis. (B, C) PET/CT performed 4 weeks later confirmed a hypermetabolic recurrent left vaginal wall nodule (*arrowheads*) with (D) a metastatic hypermetabolic mesenteric lymph node (*short arrows in B and D*), which retrospectively was present on (E) the prior CT (*arrow*). (D, E) A dilated right ureter caused by a distal ureteral stricture (*asterisks*) and a left nephrostomy tube (*long arrow in B*) are also present.

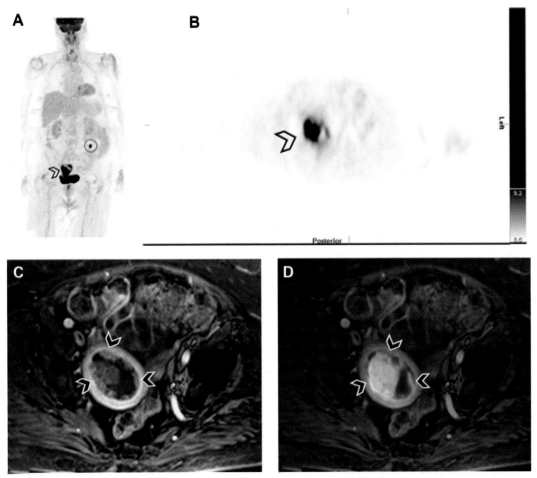

Fig. 3. A 64-year-old woman with postmenopausal vaginal bleeding. Pelvic examination showed a bulky cervix with central ulceration, and biopsy was consistent with endometrial endometrioid adenocarcinoma, International Federation of Gynecology and Obstetrics (FIGO) grade II. FDG-PET/MR imaging was performed for initial staging. (*A*) MIP and (*B*) axial attenuation-corrected PET images show a markedly hypermetabolic mass (*arrowheads*) in the endometrial cavity corresponding with a heterogeneously enhancing mass (*arrowheads*) on (*C*) axial T1-postcontrast MR imaging and (*D*) fused images. Incidentally noted was a hypermetabolic focus in the sigmoid colon (*circle in A*), corresponding with a 3-cm excised tubulovillous adenoma on subsequent colonoscopy.

reduced estrogen dependency and increased glucose metabolism. Zhao and colleagues[46] evaluated FDG and FES as noninvasive biomarkers to assess uterine tumor hormone-receptor expression, glucose metabolism, and proliferation and as a tool to differentiate between uterine leiomyomas and sarcomas. They found a similar relationship of increased FDG/FES ratio in sarcomas compared with leiomyomas of 5.9 ± 3.9 versus 0.9 ± 0.5, respectively.[46] Now that FES is approved in breast cancer, it is possible that this tracer will be available for evaluating gynecologic cancers in the future.

3′-Deoxy-3′-[18F]fluorothymidine PET

Uterine leiomyoma is a common benign endometrial tumor, whereas leiomyosarcoma is a rare malignant tumor. However, leiomyomas occasionally resemble leiomyosarcoma on MR imaging and clinical presentation. Limited data are available for using FLT to distinguish between benign and malignant leiomyomas such as leiomyosarcomas.[47] Yamane and colleagues[47] showed that, although FDG and FLT both had sensitivities and negative predictive values (NPVs) for malignancies of 100%, FLT had better specificity, positive predictive value (PPV), and accuracy of 90.0%, 83.9%, and 93.3% compared with FDG values of 70.0%, 62.5%, and 80.0%, respectively. They also noted that FLT had better correlation with Ki-67 labeling index compared with FDG, with $R^2 = 0.91$ compared with $R^2 = 0.26$. Thus, it is possible that FLT-PET will become a valuable diagnostic tool for differentiating uterine leiomyosarcoma from leiomyoma in the future.

Table 4
Summary of the revised International Federation of Gynecology and Obstetrics staging of cancer of the ovaries, fallopian tubes, and primary peritoneal cancer[52]

Stage	Description
Stage I	Carcinoma limited to the ovary (or ovaries) or fallopian tubes without spread to nearby lymph nodes or to distant sites
IA	Carcinoma in 1 ovary or 1 fallopian tube, but not on their outer surfaces. No cancer cells in the ascites or washings from the abdomen and pelvis
IB	Carcinoma in both ovaries or fallopian tubes but not on their outer surfaces. No cancer cells in the ascites or washings from the abdomen and pelvis
IC	Carcinoma in both ovaries or fallopian tubes and any of the following are present:
IC1	Surgical spill
IC2	Capsule ruptured before surgery or tumor on ovarian or fallopian tube surface
IC3	Cancer cells in the ascites or washings from the abdomen and pelvis
Stage II	Carcinoma in 1 or both ovaries or fallopian tubes with pelvic extension (below pelvic rim) or primary peritoneal cancer[a] without spread to nearby lymph nodes or to distant sites
IIA	Extension and/or implants on uterus and/or fallopian tubes and/or ovaries
IIB	Extension to other pelvic intraperitoneal tissues
Stage III	Carcinoma involves 1 or both ovaries or fallopian tubes, or primary peritoneal cancer, with cytologically or histologically confirmed spread to the peritoneum outside the pelvis and/or metastasis to the retroperitoneal lymph nodes without distant metastasis
IIIA1	Positive retroperitoneal (pelvic and/or para-aortic) lymph nodes only
IIIA2	Microscopic extrapelvic (above the pelvic rim) peritoneal involvement with or without positive retroperitoneal lymph nodes
IIIB	Macroscopic peritoneal metastasis beyond the pelvis up to 2 cm in greatest dimension, with or without metastasis to the retroperitoneal lymph nodes
IIIC	Macroscopic peritoneal metastasis beyond the pelvis more than 2 cm in greatest dimension, with or without metastasis to the retroperitoneal lymph nodes (includes extension of tumor to capsule of liver and spleen without parenchymal involvement of either organ)
Stage IV	Carcinoma has spread beyond abdomen and to distant organs
IVA	Cancer cells in the pleural fluid
IVB	Spread to distant organs

[a] There is no stage I peritoneal cancer.

OVARIAN CANCER

Ovarian cancer is classified into 3 categories based on histology: epithelial, germ cell, and sex cord–stromal tumors. Epithelial ovarian cancer accounts for 95% of ovarian malignancies[48] and originates from the surface epithelial layer of the ovaries or from the distal fallopian tubes.[49] The ovaries are also a common location of metastatic disease, with 5% to 30% of ovarian cancers being metastatic, primarily from the gastrointestinal tract.[50] Early diagnosis is difficult because of the lack of screening and nonspecific symptoms, leading to advanced stage (III or IV) at the time of diagnosis in most patients.[51] Ovarian cancer is surgically staged and, thus, the FIGO staging system for this cancer, summarized in **Table 4**, is surgically based and is defined by the extent and location of disease noted on cytoreduction (ie, debulking) surgery and biopsies.[52]

Ovarian nodal metastatic pattern differs from other gynecologic malignancies because of the embryologic location and subsequent descent. Metastases first spread to retroperitoneal lymph nodes (pelvic and/or para-aortic) representing stage IIIA1.[29] Para-aortic nodal disease typically first occurs at L1 to L2 level and then spreads retrograde toward the aortic bifurcation. Pelvic pathways follow the ovarian branches of the uterine vessels laterally and extend to external iliac lymph nodes. Mesenteric and inferior phrenic pathways are less common.

2-Deoxy-2-[¹⁸F]fluoro-D-glucose PET

Benign and physiologic uptake patterns overlap, with physiologic uptake most commonly seen in corpus luteum cysts and endometriomas.[53] Benign ovarian lesions that might show increased FDG uptake also include cystadenomas, teratomas, thecomas, hydrosalpinx, and granulation tissue.[53] FDG-PET/CT can play a role in detecting malignant transformation of endometriomas, because they tend to have higher SUV, with an SUV_{max} of 4.0 being suggested as a cutoff.[54]

Epithelial ovarian cancers show variable degree of FDG uptake, and the SUV_{max} correlates positively with chemosensitivity and with Ki-67 index,[55] which is likely a macroscopic reflection of the positive correlation between GLUT-1 (glucose transporter 1) expression and tumor proliferation.[56] Although GLUT-1 overexpression is associated with epithelial malignancy, the prognostic value of SUV for FDG is not well established.[56,57] Patient survival is directly linked to successful surgical resection of all malignancy, with unsuccessful debulking and residual tumor greater than 1 cm resulting in increased morbidity without associated survival benefit.[24] FDG-PET/CT in combination with laparoscopy improves detection of disease and increases the likelihood of successful debulking.[58]

FDG-PET/CT performs better than diagnostic CT in preoperative staging, providing 69% concordance with final surgical staging, and 78% concordance when PET is combined with contrast-enhanced CT, compared with 53% by CT alone.[59,60] Fig. 4 shows the greater sensitivity of FDG-PET/CT for showing metastatic deposits compared with the corresponding contrast-enhanced CT in a patient with a high-grade serous carcinoma of the right ovary and peritoneal carcinomatosis at initial staging. Preoperative FDG-PET/CT has been consistently shown to provide high specificity for detecting sites of distant metastatic disease, may alter therapy and direct surgery in patients with advanced disease, and provides a baseline to monitor treatment.[24,61]

FDG-PET has a strong role for monitoring therapy and restaging, and outperforms conventional imaging with reported PPV greater than 90% in the setting of increased cancer antigen (CA) 125 level tumor marker,[62,63] and can also detect disease in symptomatic patients with normal CA-125 levels.[64] An example for FDG-PET detection of recurrent high-grade ovarian serous carcinoma is shown in Fig. 5. FDG-PET/CT confirmed locally recurrent left vaginal cuff disease and identified an additional unsuspected metastatic retroperitoneal lymph node.

2-Deoxy-2-[¹⁸F]fluoro-D-glucose PET/Magnetic Resonance

Similar to endometrial cancer, PET/MR is not yet officially endorsed for standard-of-care work-up. Although many groups have failed to show a significant difference between PET/MR and PET/CT results, a few groups showed advantages of PET/MR. Fiaschetti and colleagues[65] found FDG-PET/MR to have superior sensitivity, specificity, PPV, and NPV (n = 19) compared with FDG-PET/CT and MR-only imaging, with PET/MR detecting 95% of the malignant lesions (18 out of 19) compared with 74% with PET/CT (14 out of 19). Nakajo and colleagues[66] found that PET/MR, specifically PET/T2-weighting imaging, better localized disease sites compared with PET/CT (n = 31).

16α-¹⁸F-fluoro-17β-estradiol PET

Seventy percent of epithelial ovarian cancer is ERα positive,[10] but only 19% of patients show objective response to endocrine therapy, with 51% reporting clinical benefit.[67–69] In patients with epithelial ovarian cancer, van Kruchte and colleagues[10] found a significant correlation between FES uptake and the semiquantitative immunoscore for tumor ERα (r = 0.65, $P<.01$) based on a sample size of 28 lesions. They proposed a threshold of SUV_{max} greater than 1.8 resulting in a 79% sensitivity, 100% specificity, and AUC of 0.86 (95% CI, 0.70–1.00) to distinguish ERα-positive from ERα-negative lesions.[10]

CERVICAL CANCER

Papanicolaou (Pap) screening and human papillomavirus (HPV) vaccination have resulted in the marked reduction of cervical cancer. Pap screening often leads to diagnosis in premalignant or early stage. HPV types 16 and 18 are responsible for approximately 75% of HPV-related cancers. Risk factors include smoking, number of sexual partners, early age of first coitus, diethylstilbestrol exposure, compromised immune system, long-term oral contraceptive use, and HPV infection.[70] Early-stage cancer has a good prognosis of nearly 90% survival at 5 years and is treated

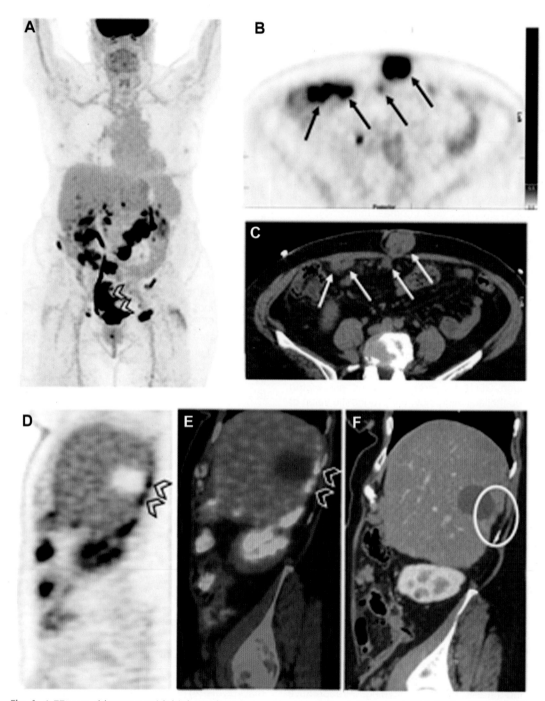

Fig. 4. A 77-year-old woman with high-grade serous carcinoma of the right ovary. Initial staging FDG-PET/CT was performed after contrast-enhanced CT of the abdomen and pelvis. (A) MIP PET images show a large hypermetabolic right pelvic primary malignancy (*arrowheads*) and peritoneal carcinomatosis, which is better appreciated on (B) axial attenuation-corrected PET and (C) CT images (*arrows*), extending into an umbilical hernia. Metastatic deposits posterior to the liver (*arrowheads*) can also be visualized on the (D) sagittal PET image and (E) fused PET/CT image. These deposits are harder to appreciate on (F) corresponding sagittal contrast-enhanced CT image (*circle*); the CT scan was performed 10 days after the PET/CT.

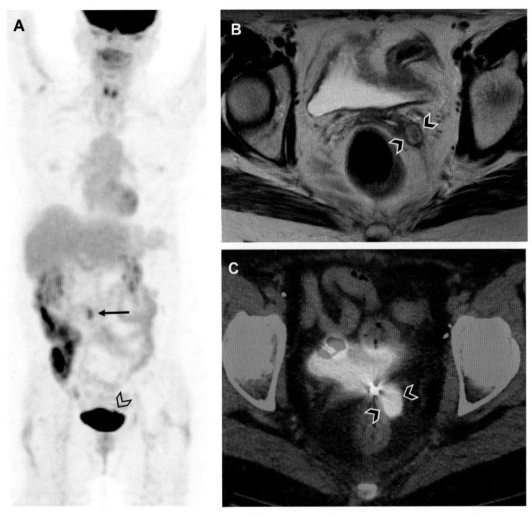

Fig. 5. FDG-PET/CT of a 66-year-old woman with recurrent ovarian high-grade serous carcinoma after hysterectomy, salpingo-oophorectomy, and adjuvant intraperitoneal chemotherapy. (*A*) PET MIP and (*B*) axial T2-weighted MR imaging show a recurrent nodule in the left vaginal cuff (*arrowheads*). MIP and (*C*) axial-fused PET/CT images confirm intense hypermetabolic activity within the recurrent left vaginal cuff nodule (*arrowheads*) posterior to the urinary bladder, and an additional metastatic retroperitoneal lymph node (*arrow* on MIP).

with surgical resection, whereas more advanced locally invasive cancers may need definitive chemoradiation. Neoadjuvant therapy is uncommon; advanced stage IV cancer has a 5-year survival rate of only 16%.[24]

Although FIGO staging originally did not incorporate imaging, revised FIGO staging now enables stage IIIC involvement of pelvic and/or para-aortic lymph nodes to be documented by imaging and/or pathology, and is summarized in **Table 5**,[71] highlighting the importance of nodal status in disease staging. Typical progress of cervical cancer is invasion into the cervical stroma, followed by direct invasion into adjacent parametrium, uterine body, and vagina, and then lymphatic spread. Lymph node metastatic pattern progresses from pelvic

to para-aortic lymph nodes, before distant supraclavicular nodal spread. Hematogenous spread is more typical with advanced disease. An example of an initial staging FDG-PET/CT is presented in **Fig. 6**, which shows a hypermetabolic primary cervical lesion as well as metastatic left iliac chain lymph nodes; difficulty in assessing local invasion on FDG-PET/CT, requiring MR imaging, is also shown in this example. Prognosis is largely determined by the presence and extent of lymph node involvement, and the presence of metastatic supraclavicular nodes typically indicates an extremely poor prognosis. In patients who undergo surgery, the parametrial surgical margins are also an important prognostic factor.[72]

Table 5
Revised International Federation of Gynecology and Obstetrics staging of cervical cancer, 2018[71]

Stage	Description
Stage I	Carcinoma limited to the uterine cervix
IA	Invasive carcinoma that can be diagnosed only with microscopy, with maximum depth of invasion <5 mm
IA1	Stromal invasion <3 mm in depth
IA2	Stromal invasion ≥3 mm and <5 mm in depth
IB	Invasive carcinoma confined to the uterine cervix, with measured deepest invasion ≥5 mm
IB1[a]	Tumor measures <2 cm in greatest dimension
IB2[a]	Tumor measures ≥2 cm and <4 cm in greatest dimension
IB3[a]	Tumor measures ≥4 cm in greatest dimension
Stage II	Cervical carcinoma invades beyond uterus but not to pelvic wall or to lower third of vagina
IIA	Involvement of the upper two-thirds of the vagina, without parametrial involvement
IIA1	Tumor measures <4 cm in greatest dimension
IIA2	Tumor measures ≥4 cm in greatest dimension
IIB	Parametrial involvement but not up to the pelvic wall
Stage III	Carcinoma extends to pelvic wall, and/or involves lower third of vagina, and/or causes hydronephrosis or nonfunctional kidney, and/or involves para-aortic lymph nodes
IIIA	Involves lower third of vagina, but no extension to pelvic wall
IIIB	Extension to pelvic wall and/or hydronephrosis or nonfunctional kidney from tumor
IIIC[a]	Involvement of pelvic and/or para-aortic lymph nodes, irrespective of tumor size and extent
IIIC1[a]	Pelvic lymph node metastasis only
IIIC2[a]	Para-aortic lymph node metastasis
Stage IV	Carcinoma has extended beyond the true pelvis or has involved (biopsy-proven) mucosa of bladder or rectum
IVA	Spread to adjacent pelvic organs
IVB	Spread to distant organs

Uterine sarcomas have a different FIGO staging.
[a] Indicates stages that are new from the 2009 FIGO system. Stage IIIC can be documented by imaging and/or pathology.

FDG-PET

FDG-PET has a limited role in diagnosis and staging of early cervical cancer, because it suffers from poor sensitivity in the detection of pelvic and para-aortic lymph nodes in early-stage disease; lymphadenectomy is required for disease confirmation and staging, although it is not routinely performed because of its high morbidity.[73,74] Nonetheless, sensitivity of FDG-PET for detection of lymph node metastasis increases with more advanced disease. There are many studies in the literature that evaluated the utility of FDG-PET in cervical cancer. In an early study, Grigsby and colleagues[75] showed that FDG-PET was superior to CT in the detection of abnormal nodes and prediction of treatment outcome. In a later study, they showed that the frequency of FDG-avid lymph nodes correlates with disease stage.[76] Patients with FDG-avid lymph nodes have poorer outcomes compared with patients without FDG-avid lymph nodes within the same stage.[76] A meta-analysis performed by Choi and colleagues[73] showed that FDG-PET/CT significantly outperformed CT and MR imaging with a pooled sensitivity and specificity of 82% and 95%, respectively, with region-based or lymph node–based sensitivity and specificity of 54% and 97%, respectively.

Although FDG-PET may not play a substantial role in disease staging at early stages, it is used to help optimize therapy planning, particularly in radiation therapy planning, and it also provides prognostic information.[77] Pretreatment disease showing greater SUV_{max} in the primary or locoregional lymph node metastases is associated with poor outcomes. Pan and colleagues[78] reported that an SUV_{max} greater than or equal to 11.2 of the primary tumor significantly ($P = .0099$) predicted worse prognosis. In addition, other FDG parameters of the primary tumor, such as MTV and

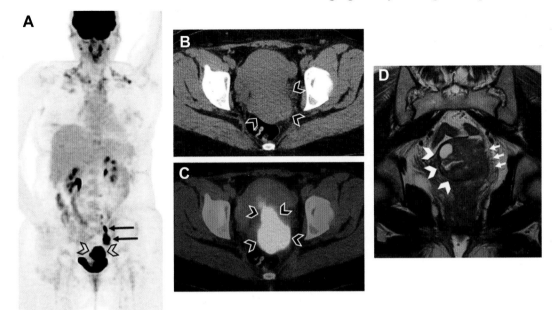

Fig. 6. Initial staging FDG-PET/CT of a 39-year-old woman presenting with abnormal vaginal bleeding caused by cervical cancer. Pelvic examination revealed a cervical mass, and biopsy confirmed invasive squamous cell carcinoma. (*A*) PET MIP, (*B*) axial CT, and (*C*) fused axial PET/CT images show a hypermetabolic primary mass in the uterine cervix (*arrowheads*) with metastatic left iliac chain lymph nodes (*arrows*). (*D*) Coronal T2-weighted MR imaging shows left parametrial invasion, which is hard to appreciate on PET/CT, as shown by infiltrative intermediate signal intensity lines (*short arrows*) causing disruption of the low signal intensity of the left cervical stromal ring compared with the normal right side (*white arrowheads*).

TLG, have been shown to correlate with patient outcome and survival.[79]

FDG-PET also has a role in monitoring therapy response and restaging, with sensitivity ranging between 85% and 100% for recurrent or persistent tumors, including asymptomatic patients.[80,81] Grigsby and colleagues[82] determined that post-treatment abnormal FDG uptake (persistent or new) was the most significant prognostic factor ($P<.0001$) for death from cervical cancer. In a multivariate analysis of prognostic factors, they found a 2-year progression-free survival of 86% for patients without abnormal FDG uptake at any site, but only 40% for those with persistent abnormal uptake. Moreover, there were no survivors at 2 years among patients who developed new sites of abnormal FDG uptake ($P<.0001$).[82] Siva and colleagues[83] had similar findings and calculated a distant failure rate 36-fold lower in patients with complete metabolic response compared with those with only partial response.

2-Deoxy-2-[18F]fluoro-D-glucose PET/ Magnetic Resonance

Although separate MR anatomic imaging and PET/CT both play a role in staging, data on PET/MR remain limited. The investigation of gynecologic malignancies with PET/MR has generally combined endometrial, ovarian, and cervical cancers, and findings have been generalized across different malignancies. There are a few reports of particular cases where PET/MR changed staging compared with PET/CT. Schwartz and colleagues[84] noted 6 of 18 patients with parametrial invasion and 1 patient with bladder invasion on PET/MR that was not detected on PET/CT. In addition, 5 patients had discordant PET/MR staging compared with clinical staging, of whom 2 patients had management changes because of IIB radiographic staging compared with the original IB1 clinical staging. PET/MR has been shown to have high accuracy in determining T stage and lymph node status in cervical cancer. Grueneisen and colleagues[85] reported that PET/MR imaging was 85% accurate (23 of 27 patients) in determination of the T stage and 93% accurate for nodal detection. Mayerhoefer and colleagues[36] also described change in management of a patient with cervical cancer (9 of 330 patients had gynecologic malignancies) by showing lack of urinary bladder infiltration on PET/MR, which was unclear on the correlating PET/CT, and resulted in the patient receiving both surgery and chemotherapy rather than only chemotherapy. Several studies reported significant associations between PET/MR biomarkers and several prognostic factors, including tumor size, grade, stage, and lymph node metastasis.[85–87] In a recent study, Shih and colleagues[88] reported that PET/MR biomarkers of cervical cancer are associated with tumor stage and survival; SUV_{max} and minimum ADC were independent predictors of progression-free survival and overall survival, respectively.

3'-Deoxy-3'-[^{18}F]fluorothymidine PET

Concurrent use of radiation therapy with chemotherapy is the standard-of-care therapy for most patients with cervical cancers, but increased hematologic toxicity caused by irradiation of physiologic active bone marrow is a common problem.[89,90] FLT-PET has been proposed to identify active bone marrow distribution, enabling tailoring radiation treatment to minimize collateral damage. McGuire and colleagues[16] studied a combination of patients with cervical and head/neck cancers. They showed that reducing bone marrow radiation dose with the aid of FLT-PET enabled a higher proportion of patients to complete a full course of treatment and reduced bone marrow toxicity.[16] Although FDG can also identify active bone marrow, a small study by Wyss and colleagues[91] showed that FLT had a higher interpatient consistency, and therefore may be the better imaging agent.

Copper-labeled Diacetyl-bis(N4-ethylthiosemicarbazone) PET

Dehdashti and colleagues[21,22] evaluated pretreatment cervical cancer hypoxia by ^{60}Cu-ATSM and found an inverse correlation between tracer

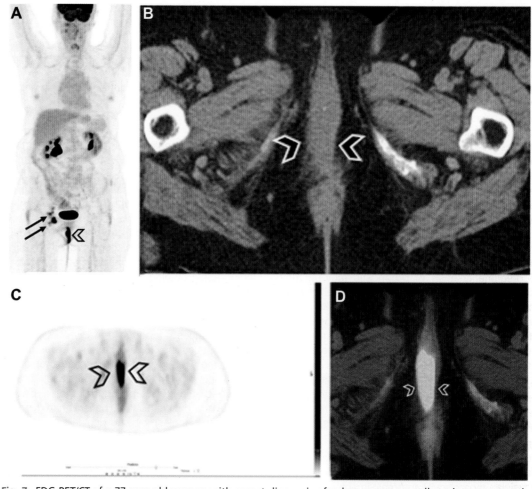

Fig. 7. FDG-PET/CT of a 77-year-old woman with recent diagnosis of vulvar squamous cell carcinoma presenting for initial staging. (A) PET MIP image shows a markedly hypermetabolic primary vulvar lesion (arrowhead) with metastatic right inguinal lymph nodes (arrows). (B) Axial CT, (C) axial attenuation-corrected PET, and (D) fused PET/CT images show the primary hypermetabolic carcinoma (arrowheads). Surgical pathology confirmed 7 metastatic right inguinal lymph nodes.

uptake and progression-free survival. A tumor/muscle uptake (T/M) ratio greater than 3.5 correlated with hypoxic tumors, and these patients were likely to develop recurrence with only a 28% 3-year progression-free survival compared with 71% in normoxic tumors with T/M less than or equal to 3.5. However, there was no significant difference between hypoxic and normoxic FDG uptake, and FDG uptake did not correlate with ^{60}Cu-ATSM uptake. ^{60}Cu-ATSM uptake has been shown to correlate with FDG-positive lymph nodes and hypoxia-related tumor molecular markers, including vascular endothelial growth factor, cyclooxygenase-2, EGFR, carbonic anhydrase IX (CA-9), and apoptotic index.[92] Subsequent studies comparing ^{60}Cu-ATSM and ^{64}Cu-ATSM showed similar findings but lower noise, resulting in better image quality with ^{64}Cu-ATSM.[23]

VAGINAL CANCER

Vaginal cancer is rare, representing only 10% of all vaginal malignant neoplasms, and most commonly affects elderly postmenopausal women. Typical presentation is vaginal bleeding or an odorous discharge. Nearly 90% of cases are squamous cell carcinoma, and 8% to 10% of cases are adenocarcinoma. Surgery is limited to early-stage small cancers less than 2 cm, with chemoradiation therapy required for more advanced cases.[93]

Nodal involvement at the time of diagnosis is less common, involving 16% to 40% of cases, but is important because it is associated with worse prognosis and influences management. Vaginal cancer with nodal involvement is typically treated with radiation therapy.[29] Pelvic and inguinal lymph node involvement is considered locoregional disease, with spread via the superficial inguinal pathway, and secondary drainage to the external iliac lymph nodes; confluence of pathways can result in contralateral spread, and laterality is therefore not taken into account for staging.

2-Deoxy-2-[^{18}F]fluoro-ᴅ-glucose PET

Data on the role of FDG-PET in vaginal cancers are much sparser compared with endometrial, cervical, and ovarian. Lamoreaux and colleagues[94] showed that FDG-PET detects the primary tumor and abnormal lymph nodes more often than diagnostic CT. Robertson and colleagues[95] studied 29 patients with vaginal cancer and found that the physician's prognostic impression changed in 13 of the 29 cases (45%) based on the FDG-PET/CT, 7 patients receiving a better prognosis and 6 receiving a worse prognosis. They also suggested that PET/CT was able to identify abnormalities not

seen on diagnostic CT, but the limited number of patients in the study precludes meaningful statistical analysis.[95] However, the ultimate role of FDG-PET in detecting and monitoring vaginal cancer still requires further studies.

VULVAR CANCER

Vulvar cancer is rare and often diagnosed in early stages. Squamous cell cancer represents 90% of cases. Risk factors included advanced age, HPV infection, cigarette smoking, inflammatory conditions of the vulva, and immunodeficiency. Standard treatment is radical surgery and sentinel lymph node biopsy with possible inguinofemoral lymphadenectomy.[96]

Nodal metastatic disease is the most important prognostic factor, with 90% survival rate for patients with negative inguinal lymph nodes compared with 50% for those with histologically positive inguinal lymph nodes.[29] One or multiple metastatic nodes, short-axis diameter, and presence of extracapsular spread or ulcerated inguinal adenopathy are all crucial details. As with vaginal cancers, laterality of the locoregional lymph nodes is not considered prognostic.

2-Deoxy-2-[^{18}F]fluoro-ᴅ-glucose PET

Although data are not as sparse as for vaginal cancer, evaluation of the role of FDG-PET remains much more limited compared with endometrial, cervical, and ovarian cancers. Several studies have suggested that FDG-PET is useful for detecting nodal and distant metastases.[97,98] In particular, Cohn and colleagues[98] reported a sensitivity of 80%, specificity of 90%, PPV of 80%, and NPV of 90% on a patient-by-patient basis. More recently, Kamran and colleagues[99] reported a sensitivity of 50%, specificity of 100%, PPV of 100%, and NPV of 57.1% for detection of lymph node metastases. They concluded that the poor sensitivity makes it unsuitable as a substitute for lymphadenectomy. Similar to their findings on vaginal cancer, Robertson and colleagues[95] found that the physician's prognostic impression changed in 29 of the 54 cases of vulvar cancer (54%). Although ultimately still to be proved, identification of metastatic pelvic nodes on FDG-PET may allow patients to avoid morbidity with unnecessarily extensive surgery in favor of chemoradiation.[100] Investigators such as Lin and colleagues[101] showed that false-positive locoregional and distant metastases on PET are common, and recommended caution with interpretations. **Fig. 7** shows FDG-PET/CT at initial staging of vulvar squamous cell carcinoma with metastatic inguinal lymph nodes.

FUTURE DIRECTIONS

Several non-FDG tracers have shown promise in evaluating specific phenotypes of gynecologic cancers. These tracers may have a future role in gynecologic imaging. Somatostatin receptor imaging, typically performed with ^{68}Ga-1, 4, 7, 10-tetraazacyclododecane- N, N′, N″, N‴-tetraacetic acid-D-Phe 1-Tyr 3-octreotide (DOTATOC) and ^{64}Cu-1, 4, 7, 10-tetraazacyclododecane-N, N′, N″, N‴-tetraacetic acid-D-Phe 1, Tyr 3-octreotate (DOTATATE), can be used to be evaluate rare neuroendocrine variants of cervical and ovarian cancers.[102–106] Vaginal and vulvar human epidermal growth factor receptor (HER) imaging targets HER2 and HER3, using [89]Zr-labeled and ^{64}Cu-labeled antibodies, is another class of tracers. HER3 overexpression is strongly associated with poor prognosis and could play a role in prediction and monitoring of response to HER3-directed therapy in gynecologic cancers, particularly ovarian cancer.[107,108] Poly(ADP-ribose) polymerase (PARP) inhibitors are an emerging therapeutic class of anticancer drugs with the potential to treat cancers that are deficient in DNA repair machinery. ^{18}F-FluorThanatrace (FTT), a PARP imaging tracer, is a radiolabeled analogue of the PARP inhibitor rucaparib. FTT is currently in clinical trials in several cancers and has the potential for predicting patient response to PARP-inhibiting therapy, particularly in patients with ovarian cancer.[109,110] FLT, a marker of cell proliferation rate, may be useful in patients with ovarian cancers, identifying malignant lesions and predicting response to therapy.[111–113]

SUMMARY

Gynecologic cancer staging and management require a multidisciplinary approach with primary oncological and surgical teams working in conjunction with radiology and nuclear medicine physicians to provide patients with optimal care. PET plays a limited role in early-stage disease because this is governed by local disease extent and spread, and is better evaluated with diagnostic CT and MR imaging, and confirmed after possible surgical intervention. FDG-PET plays a role in advanced disease, has been proven to have greater sensitivity compared with CT and MR imaging alone for many of the gynecologic malignancies, and can spare patients unnecessary surgeries. FIGO staging is starting to acknowledge the role and advantage of imaging, and the recent update for cervical cancer now allows for upstaging of cervical cancer based on radiologic identification of pelvic and/or para-aortic lymph node disease.

FDG-PET/MR remains an emerging technology with data currently insufficient to show superiority compared with PET/CT, but several reports suggest superior information of PET/MR on local spread compared with FDG-PET/CT, ultimately leading to change in management. DOTATATE-PET/CT can be a useful tool in mapping disease of rare gynecologic neuroendocrine malignancies of the cervix and ovaries. A brief introduction of other emerging PET tracers is also provided, and although many of these tracers show promise for specialized cancer imaging and characterization, they are currently only used in research settings. Additional studies and data are required to confirm their utility and role in clinical management.

CLINICS CARE POINTS

- FDG-PET/CT has a limited role in initial staging of gynecologic cancers and is insufficient to replace lymphadenectomy.
- FDG-PET/CT can play a role in identification of distant metastases and treatment planning for gynecologic cancers.
- SUV_{max} has been correlated with greater endometrial tumor aggressiveness.
- No statistically significant advantage of PET/MR compared with PET/CT has been ascertained, but data remain limited.
- PET/CT is superior to PET/MR for detecting lung metastases.
- FDG-PET/MR has superior accuracy for detecting myometrial invasion in endometrial cancer, which is an important prognostic factor.
- Ovarian nodal metastatic pattern differs from other gynecologic malignancies because of their embryology, with metastases first spreading to retroperitoneal lymph nodes (pelvic and/or para-aortic).
- FDG-PET/CT ovarian cancer uptake patterns overlap with physiologic uptake most commonly seen in corpus luteum cysts and endometriomas.
- Ovarian cancer SUV_{max} for FDG correlates positively with chemosensitivity and with Ki-67 index.
- FDG-PET/CT in combination with laparoscopy improves detection of ovarian cancer disease and increases the likelihood of successful debulking.
- FDG-PET/CT performs better than CT in preoperative staging of ovarian cancer.

- FDG-PET/CT outperforms conventional imaging for monitoring therapy and restating of ovarian and cervical cancers.

- Revised cervical cancer FIGO staging now enables stage IIIC involvement of pelvic and/or para-aortic lymph node disease to be documented by imaging and/or pathology.

- FDG-PET/CT sensitivity for metastatic cervical cancer increases with more advanced disease, and outperforms CT and MR imaging in the detection of abnormal nodes and prediction of treatment outcome.

- FDG-avid lymph nodes in cervical cancer correlate with poorer outcomes compared with patients without FDG-avid lymph nodes within the same stage of disease.

- FDG-PET/CT data for vaginal and vulvar cancers are sparse, and more studies are required to determinate its ultimate role.

DISCLOSURE

The authors have nothing to disclose.

REFERENCES

1. Center for Disease Control and Prevention. Gynecologic cancer Incidence, United States—2012–2016. USCS data brief, vol. 11. Atlanta, GA: Centers for Disease Control and Prevention: US Department of Health and Human Services; 2019.
2. Alt CD, Brocker KA, Eichbaum M, et al. Imaging of female pelvic malignancies regarding MRI, CT, and PET/CT: Part 2. Strahlenther Onkol 2011;187(11):705–14.
3. Brocker KA, Alt CD, Eichbaum M, et al. Imaging of female pelvic malignancies regarding MRI, CT, and PET/CT : part 1. Strahlenther Onkol 2011;187(10):611–8.
4. Hricak H. MRI of the female pelvis: a review. AJR Am J Roentgenol 1986;146(6):1115–22.
5. Hameeduddin A, Sahdev A. Diffusion-weighted imaging and dynamic contrast-enhanced MRI in assessing response and recurrent disease in gynaecological malignancies. Cancer Imaging 2015;15(1):3.
6. Ratner ES, Staib LH, Cross SN, et al. The clinical impact of gynecologic MRI. AJR Am J Roentgenol 2015;204(3):674–80.
7. Eiber M, Martinez-Möller A, Souvatzoglou M, et al. Value of a Dixon-based MR/PET attenuation correction sequence for the localization and evaluation of PET-positive lesions. Eur J Nucl Med Mol Imaging 2011;38(9):1691–701.
8. Keller SH, Holm S, Hansen AE, et al. Image artifacts from MR-based attenuation correction in clinical, whole-body PET/MRI. Magma 2013;26(1):173–81.
9. Gustafsson JA. Estrogen receptor beta–a new dimension in estrogen mechanism of action. J Endocrinol 1999;163(3):379–83.
10. van Kruchten M, de Vries EFJ, Arts HJG, et al. Assessment of estrogen receptor expression in epithelial ovarian cancer patients using 16α-18F-fluoro-17β-estradiol PET/CT. J Nucl Med 2015;56(1):50–5.
11. Antunes IF, van Waarde A, Dierckx RAJO, et al. Synthesis and Evaluation of the Estrogen Receptor β-Selective Radioligand 2-[18F]-Fluoro-6-(6-Hydroxy-naphthalen-2-yl)Pyridin-3-ol: Comparison with 16α-[18F]-Fluoro-17β-Estradiol. J Nucl Med 2017;58(4):554–9.
12. McKinley ET, Ayers GD, Smith RA, et al. Limits of [18F]-FLT PET as a biomarker of proliferation in oncology. PLoS One 2013;8(3):e58938.
13. Dittmann H, Dohmen BM, Kehlbach R, et al. Early changes in [18F]FLT uptake after chemotherapy: an experimental study. Eur J Nucl Med Mol Imaging 2002;29(11):1462–9.
14. Plotnik DA, Emerick LE, Krohn KA, et al. Different modes of transport for 3H-thymidine, 3H-FLT, and 3H-FMAU in proliferating and nonproliferating human tumor cells. J Nucl Med 2010;51(9):1464–71.
15. Shields AF. Positron emission tomography measurement of tumor metabolism and growth: its expanding role in oncology. Mol Imaging Biol 2006;8(3):141–50.
16. McGuire SM, Menda Y, Ponto LLB, et al. Spatial mapping of functional pelvic bone marrow using FLT PET. J Appl Clin Med Phys 2014;15(4):129–36.
17. Turcotte E, Wiens LW, Grierson JR, et al. Toxicology evaluation of radiotracer doses of 3'-deoxy-3'-[18F] fluorothymidine (18F-FLT) for human PET imaging: Laboratory analysis of serial blood samples and comparison to previously investigated therapeutic FLT doses. BMC Nucl Med 2007;7:3.
18. Lopci E, Grassi I, Chiti A, et al. PET radiopharmaceuticals for imaging of tumor hypoxia: a review of the evidence. Am J Nucl Med Mol Imaging 2014;4(4):365–84.
19. Lee ST, Scott AM. Hypoxia positron emission tomography imaging with 18f-fluoromisonidazole. Semin Nucl Med 2007;37(6):451–61.
20. Koh WJ, Rasey JS, Evans ML, et al. Imaging of hypoxia in human tumors with [F-18]fluoromisonidazole. Int J Radiat Oncol Biol Phys 1992;22(1):199–212.
21. Dehdashti F, Grigsby PW, Mintun MA, et al. Assessing tumor hypoxia in cervical cancer by positron emission tomography with 60Cu-ATSM: relationship to therapeutic response-a preliminary report. Int J Radiat Oncol Biol Phys 2003;55(5):1233–8.

22. Dehdashti F, Grigsby PW, Lewis JS, et al. Assessing tumor hypoxia in cervical cancer by PET with 60Cu-labeled diacetyl-bis(N4-methylthiosemicarbazone). J Nucl Med 2008;49(2):201–5.

23. Lewis JS, Laforest R, Dehdashti F, et al. An imaging comparison of 64Cu-ATSM and 60Cu-ATSM in cancer of the uterine cervix. J Nucl Med 2008;49(7): 1177–82.

24. Brunetti J. PET/CT in gynecologic malignancies. Radiol Clin North Am 2013;51(5):895–911.

25. Cramer DW. The epidemiology of endometrial and ovarian cancer. Hematol Oncol Clin North Am 2012;26(1):1–12.

26. Pecorelli S. Revised FIGO staging for carcinoma of the vulva, cervix, and endometrium. Int J Gynaecol Obstet 2009;105(2):103–4.

27. Freeman SJ, Aly AM, Kataoka MY, et al. The revised FIGO staging system for uterine malignancies: implications for MR imaging. Radiographics 2012;32(6):1805–27.

28. Meissnitzer M, Forstner R. MRI of endometrium cancer - how we do it. Cancer Imaging 2016;16:11.

29. Paño B, Sebastià C, Ripoll E, et al. Pathways of lymphatic spread in gynecologic malignancies. Radiographics 2015;35(3):916–45.

30. Chang MC, Chen JH, Liang JA, et al. 18F-FDG PET or PET/CT for detection of metastatic lymph nodes in patients with endometrial cancer: a systematic review and meta-analysis. Eur J Radiol 2012; 81(11):3511–7.

31. Bollineni VR, Ytre-Hauge S, Bollineni-Balabay O, et al. High Diagnostic Value of 18F-FDG PET/CT in Endometrial Cancer: Systematic Review and Meta-Analysis of the Literature. J Nucl Med 2016; 57(6):879–85.

32. Kitajima K, Kita M, Suzuki K, et al. Prognostic significance of SUVmax (maximum standardized uptake value) measured by [18F]FDG PET/CT in endometrial cancer. Eur J Nucl Med Mol Imaging 2012;39(5):840–5.

33. Ryu SY, Kim K, Kim Y, et al. Detection of recurrence by 18F-FDG PET in patients with endometrial cancer showing no evidence of disease. J Korean Med Sci 2010;25(7):1029–33.

34. Sharma P, Kumar R, Singh H, et al. Role of FDG PET-CT in detecting recurrence in patients with uterine sarcoma: comparison with conventional imaging. Nucl Med Commun 2012;33(2):185–90.

35. Martin O, Schaarschmidt BM, Kirchner J, et al. PET/MRI Versus PET/CT for Whole-Body Staging: Results from a Single-Center Observational Study on 1,003 Sequential Examinations. J Nucl Med 2020;61(8):1131–6.

36. Mayerhoefer ME, Prosch H, Beer L, et al. PET/MRI versus PET/CT in oncology: a prospective single-center study of 330 examinations focusing on implications for patient management and cost considerations. Eur J Nucl Med Mol Imaging 2020;47(1):51–60.

37. Morsing A, Hildebrandt MG, Vilstrup MH, et al. Hybrid PET/MRI in major cancers: a scoping review. Eur J Nucl Med Mol Imaging 2019;46(10):2138–51.

38. Tsuyoshi H, Tsujikawa T, Yamada S, et al. Diagnostic value of 18F-FDG PET/MRI for staging in patients with endometrial cancer. Cancer Imaging 2020;20(1):75.

39. Tsuyoshi H, Tsujikawa T, Yamada S, et al. FDG-PET/MRI with high-resolution DWI characterises the distinct phenotypes of endometrial cancer. Clin Radiol 2020;75(3):209–15.

40. Bian LH, Wang M, Gong J, et al. Comparison of integrated PET/MRI with PET/CT in evaluation of endometrial cancer: a retrospective analysis of 81 cases. PeerJ 2019;7:e7081.

41. Takeuchi M, Matsuzaki K, Harada M. Evaluating Myometrial Invasion in Endometrial Cancer: Comparison of Reduced Field-of-view Diffusion-weighted Imaging and Dynamic Contrast-enhanced MR Imaging. Magn Reson Med Sci 2018;17(1):28–34.

42. Bokhman JV. Two pathogenetic types of endometrial carcinoma. Gynecol Oncol 1983;15(1):10–7.

43. Singh M, Zaino RJ, Filiaci VJ, et al. Relationship of estrogen and progesterone receptors to clinical outcome in metastatic endometrial carcinoma: a Gynecologic Oncology Group Study. Gynecol Oncol 2007;106(2):325–33.

44. Tsujikawa T, Yoshida Y, Kudo T, et al. Functional images reflect aggressiveness of endometrial carcinoma: estrogen receptor expression combined with 18F-FDG PET. J Nucl Med 2009;50(10): 1598–604.

45. Tsujikawa T, Yoshida Y, Mori T, et al. Uterine tumors: pathophysiologic imaging with 16alpha-[18F]fluoro-17beta-estradiol and 18F fluorodeoxyglucose PET–initial experience. Radiology 2008;248(2): 599–605.

46. Zhao Z, Yoshida Y, Kurokawa T, et al. 18F-FES and 18F-FDG PET for differential diagnosis and quantitative evaluation of mesenchymal uterine tumors: correlation with immunohistochemical analysis. J Nucl Med 2013;54(4):499–506.

47. Yamane T, Takaoka A, Kita M, et al. 18F-FLT PET performs better than 18F-FDG PET in differentiating malignant uterine corpus tumors from benign leiomyoma. Ann Nucl Med 2012;26(6):478–84.

48. Desai A, Xu J, Aysola K, et al. Epithelial ovarian cancer: An overview. World J Transl Med 2014;3(1):1–8.

49. Erickson BK, Conner MG, Landen CN. The role of the fallopian tube in the origin of ovarian cancer. Am J Obstet Gynecol 2013;209(5):409–14.

50. Lee SJ, Bae JH, Lee AW, et al. Clinical characteristics of metastatic tumors to the ovaries. J Korean Med Sci 2009;24(1):114–9.

51. Copeland LJ. Epithelial Ovarian Cancer. In: DiSaia PJ, Creasman WT, editors. Clinical gynecologic oncology. 7th edition. Philadelphia: Elsevier; 2007. p. 313–67.

52. Prat J, FIGO Committee on Gynecologic Oncology. Staging classification for cancer of the ovary, fallopian tube, and peritoneum. Int J Gynaecol Obstet 2014;124(1):1–5.

53. Fenchel S, Grab D, Nuessle K, et al. Asymptomatic adnexal masses: correlation of FDG PET and histopathologic findings. Radiology 2002;223(3):780–8.

54. Kusunoki S, Ota T, Kaneda H, et al. Analysis of positron emission tomography/computed tomography in patients to differentiate between malignant transformation of endometrioma and endometrioma. Int J Clin Oncol 2016;21(6):1136–41.

55. Liu S, Feng Z, Wen H, et al. 18F-FDG PET/CT can predict chemosensitivity and proliferation of epithelial ovarian cancer via SUVmax value. Jpn J Radiol 2018;36(9):544–50.

56. Semaan A, Munkarah AR, Arabi H, et al. Expression of GLUT-1 in epithelial ovarian carcinoma: correlation with tumor cell proliferation, angiogenesis, survival and ability to predict optimal cytoreduction. Gynecol Oncol 2011;121(1):181–6.

57. Risum S, Loft A, Høgdall C, et al. Standardized FDG uptake as a prognostic variable and as a predictor of incomplete cytoreduction in primary advanced ovarian cancer. Acta Oncol 2011;50(3):415–9.

58. De Iaco P, Musto A, Orazi L, et al. FDG-PET/CT in advanced ovarian cancer staging: value and pitfalls in detecting lesions in different abdominal and pelvic quadrants compared with laparoscopy. Eur J Radiol 2011;80(2):e98–103.

59. Castellucci P, Perrone AM, Picchio M, et al. Diagnostic accuracy of 18F-FDG PET/CT in characterizing ovarian lesions and staging ovarian cancer: correlation with transvaginal ultrasonography, computed tomography, and histology. Nucl Med Commun 2007;28(8):589–95.

60. Nam EJ, Yun MJ, Oh YT, et al. Diagnosis and staging of primary ovarian cancer: correlation between PET/CT, Doppler US, and CT or MRI. Gynecol Oncol 2010;116(3):389–94.

61. Han S, Woo S, Suh CH, et al. Performance of pre-treatment ^{18}F-fluorodeoxyglucose positron emission tomography/computed tomography for detecting metastasis in ovarian cancer: a systematic review and meta-analysis. J Gynecol Oncol 2018;29(6):e98.

62. Palomar A, Nanni C, Castellucci P, et al. Value of FDG PET/CT in patients with treated ovarian cancer and raised CA125 serum levels. Mol Imaging Biol 2012;14(1):123–9.

63. Peng NJ, Liou WS, Liu RS, et al. Early detection of recurrent ovarian cancer in patients with low-level increases in serum CA-125 levels by 2-[F-18]fluoro-2-deoxy-D-glucose-positron emission tomography/computed tomography. Cancer Biother Radiopharm 2011;26(2):175–81.

64. Bhosale P, Peungjesada S, Wei W, et al. Clinical utility of positron emission tomography/computed tomography in the evaluation of suspected recurrent ovarian cancer in the setting of normal CA-125 levels. Int J Gynecol Cancer 2010;20(6):936–44.

65. Fiaschetti V, Calabria F, Crusco S, et al. MR-PET fusion imaging in evaluating adnexal lesions: a preliminary study. Radiol Med 2011;116(8):1288–302.

66. Nakajo K, Tatsumi M, Inoue A, et al. Diagnostic performance of fluorodeoxyglucose positron emission tomography/magnetic resonance imaging fusion images of gynecological malignant tumors: comparison with positron emission tomography/computed tomography. Jpn J Radiol 2010;28(2):95–100.

67. Hasan J, Ton N, Mullamitha S, et al. Phase II trial of tamoxifen and goserelin in recurrent epithelial ovarian cancer. Br J Cancer 2005;93(6):647–51.

68. Bowman A, Gabra H, Langdon SP, et al. CA125 response is associated with estrogen receptor expression in a phase II trial of letrozole in ovarian cancer: identification of an endocrine-sensitive subgroup. Clin Cancer Res 2002;8(7):2233–9.

69. Papadimitriou CA, Markaki S, Siapkaras J, et al. Hormonal therapy with letrozole for relapsed epithelial ovarian cancer. Long-term results of a phase II study. Oncology 2004;66(2):112–7.

70. Duarte-Franco E, Franco EL. Cancer of the Uterine Cervix. BMC Womens Health 2004;4(Suppl 1):S13.

71. Bhatla N, Berek JS, Cuello Fredes M, et al. Revised FIGO staging for carcinoma of the cervix uteri. Int J Gynaecol Obstet 2019;145(1):129–35.

72. Tran BN, Grigsby PW, Dehdashti F, et al. Occult supraclavicular lymph node metastasis identified by FDG-PET in patients with carcinoma of the uterine cervix. Gynecol Oncol 2013;90(3):572–6.

73. Choi HJ, Ju W, Myung SK, et al. Diagnostic performance of computer tomography, magnetic resonance imaging, and positron emission tomography or positron emission tomography/computer tomography for detection of metastatic lymph nodes in patients with cervical cancer: meta-analysis. Cancer Sci 2010;101(6):1471–9.

74. Ferrandina G, Petrillo M, Restaino G, et al. Can radicality of surgery be safely modulated on the basis of MRI and PET/CT imaging in locally advanced cervical cancer patients administered preoperative treatment? Cancer 2012;118(2):392–403.

75. Grigsby PW, Siegel BA, Dehdashti F. Lymph node staging by positron emission tomography in patients with carcinoma of the cervix. J Clin Oncol 2001;19(17):3745–9.

76. Kidd EA, Siegel BA, Dehdashti F, et al. Lymph node staging by positron emission tomography in cervical cancer: relationship to prognosis. J Clin Oncol 2010;28(12):2108–13.

77. Kidd EA, Siegel BA, Dehdashti F, et al. Pelvic lymph node F-18 fluorodeoxyglucose uptake as a prognostic biomarker in newly diagnosed patients with locally advanced cervical cancer. Cancer 2010;116(6):1469–75.

78. Pan L, Cheng J, Zhou M, et al. The SUVmax (maximum standardized uptake value for F-18 fluorodeoxyglucose) and serum squamous cell carcinoma antigen (SCC-ag) function as prognostic biomarkers in patients with primary cervical cancer. J Cancer Res Clin Oncol 2012;138(2):239–46.

79. Viswanathan C, Faria S, Devine C, et al. [18F]-2-Fluoro-2-Deoxy-D-glucose-PET Assessment of Cervical Cancer. PET Clin 2018;13(2):165–77.

80. Chung HH, Kim SK, Kim TH, et al. Clinical impact of FDG-PET imaging in post-therapy surveillance of uterine cervical cancer: from diagnosis to prognosis. Gynecol Oncol 2006;103(1):165–70.

81. Cetina L, Serrano A, Cantú-de-León D, et al. F18-FDG-PET/CT in the evaluation of patients with suspected recurrent or persistent locally advanced cervical carcinoma. Rev Invest Clin 2011;63(3):227–35.

82. Grigsby PW, Siegel BA, Dehdashti F, et al. Posttherapy surveillance monitoring of cervical cancer by FDG-PET. Int J Radiat Oncol Biol Phys 2003;55(4):907–13.

83. Siva S, Herschtal A, Thomas JM, et al. Impact of post-therapy positron emission tomography on prognostic stratification and surveillance after chemoradiotherapy for cervical cancer. Cancer 2011;117(17):3981–8.

84. Schwartz M, Gavane SC, Bou-Ayache J, et al. Feasibility and diagnostic performance of hybrid PET/MRI compared with PET/CT for gynecological malignancies: a prospective pilot study. Abdom Radiol (Ny) 2018;43(12):3462–7.

85. Grueneisen J, Schaarschmidt BM, Heubner M, et al. Integrated PET/MRI for whole-body staging of patients with primary cervical cancer: preliminary results. Eur J Nucl Med Mol Imaging 2015;42(12):1814–24.

86. Gong J, Wang N, Bian L, et al. Cervical cancer evaluated with integrated 18F-FDG PET/MR. Oncol Lett 2019;18(2):1815–23.

87. Surov A, Meyer HJ, Schob S, et al. Parameters of simultaneous 18F-FDG-PET/MRI predict tumor stage and several histopathological features in uterine cervical cancer. Oncotarget 2017;8(17):28285–96.

88. Shih IL, Yen RF, Chen CA, et al. PET/MRI in Cervical Cancer: Associations Between Imaging Biomarkers and Tumor Stage, Disease Progression, and Overall Survival. J Magn Reson Imaging 2021;53(1):305–18.

89. Abu-Rustum NR, Lee S, Correa A, et al. Compliance with and acute hematologic toxic effects of chemoradiation in indigent women with cervical cancer. Gynecol Oncol 2001;81(1):88–91.

90. Torres MA, Jhingran A, Thames HD, et al. Comparison of treatment tolerance and outcomes in patients with cervical cancer treated with concurrent chemoradiotherapy in a prospective randomized trial or with standard treatment. Int J Radiat Oncol Biol Phys 2008;70(1):118–25.

91. Wyss JC, Carmona R, Karunamuni RA, et al. [(18)F]Fluoro-2-deoxy-2-d-glucose versus 3'-deoxy-3'-[(18)F]fluorothymidine for defining hematopoietically active pelvic bone marrow in gynecologic patients. Radiother Oncol 2016;118(1):72–8.

92. Grigsby PW, Malyapa RS, Higashikubo R, et al. Comparison of molecular markers of hypoxia and imaging with (60)Cu-ATSM in cancer of the uterine cervix. Mol Imaging Biol 2007;9(5):278–83.

93. Adams TS, Cuello MA. Cancer of the vagina. Int J Gynaecol Obstet 2018;143(Suppl 2):14–21.

94. Lamoreaux WT, Grigsby PW, Dehdashti F, et al. FDG-PET evaluation of vaginal carcinoma. Int J Radiat Oncol Biol Phys 2005;62(3):733–7.

95. Robertson NL, Hricak H, Sonoda Y, et al. The impact of FDG-PET/CT in the management of patients with vulvar and vaginal cancer. Gynecol Oncol 2016;140(3):420–4.

96. Koh WJ, Greer BE, Abu-Rustum NR, et al. Vulvar Cancer, Version 1.2017, NCCN Clinical Practice Guidelines in Oncology. J Natl Compr Canc Netw 2017;15(1):92–120.

97. Peiró V, Chiva L, González A, et al. [Utility of the PET/CT in vulvar cancer management]. Rev Esp Med Nucl Imagen Mol 2014;33(2):87–92.

98. Cohn DE, Dehdashti F, Gibb RK, et al. Prospective evaluation of positron emission tomography for the detection of groin node metastases from vulvar cancer. Gynecol Oncol 2002;85(1):179–84.

99. Kamran MW, O'Toole F, Meghen K, et al. Whole-body [18F]fluoro-2-deoxyglucose positron emission tomography scan as combined PET-CT staging prior to planned radical vulvectomy and inguinofemoral lymphadenectomy for squamous vulvar cancer: a correlation with groin node metastasis. Eur J Gynaecol Oncol 2014;35(3):230–5.

100. Viswanathan C, Kirschner K, Truong M, et al. Multimodality imaging of vulvar cancer: staging, therapeutic response, and complications. AJR Am J Roentgenol 2013;200(6):1387–400.

101. Lin G, Chen CY, Liu FY, et al. Computed tomography, magnetic resonance imaging and FDG positron emission tomography in the management of

vulvar malignancies. Eur Radiol 2015;25(5): 1267–78.

102. Antunes P, Ginj M, Zhang H, et al. Are radiogallium-labelled DOTA-conjugated somatostatin analogues superior to those labelled with other radiometals? Eur J Nucl Med Mol Imaging 2007;34(7):982–93.

103. Virgolini I, Ambrosini V, Bomanji JB, et al. Procedure guidelines for PET/CT tumour imaging with 68Ga-DOTA-conjugated peptides: 68Ga-DOTA-TOC, 68Ga-DOTA-NOC, 68Ga-DOTA-TATE. Eur J Nucl Med Mol Imaging 2013;37(10):2004–10.

104. Miller B, Dockter M, el Torky M, et al. Small cell carcinoma of the cervix: a clinical and flow-cytometric study. Gynecol Oncol 1991;42(1):27–33.

105. Damian A, Lago G, Rossi S, et al. Early Detection of Bone Metastasis in Small Cell Neuroendocrine Carcinoma of the Cervix by 68Ga-DOTATATE PET/CT Imaging. Clin Nucl Med 2017;42(3):216–7.

106. Delpassand ES, Ranganathan D, Wagh N, et al. 64Cu-DOTATATE PET/CT for Imaging Patients with Known or Suspected Somatostatin Receptor-Positive Neuroendocrine Tumors: Results of the First U.S. Prospective, Reader-Masked Clinical Trial. J Nucl Med 2020;61(6):890–6.

107. Neve RM, Lane HA, Hynes NE. The role of overexpressed HER2 in transformation. Ann Oncol 2001; 12(Suppl 1):S9–13.

108. Bensch F, Lamberts LE, Smeenk MM, et al. 89Zr-Lumretuzumab PET Imaging before and during HER3 Antibody Lumretuzumab Treatment in Patients with Solid Tumors. Clin Cancer Res 2017;23(20):6128–37.

109. Chan CY, Tan KV, Cornelissen B. PARP Inhibitors in Cancer Diagnosis and Therapy. Clin Cancer Res 2020;10:1585–94.

110. Makvandi M, Pantel A, Schwartz L, et al. A PET imaging agent for evaluating PARP-1 expression in ovarian cancer. J Clin Invest 2018;128(5):2116–26.

111. Richard SD, Bencherif B, Edwards RP, et al. Noninvasive assessment of cell proliferation in ovarian cancer using [18F] 3'deoxy-3-fluorothymidine positron emission tomography/computed tomography imaging. Nucl Med Biol 2011;38(4):485–91.

112. Tsuyoshi H, Morishita F, Orisaka M, et al. 18F-fluorothymidine PET is a potential predictive imaging biomarker of the response to gemcitabine-based chemotherapeutic treatment for recurrent ovarian cancer: preliminary results in three patients. Clin Nucl Med 2013;38(7):560–3.

113. Aide N, Kinross K, Cullinane C, et al. 18F-FLT PET as a surrogate marker of drug efficacy during mTOR inhibition by everolimus in a preclinical cisplatin-resistant ovarian tumor model. J Nucl Med 2010;51(10):1559–64.

PET Cardiac Imaging (Perfusion, Viability, Sarcoidosis, and Infection)

Padma Priya Manapragada, MD[a], Efstathia Andrikopoulou, MD[b],
Navkaranbir Bajaj, MD[c], Pradeep Bhambhvani, MD[d],*

KEYWORDS

• PET Cardiac • Perfusion • Viability • Sarcoidosis • Infection

KEY POINTS

- Access to novel radiopharmaceuticals and technological advances has led to the increased utilization of PET in cardiac perfusion and metabolic imaging resulting in improved diagnostic certainty and patient care.
- Assessment of myocardial perfusion with PET tracers enables not only high quality relative perfusion imaging but also allows for quantification of myocardial blood flow and flow reserve.
- PET myocardial viability imaging plays a significant role in risk stratifying patients with ischemic cardiomyopathy who may benefit from revascularization.
- FDG PET for sarcoidosis is valuable in diagnosis, estimating cardiac and extracardiac disease burden, treatment monitoring and prognosis.
- Reliable hot spot FDG PET in suspected cardiac inflammation or infection is possible only when physiologic myocardial FDG uptake is suppressed. Thus optimal patient preparation is crucial.

MYOCARDIAL PERFUSION USING POSITRON EMISSION TOMOGRAPHY

Coronary artery disease (CAD) continues to be the major cause of morbidity and mortality in both developing and developed countries.[1] The American Heart Association reports approximately 16 million people greater than or equal to 20 years old in the United States have cardiovascular disease.[2] CAD leads to approximately one-third of all deaths in people older than 35 years.[3] Understanding of CAD has improved significantly over the past several decades. PET using different flow tracers has led to translation of qualitative and quantitative estimation of myocardial blood flow (MBF) to clinical practice and research. The information derived during the cardiac PET scan can aid clinicians in phenotyping myocardial perfusion abnormalities and thus help treat their patients better. This section briefly discusses MBF anatomy and physiology to understand the role of myocardial perfusion PET imaging to determine alterations in this physiology. Technical considerations, current clinical indications, and applications also are discussed.

Myocardial Blood Flow: Anatomy and Physiology

The coronary arteries arise from the right and the left coronary sinuses/cusps of the aorta. The left coronary artery divides into left anterior descending and the left circumflex artery, whereas the right coronary artery travels in the right atrioventricular

The authors have nothing to disclose.
[a] University of Alabama at Birmingham, 619 19th Street South JT 772, Birmingham, AL 35249, USA;
[b] University of Alabama at Birmingham, Tinsley Harrison Tower, Suite 311, 1900 University Boulevard, Birmingham, AL 35233, USA; [c] Asheville Cardiology Associates, 5 Vanderbilt Park Drive, Asheville, NC 28803, USA;
[d] University of Alabama at Birmingham, 619 19th Street South JT 777, Birmingham, AL 35249, USA
* Corresponding author.
E-mail address: pbhambhvani@uabmc.edu

Radiol Clin N Am 59 (2021) 835–852
https://doi.org/10.1016/j.rcl.2021.05.009

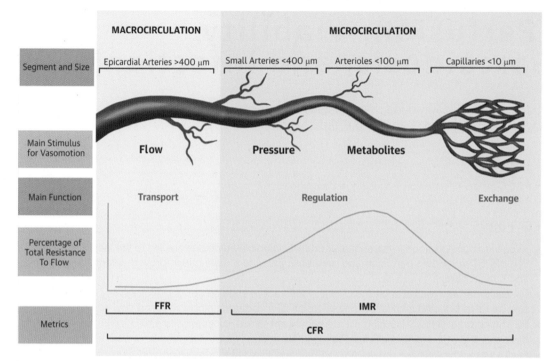

Fig. 1. Macrocirculation and microcirculation across segments and sizes of the arteries. FFR versus IMR versus CFR. (Adapted from De Bruyne B, Oldroyd KG, Pijls NHJ. Microvascular (Dys)Function and Clinical Outcome in Stable Coronary Disease. Journal of the American College of Cardiology. 2016;67(10):1170 to 1172.)

groove and commonly gives rise to posterior descending artery. These epicardial coronary arteries form the main branches of the coronary tree. These main coronary arteries then divide and subdivide into a filigree network of intramural coronary vessels, precapillary sphincters, capillaries, and coronary veins (**Fig. 1**). Different parts of coronary tree have different functions. For example, the epicardial coronary arteries contribute to the coronary capacitance, but, under most conditions, they have only a small effect on coronary vascular resistance. In contrast, the small transmural coronary vessels (<100 μm) play a dominant role in regulating total coronary vascular resistance. **Fig. 1** briefly describes the function of different segments of the coronary tree along with the commonly measured myocardial and coronary perfusion metrics, which aid in diagnosis of alterations MBF. Fractional flow reserve (FFR) measured during coronary angiography measures the transport function of epicardial coronary arteries and aids in the diagnosis of obstructive epicardial CAD, whereas index of microcirculatory resistance (IMR) measures coronary microvascular resistance; and coronary flow reserve (CFR) is a combined measure of abnormalities in the epicardial and microcirculation.[4]

Understanding Myocardial Blood Flow Physiology with Positron Emission Tomography

Myocardial perfusion imaging (MPI) with single-photon emission computed tomography (SPECT) is a widely used diagnostic and prognostic test for detection and risk stratification of patients with CAD. There is wealth of data supporting its use. MPI with SPECT and PET is limited by the relative nature of perfusion imaging, which may lead to difficulty in detection of global reduction in myocardial perfusion and thus underestimation of the extent of CAD. This fundamental limitation applies to MPI with both thallium-201–labeled and technetium-99m–labeled tracers.[5] With the use of PET, this issue with relative flow can be overcome due to better energy, spatial, temporal, and camera characteristics, allowing for global and regional MBF quantification in mL/min/g of tissue. Additional routine computed tomography (CT) attenuation correction with PET also leads to better-quality images with less artifacts.

Quantification of MBF using PET, allows assessment of peak hyperemic MBF as well as noninvasive calculation of CFR, a measure that evaluates the effects of abnormality over the entire coronary circulation (see **Fig. 1**). It, therefore, allows assessment not only of the effects of focal epicardial coronary stenosis but also of diffuse coronary atherosclerosis and microvascular dysfunction. The use of CFR measured by PET has helped diagnose balanced ischemia, atherosclerosis, and microvascular dysfunction. The CFR also appears to be a very strong prognostic measure of adverse cardiovascular events even in those without obstructive epicardial CAD.[6–8]

Technical Considerations

Perfusion tracers
The blood flow tracers used most commonly are ^{82}Rb-chloride and ^{13}N-ammonia, with a small number of centers around the world using ^{15}O-water. ^{18}F-flurpiridaz, another perfusion tracer, currently is under investigation. Because of their short half-lives, ^{13}N-ammonia and ^{15}O-water require an on-site cyclotron and ^{82}Rb, a generator. In contrast, ^{18}F-flurpiridaz, because of its longer physical half-life (110 min), can be produced in batches and distributed regionally as is done with ^{18}F-fluorodeoxyglucose (FDG).

Scanner performance
Contemporary PET scanners operate in 3-dimensional (3-D) acquisition mode, as opposed to the older 2-dimensional (2-D) (or 2-D/3-D) systems that were constructed with interplane septa designed to reduce scatter. The 3-D systems generally require lower injected activity, with a concordant reduction in patient radiation effective dose.

Image acquisition and analysis
Image acquisition consists of relative static perfusion images, gated images, and list mode acquisition for estimation of MBF after stress and rest. Quantification of MBF requires accurate measurement of the total tracer activity transported by the arterial blood and delivered to the myocardium over time. Measurements of arterial isotope activity versus time (time–activity curves) typically are acquired using image regions of interest in the arterial blood pool (eg, left ventricle [LV], atrium, or aorta).[9,10]

Stress test procedure
In the United States, regadenoson is the agent utilized most commonly for inducing hyperemia through coronary vasodilation.[10] Other agents, adenosine and dipyridamole, also are used.[9,10] Exercise stress maybe performed but is technically challenging due to short half-lives of radiotracers, smaller bores of PET gantry for supine bicycles, and motion artifacts from exercising.

Patient preparation for pharmacologic stress with PET is the same as for ^{99m}Tc SPECT MPI.[10] Patients fast for a minimum of 4 hours, avoid smoking for at least 4 hours, and avoid caffeine intake for at least 12 hours before vasodilator stress. Rest imaging should be performed before stress. Vasodilator stress with the chosen agent is followed by radiotracer injection and imaging at stress. Rest and stress images usually are performed the same day. The dose of radiotracer depends on the type of PET camera and patient weight.[11]

Image acquisition and reconstruction parameters
Images are acquired and reconstructed using standard vendor-specific parameters. Briefly, after a low-dose CT or a radionuclide-localizing scan to position the heart, a dynamic or preferably list-mode acquisition is acquired in 2-D or 3-D mode. List-mode acquisition provides comprehensive data for static images, gated images for LV volumes and ejection fraction (EF), and dynamic images for MBF quantitation. The relative and quantitative perfusion images are reconstructed from CT attenuation-corrected images.[9,10]

Indications and applications
American Society of Nuclear Cardiology[10] recommends the use of PET over SPECT myocardial perfusion when 1) Prior stress imaging study was of poor quality, equivocal or inconclusive 2) Body characteristics that commonly affect image quality. Some examples include large breasts, breast implants, obesity (BMI greater than 30), protuberant abdomen, chest wall deformities, pleural effusions, and inability for proper body positioning such as inability to position arms outside of a SPECT scanner's field of view 3) High-risk patients in whom diagnostic errors carry even greater clinical implications. Some examples include chronic kidney disease stages 3, 4 or 5; diabetes mellitus; known or suspected potentially high-risk CAD such as left main, multivessel, or proximal LAD disease or extensive coronary disease. 4) Young patients with established CAD who are anticipated to need repeated exposures to radiation-associated cardiac imaging procedures. 5) Patients in whom myocardial blood flow quantification is a needed adjunct to the imaging findings. Several investigational uses of myocardial perfusion imaging are also on the cusp of translation into clinical medicine including those suspected to have microvascular disease, cardiometabolic risk factors including those with obesity, CKD, and diabetes, heart transplant, and infiltrative cardiomyopathies.

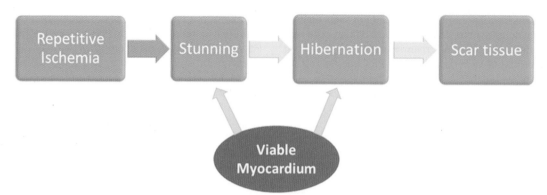

Fig. 2. Continuum of dysfunctional myocardium with subcategories of viable myocardium, that is, stunning and hibernation. Repetitive episodes of hypoperfusion and ischemia cause the development of stunned myocardium. Stunning denotes abnormal myocardial contractility in the presence of normal resting blood flow. Recurrent episodes of stunning in turn lead to hibernating myocardium, which is characterized by reduced resting blood flow and certain ultrastructural cardiomyocyte alterations, namely increased glycogen plaques and loss of their sarcoplasmic reticulum, T tubules, and contractile apparatus. Irrespective of the presence of normal or reduced resting blood flow (stunning vs hibernation), CFR is diminished, which in turn results in demand ischemia. Stunned and hibernating myocardium both are salvageable or viable, meaning that restoration of coronary perfusion may result in recovery of normal function/contractility. If no intervention is undertaken, however, to restore perfusion, hibernating myocardium evolves into scar tissue (irreversibly necrotic myocardium), characterized by alterations in gene expression, loss of mitochondrial function, increase in the myocardial extracellular space, and myocardial fibrosis. Scarred myocardium is seen as irreversibly adverse LV remodeling on cardiac imaging (echocardiography, CMR, and cardiac CT). Both scarred and hibernating myocardium may serve as substrates for ventricular arrhythmias and may increase the risk for sudden cardiac death.

PET VIABILITY
Background

Despite the advances in diagnosis, imaging, medical management, and revascularization techniques, one-third of patients following an acute myocardial infarction develop ischemic heart failure (ischemic cardiomyopathy [ICM]).[12] In 2010, the prevalence rates of ICM were 190 per 100,000 person-years and 270 per 100,000 person-years in women and men, respectively, and these rates are only expected to rise as the population ages and survival improves.[13] Viability imaging plays a significant role in risk stratifying patients with ICM who may benefit from revascularization. From an ultrastructural standpoint, viability refers to the preservation of contractile function based on cellular, metabolic, and microscopic characteristics. Clinically, the presence of viable myocardium denotes dysfunctional myocardium at rest, which may recover part or all of its contractile function following restoration of coronary perfusion.

There are 2 main categories of viable myocardium, namely hibernation and stunning, which fall on a continuum of abnormalities in myocardial perfusion and function (Fig. 2). Myocardial stunning results from transient, repetitive episodes of hypoperfusion and is characterized by reduced contractile function in the presence of normal resting blood flow. Recurrent episodes of stunning over time eventually leads to the development of hibernating myocardium characterized by reduced resting blood flow and associated alterations both at the ultrastructural cardiomyocyte level and at the macroscopic, LV level. From a macroscopic standpoint, hibernation manifests as adverse LV remodeling, LV dilation, and LV systolic and

Table 1		
Differences between myocardial stunning and hibernation		
Features	**Stunning**	**Hibernation**
Reduced flow at rest	✕	✔
Abnormal contractile function	✔	✔
Reduced CFR	✔	✔
Histopathologic abnormalities	✔	✔
Potential for recovery of LV function following revascularization	✔	✔
May progress to	Hibernation	Scar

Abbreviations: ✕, Absent; ✔, Present.

diastolic dysfunction. The main distinguishing characteristics of stunning and hibernation are listed in **Table 1**. These can be visualized by echocardiography, cardiac magnetic resonance (CMR), and cardiac CT. Myocardial radionuclide imaging, including SPECT and PET, rely on detecting changes in coronary perfusion and cardiomyocyte metabolism. Compared with SPECT, PET offers higher spatial and energy resolution and lower radiation exposure. These advantages are crucial when assessing for LV viability, when detection of scar versus hibernation is critical. The focus of this section is on providing an overview of FDG PET imaging for the evaluation of myocardial viability.

Protocols for Imaging

Normal myocardium utilizes long-chain fatty acids as its primary source of energy; however, under anaerobic conditions, for example, coronary hypoperfusion and ischemia, cardiomyocytes switch to glucose as their main energy source. The process of glucose uptake by the cardiomyocytes is active and mediated by insulin secretion. Appropriate management of glucose and insulin levels is key for generating diagnostically accurate and high-quality myocardial FDG PET studies for assessment of viability.

Evaluation of coronary perfusion and myocardial metabolism are the 2 key components of viability examination. Perfusion imaging can be performed either by SPECT tracers or by PET tracers, which are surrogates for the integrity of cardiomyocyte cellular membrane. Perfusion imaging at rest should be performed first; if there are no perfusion defects, this means that all LV segments are viable and evaluation for myocardial ischemia may be considered. If, however, there are resting perfusion defects, viability metabolic imaging can be undertaken with FDG.

The importance of patient preparation should be emphasized to provide examinations of high diagnostic quality. Following a 6-hour to 12-hour fast, plasma glucose is checked. Depending on this initial value, patients are administered an oral glucose load (25–100 mg), which leads to a transient increase in plasma glucose, stimulates pancreatic insulin secretion, and ultimately shifts myocardial consumption from fatty acids to glucose. Following the oral glucose load, intravenous insulin is administered to achieve euglycemic state prior to FDG injection.[11] An alternative to glucose loading is acipimox, a nicotinic acid derivative approved for use in Europe, which functions by inhibiting peripheral lipolysis, reducing levels of free fatty acids (FFAs), and ultimately increasing

levels of glucose. Another alternative technique is the euglycemic-hyperinsulinemic clamp, which is a rigorous and time-consuming procedure.[11] The target range for plasma glucose prior to administering FDG is 100 mg/dL to 140 mg/dL. Once glucose is within this range, FDG is injected and the patient is monitored for 45 minutes to 90 minutes prior to undergoing PET imaging. To ensure patient safety, glucose levels are monitored after FDG injection. Typically, 5 mCi to 15 mCi (185–555 MBq) of FDG is administered and image acquisition usually lasts 10 minutes to 30 minutes. An overview of the protocol is shown in **Fig. 3**.

Once both perfusion and metabolism imaging are completed, the 2 image data sets are aligned, and interpretation is based on 1 of the 4 distinct perfusion-metabolism patterns, as shown in **Fig. 4**. There are certain limitations of FDG viability assessment, namely FDG uptake, that can be impacted by the degree of underlying ischemia, coexisting abnormalities in sympathetic activity, and the severity of reduction in cardiac output/severity of underlying heart failure.[14]

Clinical Implications and Value of PET Viability Assessment

The results from multiple, single-center, observational, nonrandomized studies have shown viability imaging to be valuable in guiding decision making regarding revascularization in patients with ICM, meaning that patients with hibernating (viable) myocardium have been found to have lower mortality following revascularization. Di Carli and colleagues showed that in patients with viable myocardium detected by PET imaging, surgical revascularization compared with medical management was associated with improved 4-year survival (75% vs 30%; $P = .007$) as well as improvement in the severity of angina and symptoms of heart failure.[15–17] A more recent study on 648 patients by Ling and colleagues[18] also found that revascularization correlated with improved survival in patients with hibernating myocardium, particularly in those with more than 10% viable myocardium. These findings highlight one of the important criteria in assessing the benefits of revascularization in patients with hibernating myocardium, namely the extent of viability/hibernation. It has been shown that in patients with a higher mismatch of perfusion-metabolism (ie, larger extent of hibernation), the benefits from revascularization are larger.[19] The opposite also is true, meaning when the extent of mismatch is small (less than 7%), there is not much value in pursuing revascularization. Additional factors that should be considered when planning for

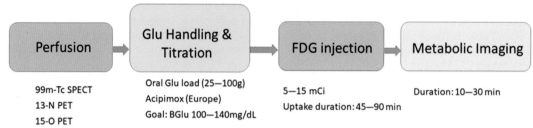

Fig. 3. Imaging protocol for ^{18}F-FDG PET viability assessment. Following administration of the perfusion tracer, perfusion imaging is performed either by means of SPECT or PET MPI. In the United States, ^{13}N-ammonia and [82]rubidium are clinically available PET tracers whereas in Europe both ^{13}N-ammonia and ^{15}O-water are available. Handling and titration of plasma glucose follow acquisition of perfusion image data set. The patient's baseline blood glucose is checked and, if less than 250 mg/dL, an oral glucose load is administered. Levels of blood glucose are checked frequently (every 10–15 min) and intravenous insulin is administered based on predefined protocols, to achieve a target plasma glucose of 100 mg/dL to 140 mg/dL. The goal is to shift myocardial energy consumption from fatty acid to glucose. Acipimox is a nicotinic acid derivative, which is an alternative to oral glucose loading. Once the plasma glucose is within the goal range of 100 mg/dL to 140 mg/dL, FDG is injected (5–15 mCi [185–555 MBq]). The patient then is monitored for 45 minutes to 90 minutes (uptake phase), during which time, blood pool concentrations of FDG decrease whereas myocardial FDG uptake increases. A higher signal-to-noise ratio can be achieved by waiting for the full 90 minutes, because blood pool FDG levels re very low while myocardial levels continue to rise. This can be beneficial particularly in diabetic patients, who pose a particular challenge due to high insulin resistance and high basal insulin requirements. Metabolic imaging is performed, which usually takes 10 minutes to 30 minutes to complete. The perfusion and metabolic image datasets then are aligned and evaluation for perfusion-metabolism patterns performed to allow for identification of viable (hibernating) myocardium versus scar versus stunning versus normal.

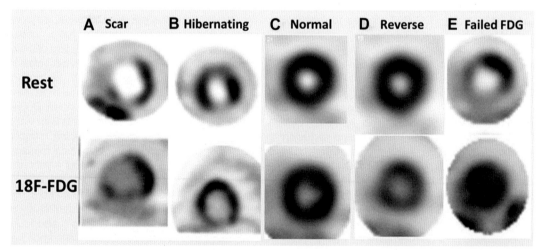

Fig. 4. Four patterns of perfusion-metabolism. (*A*) Matched perfusion and metabolism, where both are abnormal. The presence of a resting perfusion defect with accompanying defect on FDG metabolic imaging signifies absence of viability and presence of scared myocardium. There is a low likelihood this patient will experience improvement in LV dysfunction and adverse remodeling following revascularization. (*B*) Perfusion-metabolism mismatch involving the anterior wall, where a resting perfusion defect is accompanied by normal FDG uptake. This signifies the presence of viable, hibernating myocardium in the anterior wall. This patient has a high likelihood of experiencing improvement in LV systolic function and adverse remodeling following revascularization. Also note the presence of a matched perfusion-metabolism defect involving the inferior wall, which denotes scar. (*C*) Matched perfusion and metabolism where both are normal. This denotes normal myocardium at rest. If the patient experiences chest pain, angina, or other symptoms suggestive of ischemia, ischemia assessment should be considered. (*D*) Perfusion-metabolism mismatch, where there is no resting perfusion defect, but there is accompanying reduction in FDG uptake. This usually is seen in patients with left bundle branch block as a mismatch in the interventricular septum and also has been described in patients with stunning or significant insulin resistance. (*E*) Example of patient with high insulin resistance and poorly controlled diabetes mellitus resulting in poor-quality FDG images precluding accurate viability assessment.

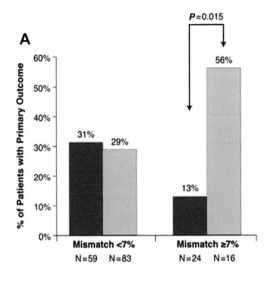

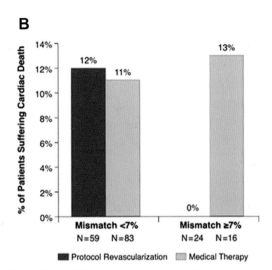

Fig. 5. (A) Proportion of patients who were randomized to either FDG-guided revascularization or medical therapy based on standard of care and who experienced the composite outcome of cardiac death, myocardial infarction, hospitalization due to unstable angina or heart failure, or heart transplantation within 1 year. The results are classified based on the size of perfusion-metabolism mismatch using 7% as the cutoff. In the subgroup with mismatch of less than 7%, revascularization was not associated with a significant improvement in the primary outcome compared with medical treatment ($P = .923$). In contrast, in the subgroup with mismatch greater than or equal to 7%, revascularization correlated with lower rates of the primary composite endpoint ($P = .015$). (B) Proportion of patients who were randomized to either FDG-guided revascularization or medical therapy based on standard of care and who experienced cardiac death within 1 year. In the subset of patients with mismatch less than 7%, revascularization was not associated with a significant difference in cardiac mortality. No cardiac deaths were noted in the subset of patients with mismatch greater than or equal to 7% who underwent FDG guided revascularization compared with 2 patients (15%) who were treated medically. (Adopted with permission from D'Egidio G, Nichol G, Williams KA, et al. JACC Cardiovasc Imaging 2009; 2:1060–1068.)

revascularization include the LVEF and the renal function.[20] Despite showing benefit of PET viability imaging to guide revascularization, these studies have undergone scrutiny due to their nonrandomized, single-center, observational design and due to the potential for including confounders and some of them only having small number of hard outcomes.[21,22]

To date the PET and Recovery Following Revascularization-2 (PARR 2) has been the only large, multicenter study that randomized 430 patients with known or suspected CAD to either FDG PET/CT viability imaging versus standard of care.[23] Over a 12-month follow-up, patients who underwent PET viability imaging showed a nonsignificant lower composite outcome of cardiac mortality, myocardial infarction, or hospitalization due to heart failure or angina.[23] In contrast, a post hoc analysis of 5-year follow-up comparing patients who adhered to PET recommendations for revascularization versus standard of care showed a significant improvement in event-free survival in the former and in those patients with a mismatch of at least 7% in extent (Fig. 5).[24,25] Two important

caveats of the PARR 2 are that only 25% of patients adhered to the PET-guided recommendations for revascularization and the variability in PET-related resources and expertise, which may have influenced decision making and patient management.[19,25] Future research for evaluation of the advantage of using advanced imaging (PET and CMR) is the focus of Alternative Imaging Modalities in Ischemic Heart Failure (AIMI-HF) trial, which itself is part of the larger, multitrial project of Imaging Modalities to Assist with Guiding Therapy and the Evaluation of Patients with Heart Failure (Fig. 6).[26]

When to Perform PET Viability Assessment

According to the most recent guidelines published by the American College of Cardiology and the American Heart Association, viability assessment using imaging is reasonable in patients with new-onset heart failure without angina and with known underlying significant CAD, provided the patient is an eligible candidate for revascularization (class IIa, level of evidence C).[27] The appropriate use criteria also are in accordance with this grading,

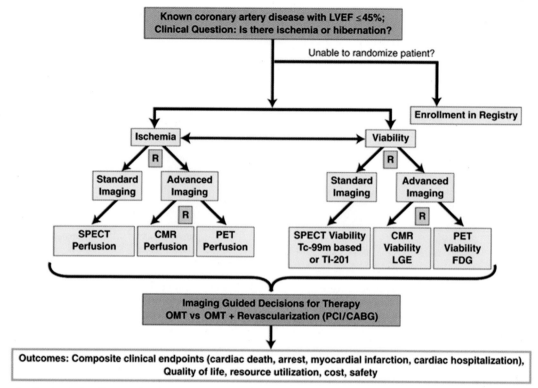

R = Randomization; Tc-99m = Technetium; TI-201 = Thallium; LGE = Late gadolinium enhancement; FDG = Fluorodexyglucose

Fig. 6. Study design of the AIMI-HF trial, is a combined randomized and registry study. Participants will be randomized either to advanced or standard imaging, depending on whether the primary clinical concern is the presence of ischemia versus viability. Patients not eligible for randomization will be assigned to a clinical registry. The primary outcome is a composite endpoint of cardiac mortality, cardiac hospitalization, myocardial infarction, or resuscitated cardiac arrest. (Adapted with permission from Mielniczuk LM, Toth GG, Xie JX et al. JACC Cardiovasc Imaging. 2017;10(3):354-64.)

that is, noninvasive imaging for viability assessment is appropriate or "may be appropriate" in most cases of LV systolic dysfunction (Table 2).[28] The most recent scientific statement from the American Heart Association on viability imaging provides algorithms for noninvasive imaging with CMR and FDG PET in patients with chronic and subacute ischemic LV systolic dysfunction.[29]

Conclusion

Noninvasive myocardial viability assessment using FDG PET so far has proved beneficial in prognosticating patients who may benefit from improved LV systolic function, quality of life, and survival following revascularization. Additional larger, randomized, multicenter studies are needed to better define the PET criteria that can be used to predict outcomes following revascularization. A heart team approach comprising cardiologists, surgeons, and imagers should be implemented to provide each patient with personalized

recommendations by integrating clinical, imaging and laboratory data.

PET FOR SARCOIDOSIS

Sarcoidosis is an immune-mediated systemic disease of unknown etiology, characterized by granulomatous inflammation of various organs.[30] Sarcoidosis first was described in 1877 by the dermatologist Jonathan Hutchinson, who described violaceous skin lesions.[31] Sarcoidosis diagnosis is made based on history, physical examination, appropriate radiologic and pathologic findings, and exclusion of other causes.[32]

Cardiac involvement often occurs with sarcoidosis (cardiac sarcoidosis [CS]); however, it produces symptoms in approximately only 5% of patients.[33] The prevalence of CS in the United States is approximately 25% for patients with sarcoidosis.[34] Clinical manifestations of CS are quite variable and range from a lack of any clinical symptoms to sudden death. Other presentations

Table 2
Indications for use of PET viability imaging in the 2013 appropriate use criteria

PET Viability Imaging in Patients Eligible for Revascularization	Rest Imaging	Stress/Rest Imaging
Severe LV systolic dysfunction (LVEF< 30%)	Appropriate	Appropriate
Moderate LV systolic dysfunction (LVEF: 30%−39%)	Appropriate	May be appropriate
Mild LV systolic dysfunction (LVEF: 40%−49%)	May be appropriate	Appropriate

Adapted from Patel MR, White RD, Abbara S, et al. 2013 ACCF/ACR/ASE/ASNC/SCCT/SCMR appropriate utilization of cardiovascular imaging in heart failure: a joint report of the American College of Radiology Appropriateness Criteria Committee and the American College of Cardiology Foundation Appropriate Use Criteria Task Force. J Am Coll Cardiol. 2013;61(21):2207-2231.

include dizziness, palpitations, syncope or near syncope, dyspnea, orthopnea, peripheral edema, chest pain, conduction abnormalities, and cardiac failure. Inflammatory granulomas or postinflammatory scarring may lead to conduction abnormalities, arrhythmias, sudden cardiac death, and congestive heart failure.[35] The myocardium is the region affected most frequently, especially the ventricular septum and LV free wall. Sarcoidosis also can involve the coronary arteries, pericardium, and valves.[34,36]

Isolated CS (ICS) is a distinct clinical phenotype. Established criteria for the diagnosis of CS are insensitive for ICS because they require either evidence of extracardiac disease or a positive endomyocardial biopsy (EMB). EMB is highly limited in its sensitivity of approximately 20% to 30%, because it often misses areas of patchy myocardial involvement.[37] As many as 25% of patients with CS may have ICS. Patients with ICS have worse LV systolic function and event-free survival and more ventricular arrhythmias compared with patients with systemic sarcoidosis and CS.[38]

Because of the potential life-threatening complications and potential benefit of treatment, all patients diagnosed with sarcoidosis should be screened for cardiac involvement. CMR and FDG PET/CT have nearly replaced other imaging techniques due to their higher accuracy for diagnosing CS.[35] PET/CT has been included in the diagnostic algorithm for CS by the Heart Rhythm Society in 2014[39] and the revised Japanese Society of Cardiac Sarcoidosis in 2017.[40]

A joint expert consensus document of the Society of Nuclear Medicine and Molecular Imaging (SNMMI) and ASNC by Chareonthaitawee and colleagues recommend PET/CT for the assessment of CS in (1) patients with histologic evidence of extra CS and 1 or more abnormal screening results for CS, (2) new-onset sustained second-degree or third degree atrioventricular block and age less than 60 years, (3) idiopathic sustained ventricular tachycardia, and (4) serial studies to assess response to treatment.[41,42]

Optimal patient preparation is essential when using FDG PET/CT to evaluate CS. It is imperative that physiologic myocardial uptake FDG be suppressed to identify areas of pathologic involvement. Standardized guidelines developed by SNMMI and ASNC recommend at least 2 high-fat (>35 g) and low-carbohydrate (<3 g) meals the day prior to the FDG PET/CT, followed by a fast of 4 hours to 12 hours prior to the study. An alternative option (for patients who cannot follow the diet) is fasting for greater than of equal to 18 h before the study.[42,43]

All CS patients scheduled for FDG PET should undergo rest MPI to compare perfusion images

Table 3
Classification of cardiac sarcoidosis stage based on perfusion and metabolism pattern

Disease Stage	Perfusion and Metabolism Pattern
Stage 1	Normal perfusion and no FDG uptake
Stage 2: mild or early disease	Patchy FDG uptake in an area with normal or only mildly decreased perfusion
Stage 3: moderate or progressive disease	FDG uptake in an area with a corresponding moderate perfusion defect
Stage 4: severe or fibrous disease	Severe perfusion defect but no or minimal corresponding FDG uptake

Data from Bokhari S, Lin JC, Julien HM. FDG-PET is a superior tool in the diagnosis and management of cardiac sarcoidosis https://www.acc.org/latest-in-cardiology/articles/2017/04/10/08/43/fdg-pet-is-a-superior-tool. Published April 10, 2017.

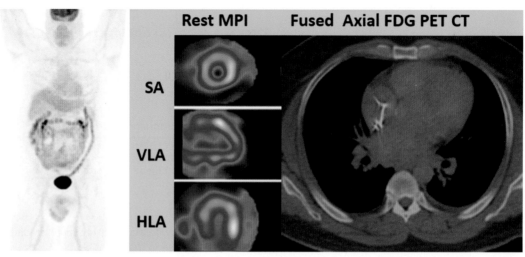

Fig. 7. A 49-year-old man with sarcoidosis and complete heart block, post-pacemaker placement, on immunosuppressive treatment. Stage 1 CS with normal Technetium-99m (99mTc) rest myocardial perfusion (*center panel*) and no active cardiac or extracardiac inflammation on MIP (*left panel*) and fused FDG PET/CT images (*right panel*). SA: Short Axis, VLA: vertical Long Axis, HLA: horizontal long axis.

with FDG PET images. After perfusion imaging, approximately 10 mCi (370 MBq) of FDG is injected intravenously to perform dedicated cardiac and optional whole-body FDG PET/CT scans. CS is categorized into stage I to stage IV, based on perfusion and metabolism patterns (**Table 3**). Rest perfusion images are classified as normal or abnormal. Regional myocardial perfusion is categorized further as normal (**Figs. 7 and 8**) or mildly, moderately, or severely reduced.[44] A resting myocardial perfusion defect in these patients could be attributed to microvascular compression from inflammation or may be due to scar. FDG images are considered normal when there is no myocardial FDG uptake (see **Fig. 7**). If concurrent FDG is noted in the same territory, then the perfusion defect likely is secondary to inflammation (**Fig. 9**). Myocardial scar is favored if FDG uptake is lacking in this territory with associated regional wall motion abnormality. Comparison of rest myocardial perfusion and FDG PET is essential to identify disease patterns (no inflammation, active inflammation, and scarring) and to evaluate response to therapy.[45]

FDG images are considered abnormal when there is a focal, heterogeneous, or focal on diffuse

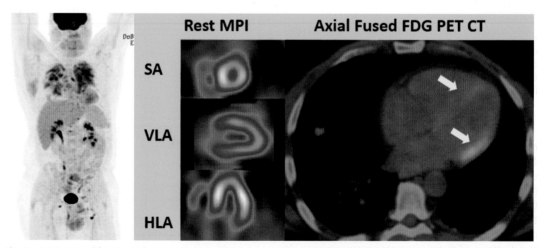

Fig. 8. A 57-year-old man with systemic sarcoidosis and right bundle-branch block. Rest perfusion is normal. FDG PET MIP shows extensive active pulmonary disease and hypermetabolic lymph nodes. Fused PET/CT images show active bilateral lung inflammation and patchy areas of FDG uptake involving the septal, anterior, and lateral myocardium, (*arrows*) from early myocardial sarcoid involvement (stage 2).

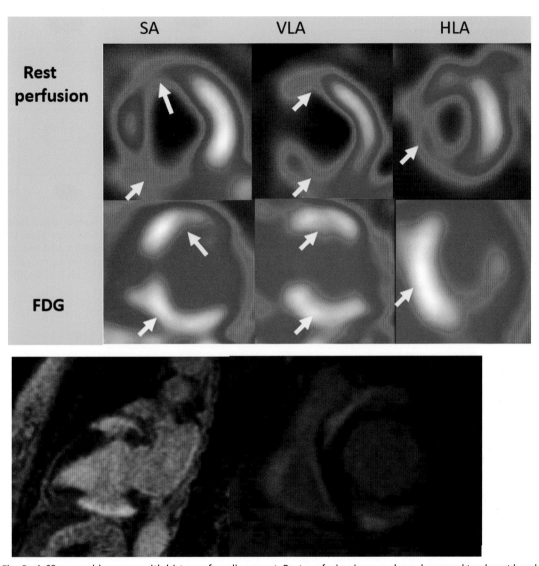

Fig. 9. A 62 -year-old woman with history of cardiac arrest. Rest perfusion images show decreased to absent basal to midanterior, anteroseptal, inferior, and inferoseptal myocardium, with corresponding FDG uptake (*arrows*)—moderate/progressive disease (stage 3). No extracardiac inflammation was identified, suggestive of ICS. CMR 2-chamber and short-axis images show subepicardial and midmyocardial late gadolinium enhancement along the anterior and inferior walls of LV, consistent with CS. HLA, horizontal long axis; SA, short axis; VLA, vertical long axis.

myocardial FDG uptake.[46] PET also helps in assessment of disease activity visually and with semiquantitative standardized uptake value (SUV) and in monitoring treatment response (Fig. 10); however, there is no specific SUV threshold that can be used to reliably delineate inflamed from normal myocardial tissue.[41] Whole-body FDG PET also is useful to evaluate the extent of systemic disease (see Fig. 8). FDG PET/CT is preferred in patients where CMR is contraindicated, in patients with implantable metallic devices (see Fig. 10), and in impaired renal function.[36] Blankstein and colleagues[46] have demonstrated the relationship between FDG uptake and focal perfusion defects, as shown by cardiac PET for identifying patients who are at higher risk of lethal arrhythmias and death.

Gallium-68 (^{68}Ga) DOTATATE, a somatostatin receptor–targeted radiotracer, is a potential alternative to FDG in imaging the CS patient. It is a commonly used tracer in neuroendocrine tumor imaging. ^{68}Ga-DOTATATE also targets activated

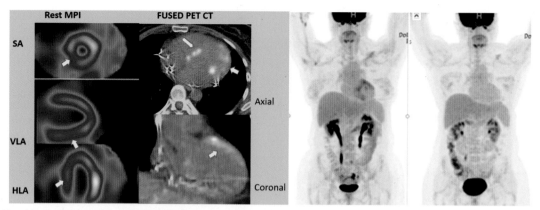

Fig. 10. A 54-year-old woman with CS. Rest perfusion images with abnormal perfusion in septum and inferior wall (*arrows*, left/1st column). Fused FDG PET-CT and MIP images with focal on diffuse uptake, notable in the anterior, inferior, anterolateral, and septal myocardium, consistent with active inflammation (2nd and 3rd column). Follow-up PET CT showing significant improvement after patient placed on steroids and immunosuppression, as shown on MIP images (right/4th column). This patient could not undergo CMR due to an incompatible defibrillator. HLA, horizontal long axis; SA, short axis; VLA, vertical long axis.

macrophages and multinucleated cells, which express somatostatin receptors. It does not target normal myocardial tissue, which lacks somatostatin receptors, and therefore possibly is suitable for patients with limitations to the adherence of FDG myocardial suppression protocols. ^{68}Ga-DOTATATE has a role in evaluating disease extent of sarcoidosis and can be used as guidance to different therapeutic options or prognosis, as proposed by Vachatimanont and colleagues.[47]

Integrated PET/MR imaging is promising. The integration of the metabolic PET imaging along with the morphologic, functional, and tissue imaging characteristics of MR imaging would improve diagnostic accuracy and potentially provide further prognostic and therapeutic insight in CS patients.[48] Wicks and colleagues[49] showed that hybrid PET/MR imaging was superior for detecting CS with sensitivity, specificity, positive, and negative predictive values of 0.94, 0.44, 0.76, and 0.80, respectively and abnormalities found on both PET and MR imaging was the strongest predictor of major adverse cardiac events.

Corticosteroid therapy is the first-line treatment of CS to reduce inflammation and prevent progression to fibrosis.[50] Starting therapy before LV dysfunction results in an excellent clinical outcome and is the mainstay in the treatment of CS. When CS patients present with sustained ventricular arrhythmias, use of implantable cardioverter-defibrillators (ICDs) is crucial.[51] Pacemaker implantation is recommended in patients with a high-grade or complete atrioventricular block.[52] Immunosuppressive therapies have been used in patients refractory to corticosteroids or in those who cannot tolerate their side effects. Treatment with methotrexate, azathioprine, or cyclophosphamide also is used as a steroid-sparing agent. In patients for whom corticosteroids are contraindicated, immunosuppressive agents are chosen for the initial treatment.[53] Orthotopic heart transplant is used increasingly for end-stage heart failure due to CS.[54]

18F-FLUORODEOXYGLUCOSE PET IMAGING OF CARDIAC AND CARDIAC DEVICE INFECTIONS

Early and accurate diagnosis of cardiac valve and cardiac device infection is crucial for clinical decision making because these infections are associated with significant morbidity and mortality, especially when there is a delay in diagnosis and treatment. Cardiac implantable electronic devices (CIEDs) include pacemakers, ICDs, and cardiac resynchronization therapy devices with or without defibrillator. Cardiac device infections can be pocket and/or systemic infection. Pocket infection involves the subcutaneous pocket containing the generator and the subcutaneous portion of the leads. Systemic infection involves the transvenous segment of the lead (**Fig. 11**) or an epicardial electrode. Infection rates are lowest during initial implantation and 1.5-fold to 3-fold higher during revision or replacement.[55]

Diagnosis of cardiac and cardiac device infection is based on clinical manifestations, blood cultures (and other microbiologic data), and first-line

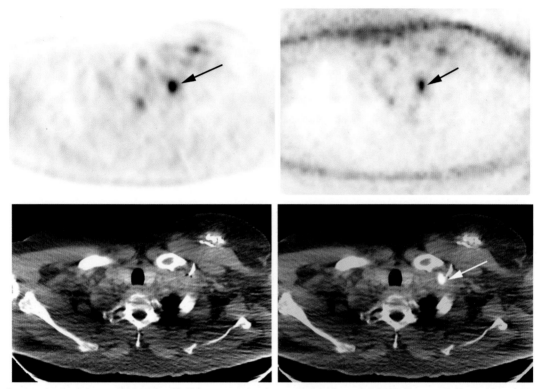

Fig. 11. Attenuation-corrected (*top left*), non-attenuation-corrected (*top right*), CT (*bottom left*), and fused PET/CT images (bottom right) show prominent focal hypermetabolic activity associated with left chest wall ICD lead infection (*arrows*) in the subclavian vein with tiny air bubbles in a patient with methicillin-sensitive Staphylococcus aureus bacteremia.

imaging with echocardiography. Although the utility of FDG PET for diagnosis of native valve infective endocarditis is limited, it is more useful for evaluating prosthetic valve endocarditis (**Fig. 12**). FDG PET not only promptly identifies the presence and extent of cardiac infection (abscess and paravalvular spread) but also demonstrates any embolic extracardiac infection (given the wide field of view) and primary source of infection, which can affect treatment decision making. In 1 study, extracardiac infection PET findings led to treatment change in 35% of patients.[56] Recent meta-analyses report a pooled sensitivity of 61% to 81% and pooled specificity of 78% to 88% for FDG PET diagnosis of infective endocarditis, with higher sensitivity for prosthetic valve endocarditis.[57,58] The pooled sensitivity and specificity of PET/CT diagnosis of CIED infection were 83% and 89%, respectively, with diagnostic performance of pocket infection better than lead infection.[59] FDG PET/CT also has high diagnostic accuracy for LV assist device infections, with pooled sensitivity of 92% and specificity of 83%.[60] Prognostically, an abnormal FDG PET is associated with greater major adverse cardiac events in prosthetic valve endocarditis.[61] Diemberger and colleagues[62] noted increased mortality in patients with FDG PET CIED lead infection but no pocket infection. FDG PET/CT has made it into guideline recommendations for diagnosis of infective endocarditis and cardiac device infection, with FDG avidity of a greater than 3-month-old prosthetic valve a major diagnostic criterion of infection.[63,64]

Increased glucose metabolism from increased glucose transporter-1 expression to meet the higher energy demands of activated inflammatory cells (leukocytes and macrophages) is the basis of FDG PET infection and inflammation imaging.[65] Reliable hot spot FDG PET in suspected cardiac infection is possible only when physiologic myocardial FDG uptake is suppressed. The heart uses various substrates for its energy needs, including FFAs, glucose, and lactate. Thus, interventions that facilitate myocardial FFA metabolism while simultaneously suppressing physiologic glucose metabolism are imperative for successful FDG PET cardiac infection imaging.[66]

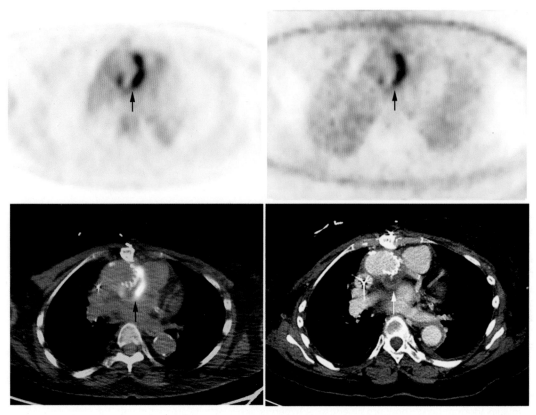

Fig. 12. Attenuation corrected (*top left*), non-attenuation-corrected (*top right*), fused PET/CT (*bottom left*), and CT (bottom right)images demonstrate prominent hypermetabolic activity involving and surrounding the infected transaortic valve prosthesis with a perivalvular fluid collection/abscess (*arrows*) in a patient with methicillin-resistant Staphylococcus aureus bacteremia.

Optimal patient preparation protocols are not well established. A combination of interventions is the norm. These include avoidance of strenuous exercise and a no-carbohydrate to very-low-carbohydrate (<3 g), high-protein, and high-fat diet (>35 g) for at least the day prior to the scan followed by an overnight fast.[11] Glucose-containing intravenous medications or fluids are prohibited. An alternative option (for patients who cannot follow the diet) is fasting for greater than or equal to 18 hours before the study.[41] The role of intravenous unfractionated heparin (induces lipolysis by lipoprotein lipase activation and increases FFA in the blood) is unclear.[41] Heparin (dose 10–50 IU/kg) is given 15 minutes before FDG injection with lower doses increasing FFA without significant partial thromboplastin time prolongation. Approximately 60 minutes after intravenous FDG injection (8–10 mCi [296–370 MBq]), whole-body (typically eyes to thighs) and dedicated cardiac PET/CT or PET/MR images are acquired.

Both CT attenuation-corrected and non–attenuation-corrected images are reviewed to differentiate real from artifactual increased tracer uptake due to high-density metal in devices. Fused PET/CT images provide anatomic localization of tracer. Focal or heterogeneous uptake favors infection, whereas diffuse mild uptake may suggest nonspecific inflammatory changes. The methodology and role of semiquantitative SUV in assessment of cardiac and cardiac device infections is unclear.[67]

Noninfectious inflammatory activity may cause false-positive results, such as early after surgery or from foreign body/granulomatous reaction. Thus, it can be challenging to differentiate noninfectious inflammation from infection on FDG-PET for up to 3 months postintervention.[67] The surgical adhesive used to seal an aortic root graft may produce inflammation resulting in false-positive tracer uptake.[11] Other false positives include active thrombi, soft atherosclerotic plaques, vasculitis, primary cardiac tumors, and metastasis.[63] False-negative FDG PET (no or low uptake) may be seen in mild infection with a low bacterial load, small vegetations, chronic or indolent infection with slow-growing bacteria, infection with fastidious or biofilm-forming bacteria, and partially treated infection. Abnormal noncardiac FDG uptake may be potential sites of embolic infection (osteomyelitis, intra-abdominal abscess, and so forth). Brain septic emboli identification is limited by high physiologic brain cortical FDG uptake. Compared with alternative leukocyte scintigraphy, FDG PET has the advantage of shorter procedure duration (<2 hours), high sensitivity, and better spatial and contrast resolution but suffers from lower specificity because FDG also can accumulate in noninfectious inflammatory cells.

In conclusion, FDG PET is a promising and emerging adjunctive diagnostic tool that can help in the diagnosis, disease severity assessment, and evaluation of embolic complications and prognosis of potentially life-threatening cardiac and cardiac device infections.

CLINICS CARE POINTS

- PET myocardial perfusion imaging has distinct advantages over SPECT, specifically in patient subgroups including obesity, high risk anatomy (multivessel and left main disease), diabetes and chronic kidney disease.

- PET viability assessment is reasonable in most patients with LV systolic dysfunction and known significant underlying coronary artery disease.

- Patient preparation protocols for assessment of cardiac inflammation with FDG PET involves a combination of fasting, high fat and no to low carbohydrate diet, and avoidance of exercise. Role of intravenous unfractionated heparin is unclear.

REFERENCES

1. Roger VL. Epidemiology of myocardial infarction. Med Clin North Am 2007;91(4):537–52, ix.
2. Mozaffarian D, Benjamin EJ, Go AS, et al. Executive summary: heart disease and stroke statistics–2016 update: a report from the American Heart Association. Circulation 2016;133(4):447–54.
3. Rosamond W, Flegal K, Furie K, et al. Heart disease and stroke statistics–2008 update: a report from the American Heart Association Statistics Committee and Stroke Statistics Subcommittee. Circulation 2008;117(4):e25–146.
4. De Bruyne B, Oldroyd KG, Pijls NHJ. Microvascular (Dys)Function and clinical outcome in stable coronary disease. J Am Coll Cardiol 2016;67(10):1170–2.
5. Bateman TM, Maddahi J, Gray RJ, et al. Diffuse slow washout of myocardial thallium-201: a new scintigraphic indicator of extensive coronary artery disease. J Am Coll Cardiol 1984;4(1):55–64.
6. Gupta A, Taqueti VR, van de Hoef TP, et al. Integrated noninvasive physiological assessment of coronary circulatory function and impact on cardiovascular mortality in patients with stable coronary artery disease. Circulation 2017;136(24):2325–36.
7. Bajaj NS, Bhambhvani P. SPECT-derived absolute myocardial perfusion measures: a step in the right direction. J Nucl Cardiol 2019. https://doi.org/10.1007/s12350-019-01972-w.
8. Bajaj NS, Osborne MT, Gupta A, et al. Coronary microvascular dysfunction and cardiovascular risk in obese patients. J Am Coll Cardiol 2018;72(7):707–17.
9. Murthy VL, Bateman TM, Beanlands RS, et al. Clinical quantification of myocardial blood flow using PET: joint position paper of the SNMMI cardiovascular Council and the ASNC. J Nucl Cardiol 2018;25(1):269–97.
10. Bateman TM, Dilsizian V, Beanlands RS, et al. American Society of Nuclear Cardiology and Society of Nuclear Medicine and molecular imaging joint position statement on the clinical indications for myocardial perfusion PET. J Nucl Cardiol 2016;23(5):1227–31.
11. Dilsizian V, Bacharach SL, Beanlands RS, et al. ASNC imaging guidelines/SNMMI procedure standard for positron emission tomography (PET) nuclear cardiology procedures. J Nucl Cardiol 2016;23(5):1187–226.
12. Cahill TJ, Kharbanda RK. Heart failure after myocardial infarction in the era of primary percutaneous coronary intervention: mechanisms, incidence and identification of patients at risk. World J Cardiol 2017;9(5):407–15.
13. Moran AE, Forouzanfar MH, Roth GA, et al. The global burden of ischemic heart disease in 1990 and 2010: the Global Burden of Disease 2010 study. Circulation 2014;129(14):1493–501.
14. Löffler AI, Kramer CM. Myocardial viability testing to guide coronary revascularization. Interv Cardiol Clin 2018;7(3):355–65.
15. Di Carli MF, Asgarzadie F, Schelbert HR, et al. Quantitative relation between myocardial viability and improvement in heart failure symptoms after

revascularization in patients with ischemic cardio-myopathy. Circulation 1995;92(12):3436–44.

16. Di Carli MF, Maddahi J, Rokhsar S, et al. Long-term survival of patients with coronary artery disease and left ventricular dysfunction: implications for the role of myocardial viability assessment in management decisions. J Thorac Cardiovasc Surg 1998;116(6): 997–1004.

17. Sheikine Y, Di Carli MF. Integrated PET/CT in the assessment of etiology and viability in ischemic heart failure. Curr Heart Fail Rep 2008;5(3): 136–42.

18. Ling LF, Marwick TH, Flores DR, et al. Identification of therapeutic benefit from revascularization in patients with left ventricular systolic dysfunction: inducible ischemia versus hibernating myocardium. Circ Cardiovasc Imaging 2013;6(3):363–72.

19. D'Egidio G, Nichol G, Williams KA, et al. Increasing benefit from revascularization is associated with increasing amounts of myocardial hibernation: a substudy of the PARR-2 trial. JACC Cardiovasc Imaging 2009;2(9):1060–8.

20. Anavekar NS, Chareonthaitawee P, Narula J, et al. Revascularization in patients with severe left ventricular dysfunction: is the assessment of viability still viable? J Am Coll Cardiol 2016;67(24):2874–87.

21. Allman KC, Shaw LJ, Hachamovitch R, et al. Myocardial viability testing and impact of revascularization on prognosis in patients with coronary artery disease and left ventricular dysfunction: a meta-analysis. J Am Coll Cardiol 2002;39(7):1151–8.

22. Schelbert HR. PET contributions to understanding normal and abnormal cardiac perfusion and metabolism. Ann Biomed Eng 2000;28(8):922–9.

23. Beanlands RS, Nichol G, Huszti E, et al. F-18-fluoro-deoxyglucose positron emission tomography imaging-assisted management of patients with severe left ventricular dysfunction and suspected coronary disease: a randomized, controlled trial (PARR-2). J Am Coll Cardiol 2007;50(20):2002–12.

24. Mc Ardle B, Shukla T, Nichol G, et al. Long-term follow-up of outcomes with f-18-fluorodeoxyglucose positron emission tomography imaging-assisted management of patients with severe left ventricular dysfunction secondary to coronary disease. Circ Cardiovasc Imaging 2016;9(9):e004331.

25. Abraham A, Nichol G, Williams KA, et al. 18F-FDG PET imaging of myocardial viability in an experienced center with access to 18F-FDG and integration with clinical management teams: the Ottawa-FIVE substudy of the PARR 2 trial. J Nucl Med 2010;51(4): 567–74.

26. O'Meara E, Mielniczuk LM, Wells GA, et al. Alternative Imaging Modalities in Ischemic Heart Failure (AIMI-HF) IMAGE HF Project I-A: study protocol for a randomized controlled trial. Trials 2013;14:218.

27. Yancy CW, Jessup M, Bozkurt B, et al. 2017 ACC/AHA/HFSA focused update of the 2013 ACCF/AHA guideline for the management of heart failure: a report of the American College of Cardiology/American Heart Association Task Force on Clinical Practice Guidelines and the Heart Failure Society of America. Circulation 2017;136(6): e137–61.

28. Patel MR, White RD, Abbara S, et al. 2013 ACCF/ACR/ASE/ASNC/SCCT/SCMR appropriate utilization of cardiovascular imaging in heart failure: a joint report of the American College of Radiology Appropriateness Criteria Committee and the American College of Cardiology Foundation Appropriate Use Criteria Task Force. J Am Coll Cardiol 2013;61(21): 2207–31.

29. Garcia MJ, Kwong RY, Scherrer-Crosbie M, et al. State of the art: imaging for myocardial viability: a scientific statement from the American Heart Association. Circ Cardiovasc Imaging 2020;13(7):e000053.

30. Baughman RP, Lower EE, du Bois RM. Sarcoidosis. Lancet 2003;361(9363):1111–8.

31. Llanos O, Hamzeh N. Sarcoidosis. Med Clin North Am 2019;103(3):527–34.

32. Statement on sarcoidosis. Joint Statement of the American Thoracic Society (ATS), the European Respiratory Society (ERS) and the World Association of Sarcoidosis and Other Granulomatous Disorders (WASOG) adopted by the ATS Board of Directors and by the ERS Executive Committee, February 1999. Am J Respir Crit Care Med 1999; 160(2):736–55.

33. Vignaux O. Cardiac sarcoidosis: spectrum of MRI features. AJR Am J Roentgenol 2005;184(1):249–54.

34. Kim JS, Judson MA, Donnino R, et al. Cardiac sarcoidosis. Am Heart J 2009;157(1):9–21.

35. Schatka I, Bengel FM. Advanced imaging of cardiac sarcoidosis. J Nucl Med 2014;55(1):99–106.

36. Perez IE, Garcia MJ, Taub CC. Multimodality imaging in cardiac sarcoidosis: is there a winner? Curr Cardiol Rev 2016;12(1):3–11.

37. Cooper LT, Baughman KL, Feldman AM, et al. The role of endomyocardial biopsy in the management of cardiovascular disease: a scientific statement from the American Heart Association, the American College of Cardiology, and the European Society of Cardiology Endorsed by the Heart Failure Society of America and the Heart Failure Association of the European Society of Cardiology. Eur Heart J 2007; 28(24):3076–93.

38. Okada DR, Bravo PE, Vita T, et al. Isolated cardiac sarcoidosis: a focused review of an under-recognized entity. J Nucl Cardiol 2018;25(4): 1136–46.

39. Birnie DH, Sauer WH, Bogun F, et al. HRS expert consensus statement on the diagnosis and

management of arrhythmias associated with cardiac sarcoidosis. Heart Rhythm 2014;11(7):1305–23.

40. Kumita S, Yoshinaga K, Miyagawa M, et al. Recommendations for (18)F-fluorodeoxyglucose positron emission tomography imaging for diagnosis of cardiac sarcoidosis-2018 update: Japanese Society of Nuclear Cardiology recommendations. J Nucl Cardiol 2019;26(4):1414–33.

41. Chareonthaitawee P, Beanlands RS, Chen W, et al. Joint SNMMI-ASNC expert consensus document on the Role of (18)F-FDG PET/CT in cardiac sarcoid detection and therapy monitoring. J Nucl Med 2017; 58(8):1341–53.

42. Bois JP, Muser D, Chareonthaitawee P. PET/CT evaluation of cardiac sarcoidosis. PET Clin 2019;14(2): 223–32.

43. Osborne MT, Hulten EA, Murthy VL, et al. Patient preparation for cardiac fluorine-18 fluorodeoxyglucose positron emission tomography imaging of inflammation. J Nucl Cardiol 2017;24(1):86–99.

44. Tilkemeier PL, Wackers FJ. Myocardial perfusion planar imaging. J Nucl Cardiol 2006;13(6):e91–6.

45. Skali H, Schulman AR, Dorbala S. 18F-FDG PET/CT for the assessment of myocardial sarcoidosis. Curr Cardiol Rep 2013;15(4):352.

46. Blankstein R, Osborne M, Naya M, et al. Cardiac positron emission tomography enhances prognostic assessments of patients with suspected cardiac sarcoidosis. J Am Coll Cardiol 2014;63(4):329–36.

47. Vachatimanont S, Kunawudhi A, Promteangtrong C, et al. Benefits of [(68)Ga]-DOTATATE PET-CT comparable to [(18)F]-FDG in patient with suspected cardiac sarcoidosis. J Nucl Cardiol 2020.

48. White JA, Rajchl M, Butler J, et al. Active cardiac sarcoidosis: first clinical experience of simultaneous positron emission tomography–magnetic resonance imaging for the diagnosis of cardiac disease. Circulation 2013;127(22):e639–41.

49. Wicks EC, Menezes LJ, Barnes A, et al. Diagnostic accuracy and prognostic value of simultaneous hybrid 18F-fluorodeoxyglucose positron emission tomography/magnetic resonance imaging in cardiac sarcoidosis. Eur Heart J Cardiovasc Imaging 2018; 19(7):757–67.

50. Bargout R, Kelly RF. Sarcoid heart disease: clinical course and treatment. Int J Cardiol 2004;97(2):173–82.

51. Schuller JL, Zipse M, Crawford T, et al. Implantable cardioverter defibrillator therapy in patients with cardiac sarcoidosis. J Cardiovasc Electrophysiol 2012; 23(9):925–9.

52. Epstein AE, Dimarco JP, Ellenbogen KA, et al. ACC/AHA/HRS 2008 guidelines for device-based therapy of cardiac rhythm abnormalities: executive summary. Heart Rhythm 2008;5(6):934–55.

53. Lower EE, Baughman RP. The use of low dose methotrexate in refractory sarcoidosis. Am J Med Sci 1990;299(3):153–7.

54. Rosenthal DG, Anderson ME, Petek BJ, et al. Invasive hemodynamics and rejection rates in patients with cardiac sarcoidosis after heart transplantation. Can J Cardiol 2018;34(8):978–82.

55. Prutkin JM, Reynolds MR, Bao H, et al. Rates of and factors associated with infection in 200 909 Medicare implantable cardioverter-defibrillator implants: results from the National Cardiovascular Data Registry. Circulation 2014;130(13):1037–43.

56. Orvin K, Goldberg E, Bernstine H, et al. The role of FDG-PET/CT imaging in early detection of extra-cardiac complications of infective endocarditis. Clin Microbiol Infect 2015;21(1):69–76.

57. Juneau D, Golfam M, Hazra S, et al. Molecular Imaging for the diagnosis of infective endocarditis: a systematic literature review and meta-analysis. Int J Cardiol 2018;253:183–8.

58. Mahmood M, Kendi AT, Ajmal S, et al. Meta-analysis of 18F-FDG PET/CT in the diagnosis of infective endocarditis. J Nucl Cardiol 2019;26(3):922–35.

59. Mahmood M, Kendi AT, Farid S, et al. Role of (18)F-FDG PET/CT in the diagnosis of cardiovascular implantable electronic device infections: a meta-analysis. J Nucl Cardiol 2019;26(3):958–70.

60. Tam MC, Patel VN, Weinberg RL, et al. Diagnostic accuracy of FDG PET/CT in suspected LVAD infections: a case series, systematic review, and meta-analysis. JACC Cardiovasc Imaging 2020;13(5): 1191–202.

61. San S, Ravis E, Tessonier L, et al. Prognostic value of (18)F-fluorodeoxyglucose positron emission tomography/computed tomography in infective endocarditis. J Am Coll Cardiol 2019;74(8):1031–40.

62. Diemberger I, Bonfiglioli R, Martignani C, et al. Contribution of PET imaging to mortality risk stratification in candidates to lead extraction for pacemaker or defibrillator infection: a prospective single center study. Eur J Nucl Med Mol Imaging 2019; 46(1):194–205.

63. Habib G, Lancellotti P, Antunes MJ, et al. 2015 ESC Guidelines for the management of infective endocarditis: The Task Force for the Management of Infective Endocarditis of the European Society of Cardiology (ESC). Endorsed by: European Association for Cardio-Thoracic Surgery (EACTS), the European Association of Nuclear Medicine (EANM). Eur Heart J 2015;36(44):3075–128.

64. Blomstrom-Lundqvist C, Traykov V, Erba PA, et al. European Heart Rhythm Association (EHRA) international consensus document on how to prevent, diagnose, and treat cardiac implantable electronic device infections-endorsed by the Heart Rhythm Society (HRS), the Asia Pacific Heart Rhythm Society (APHRS), the Latin American Heart Rhythm Society (LAHRS), International Society for Cardiovascular Infectious Diseases (ISCVID), and the European Society of Clinical

Microbiology and Infectious Diseases (ESCMID) in collaboration with the European Association for Cardio-Thoracic Surgery (EACTS). Eur Heart J 2020;41(21):2012–32.

65. Mochizuki T, Tsukamoto E, Kuge Y, et al. FDG uptake and glucose transporter subtype expressions in experimental tumor and inflammation models. J Nucl Med 2001;42(10):1551–5.

66. Bhambhvani P. Challenges of cardiac inflammation imaging with F-18 FDG positron emission tomography. J Nucl Cardiol 2017;24(1):100–2.

67. Mahmood M, Abu Saleh O. The role of 18-F FDG PET/CT in imaging of endocarditis and cardiac device infections. Semin Nucl Med 2020;50(4):319–30.

Clinical Applications of PET/MR Imaging

Farshad Moradi, MD, PhD[a],*, Andrei Iagaru, MD[a], Jonathan McConathy, MD, PhD[b]

KEYWORDS

- PET/MR imaging • Oncologic imaging • Molecular neuroimaging

KEY POINTS

- PET/MR imaging for whole-body oncologic imaging performs at least as well as PET/CT and may have advantages for certain malignancies.
- Pelvic, liver, and soft-tissue malignancies are additional indications benefitting from the advantages offered by simultaneous PET/MR imaging.
- PET/MR imaging is well suited to brain imaging and has the potential to grow substantially for evaluation of cognitive impairment and neuro-oncology.
- PET/MR imaging can reduce radiation exposure compared with PET/CT and reduce the burden of diagnostic imaging for some oncologic and neurologic applications.

INTRODUCTION

Positron emission tomography (PET) and magnetic resonance imaging (MRI) are advanced clinical imaging modalities that in combination can provide structural, morphologic, functional, and molecular information about disease and physiologic processes in a single imaging session. Several simultaneous PET/MR imaging scanners are FDA-cleared and in clinical use although they are not as widely used as PET/CT scanners. Systems capable of acquiring PET and MR imaging data at the same time can provide unique advantages for both clinical and investigational applications. This article reviews current clinical applications of PET/MR imaging for oncologic and neurologic imaging including advantages and limitations compared with PET/CT and separately acquired PET and MR imaging.

A current challenge in clinical PET/MR imaging is establishing applications where PET/MR imaging is clearly superior to other imaging modalities, particularly PET/CT and separately acquired PET and MR imaging. Much of the available data on clinical PET/MR imaging reflect the lower bounds of utility compared with standard of care and established imaging techniques such as PET/CT. Some of the published results rely on sequences, radiopharmaceuticals, or processing techniques that are not universally available limiting their applicability in general practice settings.

PRACTICAL CONSIDERATIONS, STRENGTHS, AND CHALLENGES
Instrumentation

One of the key advances that enabled simultaneous PET/MR imaging was the development of mutually compatible PET detectors, MR coils, and MR gradients. The PET insert in current systems does not distort static magnetic field (B0), radiofrequency field (B1), or linear field gradients,[1] and the MR image quality is similar to MR-only systems.[2] PET subsystem cannot use certain crystal materials such as gadolinium orthosilicate that affect the magnetic field.[3] The PET insert reduces the diameter of the bore which can cause difficulties for obese or claustrophobic patients. Surface coils and scanner hardware between the PET insert and patient attenuate the gamma photons, but the reduction in the overall sensitivity of the PET subsystem is practically inconsequential.

[a] Department of Radiology, Stanford University, 300 Pasteur Drive, H2200, Stanford, CA 94305, USA;
[b] Department of Radiology, University of Alabama at Birmingham, 619 19th Street South, JT 773, Birmingham, AL 35249, USA
* Corresponding author.
E-mail address: fmoradi@stanford.edu

Radiol Clin N Am 59 (2021) 853–874
https://doi.org/10.1016/j.rcl.2021.05.013
0033-8389/21/© 2021 Elsevier Inc. All rights reserved.

Attenuation Correction

Attenuation of photons arising from positron anni- hilation results in reduced PET signal detection, particularly in deep tissues. Attenuation correction (AC) methods are used to produce PET images that visually and quantitatively reflect the true dis- tribution of the PET radiopharmaceutical. Attenua- tion maps derived from CT are widely accepted as the clinical standard of PET AC. Unlike CT, MR im- aging signal is not directly related to the photon- attenuating properties of tissues and cannot be used directly to estimate 511-keV photon attenua- tion. Instead, MR imaging-based AC (MRAC) uses MR imaging sequences to characterize tissue composition which can be used alone or in combi- nation with an atlas for segmentation of the body into various tissues such as fat, soft tissue, lung, air, and bone for which the attenuation coefficients are known. MRAC maps can introduce errors in standardized uptake value (SUV), particularly within or adjacent to cortical bone if bone is not represented in the attenuation-correction map. The magnitude of these errors is typically on the order of 10% to 20%, is clinically insignificant for most applications, and generally does not affect diagnosis even for osseous lesions.[4–7] During clin- ical interpretation of PET/MR imaging studies, the MRAC map should be reviewed to insure that tis- sue segmentation was performed correctly.

Continued progress and improvements in MRAC are increasing the quantitative accuracy of PET/MR imaging. Light-weight surface coils minimize attenuation that is not accounted for by the scanner, unlike embedded coils and other fixed hardware.[8,9] Ultrashort and zero echo time sequences can characterize osseous structures and assess tissue components in areas of high magnetic field inhomogeneity such as lungs or gas-filled bowel and are used to improve segmen- tation methods.[10,11] Segmentation can also be improved using a deep learning model or other machine learning approaches.[12–14] PET/MR imag- ing can surpass the quantification accuracy of AC compared with legacy PET scanners or PET/CT in areas where motion results in misalignment be- tween transmission and emission images by exploiting simultaneous acquisition and motion tracking.[15] Time-of-flight systems allow joint esti- mation of activity and attenuation based on PET data which can overcome challenges in MRAC, and when combined with MR-based systems mentioned previously, they improve the robust- ness and accuracy of PET quantification in organs and structures such as lung or bones or near- metallic hardware that conventional MRAC had been deficient.[16] Using these techniques, Rezaei

and colleagues recently reported a residual quan- tification error below 1% in brain PET/MR imaging.[17]

Workflow

Simultaneous acquisition of PET and MR imaging can provide patient convenience compared with two separate sessions.[18,19] In applications where only one PET bed position is needed (eg, brain or cardiac imaging), standard of care PET and MR imaging can be acquired very efficiently using a simultaneous PET/MR scanner with no or minimal change to well-established imaging protocols. In other applications such as whole-body oncologic imaging, a one-stop scan requires tailored proto- cols that can acquire PET and MR imaging im- ages with adequate diagnostic quality within a certain time constraint such as 60 minutes of total imaging.[20] Inclusion of dedicated sequence for pulmonary imaging such as respiratory- triggered, periodically rotated overlapping parallel T2-weighted imaging which can approach the diagnostic accuracy of low-dose CT for pulmo- nary nodules[21] reduces the need for a separate chest CT in most instances.

The z-axis coverage of the PET subsystem is fixed (eg, 25 cm or 25.8 cm in current iteration of in- tegrated PET/MR imaging system). Acquisition of skull to mid-thigh or whole-body PET requires scanning at multiple table positions (typically be- tween 4–6). The minimal PET acquisition time is relatively similar between different table positions. In contrast, the z-axis coverage and acquisition time vary significantly depending on the MR imag- ing sequence.

The Dixon sequence with volume coil is used for segmentation-based MRAC and provides phase, opposed-phase, water, and fat images which can be used for basic anatomic correlation. Using coronal acquisition covering two stations in z-axis and adding fat saturation at every other table position can be used to provide images with high soft-tissue contrast efficiently. However, additional sequences such as volumetric T2-weighted images or whole-body diffu- sion-weighted imaging (DWI) can increase MR acqui- sition time significantly. The protocol requires compromises to fit the timing and order of acquisition of different table positions for simultaneous MR imag- ing and PET,[22] and the overall clinical question should be considered in designing the protocol.

Improved Anatomical Registration

An advantage of PET/MR imaging is improved cor- registration of PET with anatomic images through simultaneous acquisition of both modalities. Changes in location of structures between anatomic (ie, CT or MR imaging) and PET image acquisition can introduce diagnostic errors such as misinterpretation of activity or mis-localization of a lesion. With simultaneous acquisition, bulk motion from patient repositioning is minimized, improving anatomic coregistration compared with sequential acquisition with PET/CT or separately acquire PET and MR imaging studies.[18,19]

PET and MR sequences are affected by movements of the diaphragm and rib cage resulting in nonrigid motion and elastic deformation of adjacent structures during respiration,[23] as well as periodic or irregular movements in other structures such as cardiac contractions and bowel peristalsis. Depending on the MR sequence, these effects manifest differently, and certain sequences require breath hold or gating or the use of navigator pulses to minimize distortions or other artifacts. Movements during PET acquisition result in blurring of the PET images and quantification errors due to lower recovery coefficient or mismatch between MRAC maps and PET.[24,25] When multiple MR sequences (eg, free breathing and single-shot breath hold sequences) are acquired during PET acquisition at each table position, or if a particular MR sequence is performed separately before or after PET acquisition (as frequently is the case for postcontrast whole-body T1W images), the position of anatomic structures on MR images may not match the position of time-averaged associated activity on PET. Combination of free-breathing PET data with breath-hold MR imaging sequences not only lead to registration errors due to nonrigid deformations in the liver and other upper abdominal organs but may also cause attenuation-correction errors.[22] With improved spatial resolution of clinical PET images, small changes in position and blurring of activity in areas of motion are becoming more noticeable. Various techniques for detection and monitoring motions are currently available and can be paired with correction algorithms in PET after processing. Gating is useful for periodic motions such as respiration or cardiac cycle and, in an application such as cardiac PET/MR imaging, improves spatial resolution, contrast-to-noise, and quantification accuracy compared with nongated PET as depicted in **Fig. 1.**[26]

Reducing Radiation Exposure

The effective exposure from low-dose CT can be as high as radiation exposure from the PET agent, and elimination of CT reduces exposure by as much as 50%.[27] Moreover, optimized workflow efficiency allows for a focused MR imaging to be performed in the same session to avoid additional exposure from a separate dedicated contrast-enhanced CT or multiphase CT. An additional 40%-50% reduction of radiation exposure (depending on BMI) compared to conventional PET/CT is feasible because of higher sensitivity of detector rings in modern hybrid PET/MR systems by reducing the injected dose.[28] With MR acquisition protocols that require longer time per bed, the injected activity can be reduced even further. Overall, with careful optimization of the protocol, PET/MR imaging can result in 70% to 80% less radiation than standard PET/CT,[29,30] which is particularly relevant in pediatric and young adult populations because of risk of secondary malignancies later in life associated with radiation exposure.[31,32]

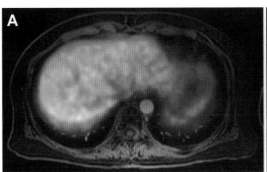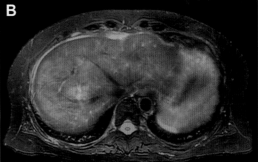

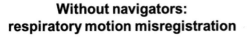

Without navigators: respiratory motion misregistration

With navigators: accurate co-registration

Fig. 1. ^{68}Ga-DOTATATE-PET/MR imaging performed in a 39-year-old woman with metastatic NET for restaging. (A) Misregistration due to respiratory images blurs the PET images of the upper abdomen and introduces AC errors. (B) Motion correction leads to accurate coregistration of the PET and MR images with decreased blurring of the PET images.

IMAGING PROTOCOLS

Simultaneous focused PET/MR imaging requires minimal change to the optimized standard of care imaging protocol if a single table position provides sufficient coverage for the field of view of PET and MR imaging. Depending on the length and type of study, the PET radiopharmaceutical can be administered before or after the patient is placed in the scanner. In most clinical applications, the PET acquisition time is shorter than that of MR imaging, and ideally the timing should be set up that PET acquisition coincide with an MR sequence that provides AC information as well as sequences that provide the highest anatomic details and most relevant diagnostic information (eg, volumetric postcontrast T1WI for brain tumors, delayed postcontrast T1WI for cardiac sarcoidosis) to maximize registration accuracy.

Whole Body PET/MRI Protocols

Protocols for multistation PET/MR imaging require optimization and often compromise to satisfy certain constraints regarding the order of acquisition, timing at each bed position, and total duration of examination. For typical doses of fludeoxyglucose (FDG) and many other clinically used radiopharmaceuticals, 2 to 5 minutes of PET scan time at each table position is sufficient. Longer acquisition in chest and abdomen can improve detection rate for small pulmonary or hepatic metastases and may be necessary for certain approaches to mitigate motion artifact. A Dixon-based MR imaging sequence for AC and up to three diagnostic MR imaging pulse sequences which typically includes T2WI fit during PET imaging acquisition.[22] A T2-weighted single-shot fast-spin echo sequence in the axial and/or coronal plane is often used in whole-body PET/MR imaging because of its good soft-tissue contrast and anatomic detail, relatively fast acquisition time, and relative insensitivity to motion. An example of typical sequences used for whole-body PET/MR imaging is shown in **Fig. 2**. Depending on the body part, additional sequences (eg, respiratory triggered periodically rotated overlapping parallel T2WI of the lungs) may be acquired either simultaneously with PET or before or after PET acquisition. As the diagnostic performance of PET/MR imaging heavily depends on MR sequences, there is ongoing interest and research in developing standardized protocols for PET/MR and incorporation of multiparametric MR imaging tailored to specific clinical applications.[33]

Intravenous Contrast

Administration of contrast is primarily helpful in focused PET/MR imaging of a specific body part.

When both focused and whole-body PET/MR imaging are performed in the same session, splitting the extracellular contrast agents into two injections may be necessary. Gadolinium-enhanced T1W imaging can achieve adequate lesion conspicuity and detection rate and good anatomic details in a more time-efficient manner than T2W and DWI.[34–36] However, the experience on redundancy between PET and contrast-enhanced MR imaging in many clinical scenarios remains limited. With hepatobiliary contrast agents such as gadoxetate disodium or gadobenate dimeglumine, skull-base to thigh PET can be acquired in the interval between initial dynamic postcontrast images of the liver and delayed imaging. Gadoxetate has high uptake by hepatocytes followed by biliary excretion by the canalicular multispecific organic anion transporter, providing excellent contrast between focal lesions and normal hepatic parenchyma on delayed images.[37]

ONCOLOGIC APPLICATIONS OF PET/MR IMAGING

In oncologic applications, beyond improving diagnostic accuracy and facilitating workflow and cost-effectiveness as a one-stop shop for staging or restaging several malignancies, a multiparametric PET/MR imaging can provide biomarkers for disease activity that contribute to precision medicine.[38] A review of more than 100 published articles between 2012 and 2018 supports the utility of PET/MR imaging and superiority to other modalities including PET/CT in several malignancies.[39] The primary disadvantage of PET/MR imaging compared with PET/CT is in assessment of primary pulmonary malignancies and small lung metastases. In many oncologic applications, the diagnostic performance of FDG PET/MR imaging is at least equivalent to PET/CT. Mayerhoefer and colleagues recently reported a significantly higher accuracy for PET/MR imaging than for PET/CT in a mixed population of cancer patients (97.3% vs 83.9%, $P < .001$) primarily because of better sensitivity for liver and brain metastases, impacting management in 8% of their patients.[40] However, the impact would be smaller if metastases to brain from non-small-cell lung cancer are excluded as these patients routinely get a brain MR imaging as a part of their workup. Another observational study of more than 1000 patients found that although PET/MR imaging revealed additional information compared with PET/CT in more than a quarter of patients, malignant findings were detected only in 5.3% of the studies and lead to a change in staging in about half of those patients (2.9%). At the same time, PET/MR imaging

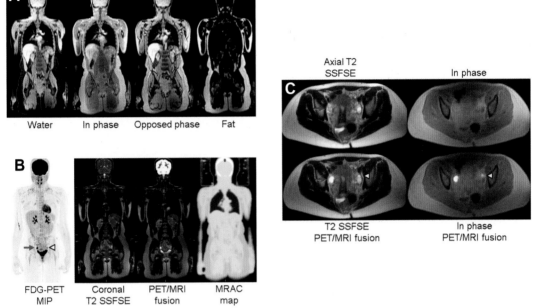

Fig. 2. Basic whole-body FDG-PET/MR imaging sequences performed in a 35-year-old woman undergoing staging after polypectomy of a rectal neuroendocrine tumor. A prior ^{68}Ga-DOTATATE-PET/CT did not demonstrate residual or metastatic SSTR-positive disease (not shown). (*A*) Dixon-derived MR sequences (water, in phase, opposed phase, fat) used for MR-based attenuation correction (MRAC) and basic anatomic localization of the PET images. (*B*) Maximum intensity projection (MIP) image from FDG-PET, coronal T2 single-shot fast-spin echo (SSFSE) MR imaging slice, fused T2 SSFSE PET/MR imaging slice, and MRAC map. Increased FDG uptake is seen in the right (*red arrow*) and in the left pelvis (*yellow arrowhead*). (*C*) Axial T2 SSFSE and in phase MR imaging images as well as corresponding PET/MR imaging fusion images of the pelvis. The higher resolution and soft tissue contrast of the T2 SSFSE images demonstrate physiologic uptake in the right and left ovaries (*red arrow* and *yellow arrowhead*, respectively) corresponding to the findings on the MIP. Note that the in-phase sequence does not provide adequate soft tissue characterization to definitively identify the ovaries as the locations of increased FDG uptake.

missed malignant lesions (compared with PET/CT) in 2.9% of studies, but the staging was affected in less than a fifth of those studies.[30] PET/MR imaging reduces the need for additional workup in 11% of patients by characterizing indeterminate lesions on PET/CT but resulted in additional studies in 26% of patients, of which less than a third were malignant. Considering limited availability of PET/MR imaging systems and concerns about cost and patient tolerability, there is interest in improving triage of patients based on histopathology and clinical stage.

Head and Neck

FDG PET/MR can have excellent diagnostic performance in staging head and neck malignancies[41,42] and has certain advantages to other available imagining modalities for initial evaluation and assessment of response to therapy.[43,44] T-staging is improved by addition of high-resolution dedicated head and neck MR sequences. Excellent soft-tissue contrast of MR imaging enables more

accurate delineation of certain cancers such as nasopharyngeal carcinoma than contrast-enhanced CT.[45] T2WI is useful for detection of necrotic or cystic lymph node metastasis.[46] Diffusion weighted imaging provides complementary information to FDG PET and can identify lesions in lymphoepithelial tissues or other areas of high background physiologic activity.[47] MR imaging has excellent sensitivity for bone marrow involvement. Ultrashort echo-time (UTE) or zero echo-time (ZTE) sequences can identify cortical bone erosions reducing the need for a separate CT. Addition of PET to MR imaging increases sensitivity and negative predictive value in detecting local recurrence and metastases.[48] In one small series, PET/MR imaging had higher accuracy than MR imaging alone in diagnosing the primary lesion at initial presentation (75% vs 50%) and local recurrence (57% vs 72%).[49]

The utility of FDG PET/CT (often in combination with contrast enhanced CT) in locally advanced head and neck malignancies is well established.[50] A few studies that have directly compared the diagnostic utility of PET/MR imaging with PET/CT have confirmed similar if not superior accuracy for PET/MR imaging for locoregional assessment[46,51] and comparable accuracy for evaluation of distant metastases or synchronous cancers.[42] MR can be used for anatomic correlation of PET findings in the oral cavity or other areas with severe streaking artifacts on CT because of dental hardware. PET/MR has shown to provide accurate staging without the use of intravenous contrast[52] which is an important consideration for patients who are unable to receive intravenous contrast because of allergy or poor renal function. An example of FDG PET/MR imaging for head and neck cancer staging is shown in **Fig. 3.**

PET/CT may be a better option for patients with hypopharyngeal or laryngeal primary cancers as CT is less degraded by motion artifact. In patients with known or suspected pulmonary metastases, PET/CT appears to be superior for assessment of small pulmonary nodules, particularly if combined with a focused chest CT. However, pulmonary nodules that are missed on PET/MR imaging are generally too small to be accurately characterized by PET, and their clinical significance remains doubtful given the relative frequency of benign incidental small pulmonary nodules.

Gastrointestinal Malignancies

Physiologic FDG uptake in the gastrointestinal tract is variable, and without accurate anatomic correlation, metabolic characterization of gastrointestinal lesions can be challenging. Single-shot spin echo sequences can depict anatomic details and provide high lesion conspicuity in gastric cancer which can improve diagnostic accuracy compared with PET/CT.[53] PET is indicated in initial evaluation of gastric adenocarcinomas and gastrointestinal stromal tumors. However, the role of PET in assessment of small bowel or colon adenocarcinoma is primarily for characterization of equivocal findings on CT or MR imaging and assessment of peritoneal disease. DWI is superior to CT and can be complementary to PET for assessment of the extent of peritoneal involvement.[54] Patients with elevated biomarkers with negative CT and endoscopy could potentially benefit most from the superior sensitivity of PET/MR imaging compared with other techniques.

In patients with rectal cancer, MR imaging and, in particular, small field of view T2WI can identify the extent of tumor beyond the muscularis propria and extension to mesorectal fascia, anal sphincter, or other pelvic structures, assess pelvic lymph nodes, and distinguish between posttreatment change and recurrence. FGD PET can help characterize small lymph nodes, and in equivocal cases, complementary information from PET improves T and N staging accuracy and detection of recurrence.[55] Detection of distant metastases on whole-body PET-MR imaging affects management. The accuracy of N and M staging or restaging on PET/MR imaging is similar if not superior to PET/CT.[56,57] In one series, PET/MR imaging was found to incrementally increase accuracy compared with MR imaging for both T staging (92% vs 89%) and N staging (92% vs 86%) compared to pathology gold standard after neoadjuvant therapy and resulted in a change in management in 11% of the patients.[58] High soft-tissue contrast of MR imaging can significantly improve diagnostic value of PET for assessment of recurrence. Plodeck and colleagues report a sensitivity and specificity of 94% and positive and negative predictive value of 97% and 90%, respectively, for detection of recurrence using a nonsimultaneous PET/MR system,[59] with PET/MR imaging leading to a change in management in 18% of their patients. Simultaneous PET/MR imaging systems provide excellent coregistration between anatomy

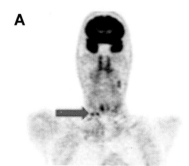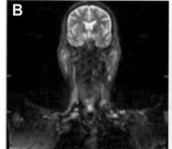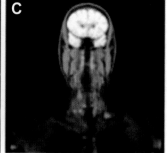

Fig. 3. FDG-PET/MR imaging performed in a 45-year-old man with head and neck squamous cell cancer undergoing presurgical staging. The coronal FDG-PET image (*A*) demonstrates focal uptake in the lower right neck ipsilateral to the primary cancer (*red arrow*) which corresponds to subcentimeter lymph nodes identified on the T2 fat saturation MR (*B*) and fusion images (*C*) which are suspicious for nodal metastases.

and metabolic activity which can be used to match individual mesorectal nodes and deposits to histopathologic samples.[60] Addition of single-bed prolonged PET acquisition over the pelvis which can be performed after voiding and simultaneous with dedicated high-resolution volumetric MR imaging increases image quality and sensitivity compared with standard-of-care PET/CT or generic multistation oncologic PET/MR imaging.[61]

The literature on clinical utility of PET/MR imaging in rectal carcinoma compared with conventional imaging has not been entirely conclusive so far. One study, for example, reported upstaging in more than 21% and downstaging in 14% that led to a change in management.[62] In contrast, the preliminary results from the REctal Cancer Trial on PET/MR imaging/CT has not yet shown a change in management for any of the patients who underwent PET/MR imaging.[63] It has been argued that the incremental added diagnostic value of PET/MR imaging compared with MR imaging alone might not be sufficient to justify its preferential clinical use in rectal cancer.[57] Liver is a frequent site of metastases in gastrointestinal malignancies (including neuroendocrine neoplasms [NENs]), and the combination of PET and MR imaging has shown to improve accuracy and diagnostics confidence for hepatic metastases detection.[64,65]

Neuroendocrine Neoplasms

[68]Ga- and ^{64}Cu-labeled somatostatin receptor (SSTR) ligand PET agents have high sensitivity and specificity for detection and localization of SSTR-expressing neoplasms including many tumors of neuroendocrine origin particularly for gastroenteropancreatic well-differentiated neuroendocrine tumors (GEP-NETs) and pheochromocytoma/paragangliomas. MR imaging is superior to CT (particularly in the absence of intravenous contrast) for identifying anatomic correlates to the PET signal. Multiparametric MR imaging of the abdomen and pelvis has excellent sensitivity for hepatic lesions and can help identify lesions in areas of high physiologic uptake that are not conspicuous on PET because of small-size and partial-volume effect and/or low somatostatin analog overexpression (Krenning score 1–2). Delayed liver MR imaging with gadoxetate has been shown to have superior sensitivity for liver lesions compared with ^{68}Ga-DOTATOC PET.[66] Complementary information on MR imaging such as growth over time or restricted water diffusion can be crucial in identifying pseudoprogression or pseudoresponse. Many patients with GEP-NETs therefore undergo both whole-body PET/

CT and abdominopelvic MR imaging at both initial evaluation and for assessment of response to therapy, particularly for liver-dominant disease as shown in **Fig. 4**.[67] Combining whole-body PET and MR imaging and dedicated abdominal MR imaging for these patients at the least achieves workflow efficiency and reduces ionizing radiation exposure. The diagnostic performance of PET/MR imaging even without administration of intravenous contrast is comparable if not superior to multiphase contrast-enhanced PET/CT,[68] and a combination of DWI and SSTR-PET was able to detect more lesions than either technique by itself.[69]

Prostate Carcinoma

The role of multiparametric MR imaging in diagnosis and staging of prostate cancer (PCa) is well established, and the recent development of several PET agents for PCa imaging make PET/MR imaging a promising modality for PCa imaging. A combination or high-resolution T2-weighted (T2W) and diffusion-weighted images can identify most clinically significant PCas particularly at with a 3-T MR imaging system.[70] T2W image delineate central and peripheral gland[71] and may detect extracapsular extension.[72,73] High b-value images ($\geq$1400 s/mm^2) facilitate detection of clinically significant cancers. Dynamic contrast-enhanced (DCE) MR imaging uses increased neovascularity and permeability of microvasculature within PCa to identify and characterize lesions that equivocal on other sequences or in areas difficult to evaluate on DWI due to artifact. Targeted biopsy of lesions seen on MR imaging improves detection of clinically significant cancers[74–76] and reduced detection of insignificant cancer compared with systematic biopsy in patients with elevated prostate-specific antigen (PSA).[77] Nonetheless, MR imaging fails to detect primary cancer or underestimates the extent of disease in a small but significant number of patients. PET using prostate-specific membrane antigen (PSMA) ligands has better diagnostic performance than multiparametric MR imaging in the detection of PCa in intermediate- or high-risk PCa patients.[78–82] In one case report, PET-guided biopsy was necessary to establish the diagnosis of cancer in *a patient* who had four negative MR imaging studies and six negative systematic biopsies despite persistently elevated PSA.[83] Combining PET with multiparametric MRI (mpMRI) is particularly useful as it enables image-guided fusion biopsy[84] and planning for targeted localized therapy.[85]

MR imaging and CT have limited sensitivity and accuracy for nodal metastases which are a poor prognostic factor [62]. Patients with nodal

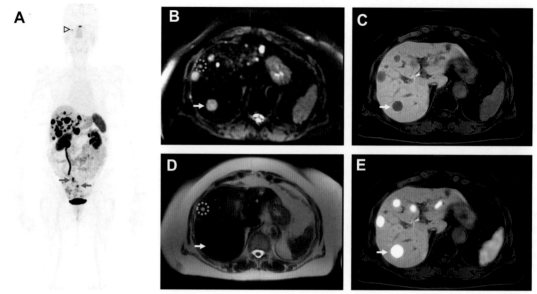

Fig. 4. DOTATATE-PET/MR imaging performed in a 73-year-old woman with a metastatic grade II NET. (*A*) Maximum intensity projection (MIP) image from the whole-body DOTATATE-PET acquisition demonstrates multiple hepatic metastases with high levels of SSTR expression as well as mesenteric nodal metastases (*red arrows*) and faint uptake in an incidental small right posterior fossa meningioma (*yellow arrowhead*). Diagnostic liver PET/MR imaging (*B–E*) demonstrates multiple hepatic metastases with restricted diffusion (B, DWI with b = 700), low signal intensity compared to normal liver on the hepatobiliary phase after IV gadoxetate contrast administration (*C*), slight hyperintensity on the whole-body T2 single-shot fast-spin echo (SSFSE) images (*D*) and high DOTATATE binding on the fused hepatobiliary phase PET/MR imaging (*E*) with an example indicated by a *white arrow*. There are also numerous hepatic cysts with hyperintensity on the DWI (*B*) and T2 SSFSE (*D*) sequences, low signal intensity on the hepatobiliary phase sequence (*C*) and no PET activity (*E*) with an example indicated by a *dashed blue circle*.

involvement may benefit from treatment options such as radiation therapy [64]. However, surgical staging with extensive nodal dissection can have high morbidity and not feasible if nonsurgical management is pursued. PET can detect metastases in subcentimeter lymph nodes [67]. Various PET radiopharmaceuticals such as choline-analogs [68], ^{18}F-fluciclovine [69], and, in particular, PSMA PET outperform anatomic imaging for nodal staging [70] [71–73]. A high negative predictive value of PSMA PET for nodal involvement in initial staging of PCa[86,87] makes it a cost-effective alternative to extended pelvic dissection[88] and has been shown in multicenter randomized studies to inform management, altering panned management in more than a quarter of patients.[89] An example of PSMA-PET/MR imaging for initial staging of PCa is shown in **Fig. 5**.

PET/MR imaging is also a promising tool for evaluation of patients with persistent elevation or rising of serum PSA from the nadir after definitive treatment (biochemical recurrence) without evidence of disease on anatomic imaging (structural recurrence). Early localization of disease with PET or MR imaging enables targeted therapies which can affect survival or prevent futile. In one series, PET was able to detect occult metastases in more than half of patients.[90] In another retrospective study of more than 1000 men with biochemical recurrence, the positivity rate of PSMA PET was close to 80%.[91] Even if anatomic imaging reveals abnormalities in patients with biochemical recurrence, accurate characterization of these abnormalities and identification of the extent of disease with PET/MR imaging can prevent futile and potentially harmful interventions. Inclusion of multiparametric pelvic MR imaging improves diagnostic accuracy in prostate bed, particularly for radiopharmaceuticals with urinary excretion. Whole-body MR imaging is an accurate and cost-effective tool in detecting distant nodal and osseous metastases[92,93] with higher sensitivity than bone scintigraphy[94] and approaching NaF-PET/CT.[95,96] Inclusion of PET, mpMRI of the prostate, and whole-body MR imaging in the same session enables a one-stop shop for evaluation of patients with biochemical recurrence. An example of fluciclovine-PET/MR imaging for PCa is shown in **Fig. 6**.

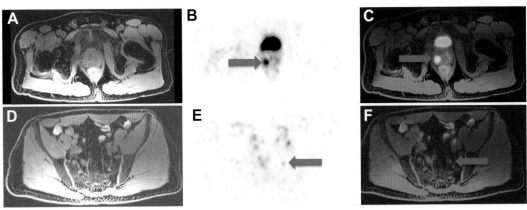

Fig. 5. PSMA-11-PET/MR imaging performed for preprostatectomy staging in a 59-year-old man with clinical stage T2b high-risk prostate cancer (Gleason 4 + 3 and serum PSA 9.7 ng/mL). PSMA-PET/MR imaging of the prostate gland (A–C) demonstrates focally increased activity (red arrows) in the prostate gland corresponding to the patient's known prostate cancer. In addition, more superior images in the pelvis (D–F) demonstrate increased PSMA-11 binding in a subcentimeter left pelvic lymph node metastasis (red arrows) confirmed after pelvic nodal dissection.

Gynecologic Malignancies

MR imaging and PET have established applications in gynecologic malignancies, with the combination of them further improving staging of cervical, endometrial, and ovarian malignancies[97,98] with more accurate characterization of lesions[99] and higher confidence in anatomic correlation for PET-positive lesions.[100] FDG PET and DWI have complementary sensitivity and specificity for nodal metastases[101] and peritoneal implants.[102] The measured biomarkers such as SUV or ADC for pelvic lesions using a hybrid scanner are equivalent to stand-alone systems (ie, PET/CT or MR imaging)[103] and can be used together to assess response during

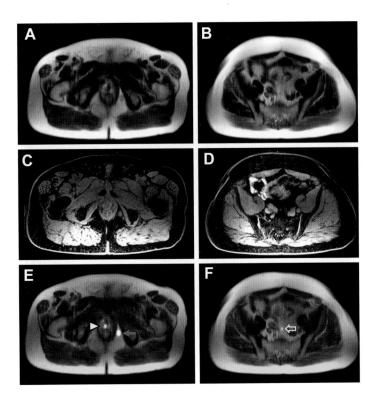

Fig. 6. 73-year-old male with biopsy-proven Gleason 8 prostate cancer and serum PSA of 19.3 ng/mL with enlarged ischiorectal fossa lymph node on initial staging that was unusual for prostate cancer metastasis. Axial T2 single-shot fast-spin echo (SSFSE) (A, B), axial T1 GRE (C, D) and fused fluciclovine-PET/MR images (E, F) demonstrate high focal uptake within the right prostate apex at the site of known malignancy (yellow arrowhead), in a left ischiorectal fossa lymph node (red arrow) (A, D) and a subcentimeter lymph node just caudal to the aortic bifurcation (open white arrow). Subsequent CT-guided biopsy of the ischiorectal fossa lymph node was consistent with metastatic prostate cancer.

concurrent chemoradiotherapy for locally advanced cervical cancer,[104] assessment of residual disease after therapy,[105] or evaluation for recurrence in various pelvic malignancies.[106] The literature overall supports favorable diagnostic performance for PET/MR imaging compared with PET/CT in both per patient and per lesion analysis,[107] although there is high variability in results reflecting the need to improve patient selection and imaging protocols.

Multiple Myeloma and Other Bone Malignancies

Evaluation of osseous malignancies on PET/MR imaging poses certain challenges due to limited assessment of cortical bone on conventional MR imaging sequences and underestimation of SUV in osseous lesions.[108] MR imaging however offers value in excellent anatomic colocalization particularly for lesions involving the spinal canal or skull base and provides complementary information to FDG PET for assessment of soft-tissue component and paramedullary and extramedullary lesions and detection of diffuse infiltrative involvement.[109–112] FDG PET and MR imaging are complementary in terms of sensitivity and specificity and contribution to management decisions.[113]

Inclusion of high-resolution T1W imaging using fast-spin echo sequences in oncologic PET/MR imaging protocols improves delineation of osseous lesions compared with PET/CT.[108] DWI improves detection and characterization of osseous lesions,[114,115] although its sensitivity for primarily sclerotic lesions may be limited. Whole-body DWI increases sensitivity for intramedullary lesions in multiple myeloma.[111] Addition of DWI to the MD Anderson bone-specific response criteria substantially increases its agreement with clinical response in multiple myeloma.[116] Administration of MR contrast is indicated in sarcomas but not in multiple myeloma.[117] In preclinical studies, DCE MR imaging is used to quantify tissue vascularity as imaging biomarkers for therapies targeting tumor angiogenesis.[118]

Pediatric Imaging

PET/MR imaging is now preferentially or exclusively used by several pediatric imaging centers for oncologic PET applications, achieving significant reduction of ionizing radiation[119] and number of general anesthesia and sedations due to workflow efficiency.[120] MR imaging is superior to CT for anatomic correlation of FDG avid lesions in pediatric patients: In one study, 98% of PET-positive lesions were visible on at least one MR imaging sequence. In contrast, more than 20% of lesions

had no clear CT correlate.[121] After treatment, MR imaging helps differentiate tumor from nonviable tissue and improves evaluation of metastatic burden in bone marrow and solid organs. Minimum apparent diffusion coefficients of target lesions are useful for assessment of response therapy with good agreement with SUV.[122]

NEUROLOGIC APPLICATIONS OF PET/MR IMAGING

PET/MR imaging has several practical advantages for brain imaging compared with PET/CT. Unlike oncologic imaging in the rest of the body, MR imaging is typically the modality of choice for the evaluation of primary or metastatic brain tumors, cognitive impairment, and epilepsy which are the most common indication for brain PET studies. Brain PET/MR imaging typically requires a single-bed position which simplifies image acquisition and limits the examination length to the longest of the 2 modalities, usually the MR imaging. Because PET can be acquired throughout the MR imaging acquisition, dynamic PET acquisition is feasible using PET radiopharmaceuticals with fast kinetics without prolonging the overall study duration. The potential roles of dynamic PET acquisition are discussed in the context of the specific applications of PET/MR imaging for brain imaging.

The primary challenge to clinical brain PET/MR imaging is the relatively low volume of brain PET studies in most practices. This low volume in the United States is in part due to the lack of FDA-approved PET radiopharmaceuticals other than FDG for brain tumors and the limited reimbursement for FDA-approved amyloid and tau PET radiopharmaceuticals for evaluation of cognitive impairment. Another issue specific to PET/MR imaging is that many patients initially have a brain MR imaging as part of their workup and may have their PET examination soon after which may preclude payer coverage of an additional diagnostic MR imaging. In addition, software fusion of separately acquired brain PET and MR imaging studies is much more straightforward than in most other body regions which somewhat reduces the importance of improved image coregistration through simultaneous acquisition.

There are also emerging techniques that take greater advantage of the simultaneous acquisition of PET and MR imaging. Motion correction of brain PET images can be achieved by using EPI or MR imaging navigator pulses[123] at the cost of increased imaging time[124,125] while sparse sampling for motion with EPI pulses embedded at the beginning of individual sequences may provide a compromise between image quality and scan time.[126,127] Although currently investigational, methods have been developed for convolutional neural network-based joint reconstruction of PET and MR imaging data to enhance the effective resolution of the PET data.[128] There are also efforts to apply automated regional brain segmentation of volumetric brain MR imaging to provide regions of interest for PET analysis of SUV, SUV ratio (SUVR), and other quantitative measures in clinical settings.[129]

Neuro-Oncology

Multiparametric MR imaging with gadolinium chelate IV contrast is the cornerstone of diagnostic imaging for primary and metastatic brain tumors. In the United States, FDG and SSTR ligands are FDA-approved radiopharmaceuticals used for clinical PET imaging of brain tumors and are typically reserved for problem-solving or specific scenarios. Radiolabeled amino acids (AAs) targeting system L AA transport including O-(2-[^{18}F]fluoroethyl)-L-tyrosine (FET), 3,4-dihydoxy-6-[^{18}F]fluoro-L-phenylalanine (FDOPA), and L-[^{11}C] methionine (MET) are investigational for brain tumor imaging in the United States but have a large body of evidence supporting their use in neuro-oncology, particularly for gliomas.[130,131]

For neuro-oncologic imaging with FDG-PET, the most common scenario is distinguishing recurrent high-grade (grade III or IV) or brain metastasis from treatment effects such as pseudoprogression or radiation necrosis based on the development of a new enhancing brain lesion. The high physiologic uptake of FDG in normal brain gray matter as well as the increased uptake of FDG by inflammatory lesions are inherent limitations to FDG-PET for evaluation of brain tumors. Fusion and correlation with contrast-enhanced postcontrast T1-weighted images are critical for accurate interpretation of FDG-PET/MR imaging studies for brain tumor evaluation. Higher lesional FDG uptake compared to normal white matter, particularly uptake higher than normal gray matter, is suspicious for viable tumor, although a wide range of diagnostic accuracies and interpretation methods have been reported in the literature.[131,132] An example of FDG-PET/MR imaging for evaluation of suspected recurrent high-grade glioma is shown in Fig. 7. The primary advantages of FDG-PET/MR imaging in neuro-oncology are a convenience for patients who need both PET and diagnostic MR imaging and coregistration of PET and MR image sets. In addition to brain imaging with FDG-PET/MR imaging, whole-body staging can be performed when there is known or suspected extracranial disease from solid tumors or lymphoma.

Where available, AA-PET agents including FET, FDOPA, and MET have superior performance to FDG for evaluation of gliomas and can complement diagnostic MR imaging.[131,133] These tracers cross the blood-brain barrier (BBB) via AA transport and accumulate preferentially in gliomas compared with normal brain. Recent studies suggest that combining AA-PET with multiparametric MR imaging provides better diagnostic performance than either modality alone for the detection of recurrent glioma, with combined PET/MR imaging providing increased specificity compared with AA-PET alone. In a retrospective study of 47 patients evaluated for recurrent glioma, FET-PET/MR imaging has a sensitivity of 78% and specificity of 92%.[134] Similarly, in a prospective study in 50 patients evaluated for recurrent glioma, MET-PET/MR imaging demonstrated a sensitivity of 97% and specificity of 93%.[135] One potential advantage for PET/MR imaging over PET/CT for FET is the ability to evaluate tracer kinetics as studies suggest that early time to peak FET uptake in lesions and rapid washout indicate recurrent glioma and may have prognostic value in low-grade gliomas.[131,136–138] This full kinetic evaluation can be performed within 45 after FET injection which can be performed during a simultaneously acquired brain tumor MR imaging protocol without lengthening the total examination time.

SSTR-PET/MR imaging can play a role in evaluation of meningiomas as the majority of these tumors have high expression of SSTR while peptide-based SSTR PET ligands do not cross the normal BBB, leading to high-contrast images. MR imaging, particularly postcontrast T1-weighted sequences, are sufficient for the detection and localization of most meningiomas, but several studies suggest that SSTR-PET can assist in detecting small meningiomas and for meningiomas located in the skull base or with intraosseous components.[139–141] As with FDG-PET, the primary advantage of PET/MR imaging appears to be the convenience of combined PET/MR imaging acquisition as small studies suggest that SSTR-PET/CT fused with separately acquired MR imaging has similar diagnostic performance as SSTR-PET/MR imaging.[142,143]

Cognitive Impairment

Techniques for molecular neuroimaging to evaluate the etiology of cognitive impairment have advanced substantially over the past decade, particularly for Alzheimer's disease (AD). Brain FDG-PET is well-established for distinguishing cognitive impairment due to AD from

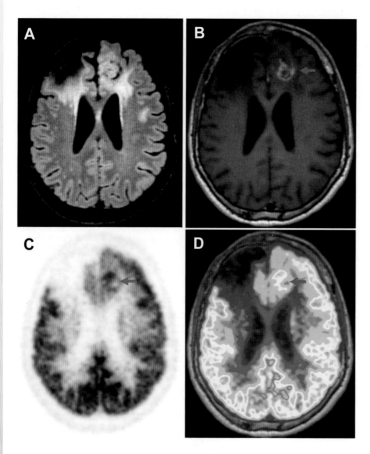

Fig. 7. FDG-PET/MR imaging performed in a 49-year-old-man previously treated for a right frontal lobe anaplastic oligodendroglioma. The patient developed recurrence in the left frontal lobe and was treated with chemoradiation 6 years prior to the PET/MR imaging study. The FLAIR (A) and post-contrast T1-weighted (B) MR imaging demonstrate extensive treatment effects and an irregular enhancing lesion in the left frontal lobe (red arrow). The FDG-PET (C) and PET/MR imaging fusion (D) images demonstrate FDG uptake similar to normal gray matter corresponding to the anteromedial aspect of this lesion, suspicious for recurrent high-grade glioma.

frontotemporal dementia (FTD) based on distinct patterns of decreased glucose metabolism.[144–146] More recently, ^{18}F-labeled PET tracers that bind to pathologic beta-amyloid and tau, two pathologic hallmarks of AD, have received FDA approval for the evaluation of patients with cognitive impairment where AD is a diagnostic consideration. These techniques are used widely in research settings, but clinical brain PET for cognitive impairment is a relatively small part of most practices in part due to limited reimbursement for amyloid and tau PET tracers. This landscape is expected to change substantially with much higher volumes if effective treatments for AD that slow or stop disease progression achieve FDA approval.

Because the pathophysiology of AD occurs over the course of years with a progression of biomarkers becoming abnormal at different times,[147,148] a single imaging biomarker is insufficient for accurately staging AD. Amyloid-PET typically becomes abnormal first, followed by tau-PET and FDG-PET, and then MR imaging measures of regional brain volumes such as the hippocampus. Abnormal amyloid PET scans can occur in cognitively normal older adults and may represent presymptomatic AD

pathophysiology while abnormal tau-PET, FDG-PET, and volumetric MR imaging are more closely associated with current cognitive impairment.

PET/MR imaging has the potential to add value to PET studies by assessing multiple imaging biomarkers in a single imaging session. In some cases, a full diagnostic brain MR imaging may be indicated as part of the PET/MR imaging study. Many patients will undergo a diagnostic MR imaging as part of their initial evaluation for cognitive impairment to exclude nondegenerative etiologies such as prior stroke or a mass lesion. In these patients, the MR imaging protocol may be modified to provide additional sequences such a volumetric T1 MR imaging for regional brain segmentation and volume measurement while other sequences previously performed are omitted. Commercially available software platforms are available for measuring regional brain volumes and comparing an individual patient's results to age- and sex-matched normal populations, with hippocampal volumes providing the greatest predictive power for progression from mild cognitive impairment to Alzheimer's dementia.[149] Volumetric assessment may also help identify patients with other

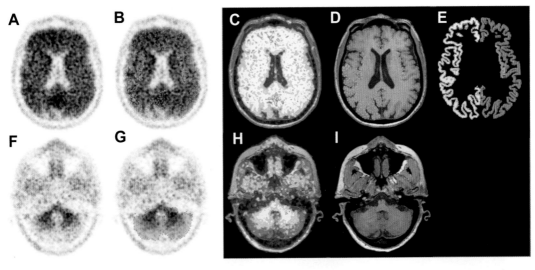

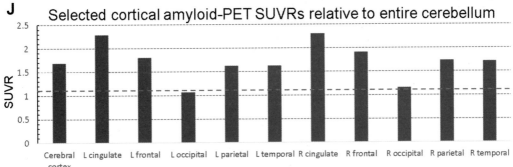

Fig. 8. ¹¹C-PiB-PET/MR imaging in a 70-year-old man with mild cognitive impairment participating in a research study. The amyloid-PET (A) and PET/MR imaging fusion (C) images at the level of the body of the lateral ventricles demonstrate abnormally increased PiB binding at in the cerebral cortex with loss of gray-white differentiation. In contrast, the amyloid-PET (F) and PET/MR imaging fusion (H) images at the level of the posterior fossa demonstrate maintained gray-white differentiation in the cerebellum. This appearance is consistent with pathologic deposition of beta-amyloid throughout the cerebral cortex as is seen in Alzheimer's disease pathophysiology. MR-based regional brain segmentation (E) is used use to generate regions of interest (ROIs) displayed on the volumetric T1-weighted MR images (D, I) as well as the amyloid-PET images (B, G). These ROIs can be used to calculate SUVRs within cortical regions with values above 1.21 indicative of elevated amyloid levels (dotted red line, J). These ROIs can also provide regional brain volume measurements (not shown).

neurodegenerative diseases such as FTD due to atrophy in regions outside of the hippocampus. MR-based segmentation maps derived from volumetric brain MR imaging can also be used to automatically define PET regions of interest in commercially available image-viewing software[129] for semi-quantitative analyses using such as SUVRs from amyloid PET studies as shown in Fig. 8.

As with brain tumors, dynamic acquisition with PET/MR imaging may provide added value in the assessment of cognitive impairment. The first few minutes after injection of amyloid PET tracers can provide surrogate measures of regional cerebral blood flow which, similar to FDG, are reduced in typical patterns in AD and FTD (REF). Recent studies suggest that early PET images from dynamic amyloid-PET/MR imaging studies may provide additional diagnostic information including evidence of neurodegeneration and prediction of pathologic tau on tau-PET studies[150,151] In addition, deep learning techniques can use MR imaging to assist in generating diagnostic quality amyloid PET images using very low amounts of administered activity (on the order of 1% of standard dosages).[152]While radiation exposure from diagnostic PET is not a major concern in older populations, there is potential cost-savings if the number of patients imaged from a single-batch production of an amyloid PET radiopharmaceutical can be increased.

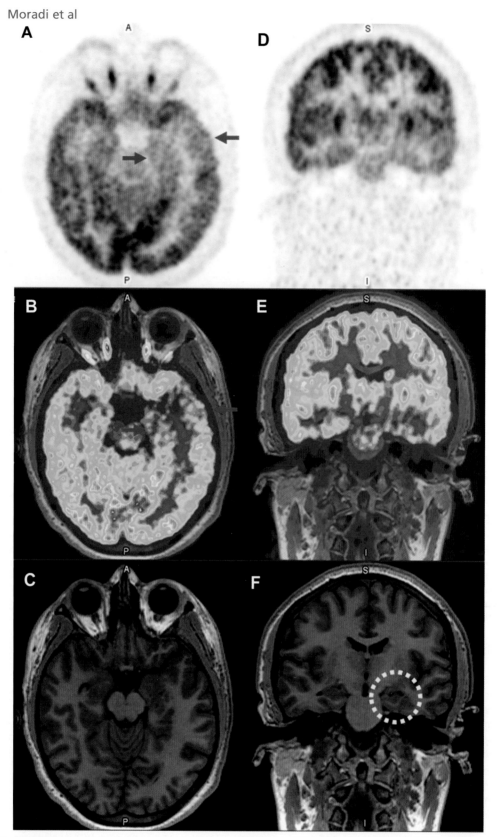

Fig. 9. FDG-PET/MR imaging performed in a woman undergoing presurgical evaluation for treatment of intractable epilepsy. Axial (*A*) and coronal (*D*) grayscale PET images demonstrate decreased FDG uptake in the medial and lateral aspects of the left temporal lobe (*red arrows*) which is more apparent on the corresponding color scale PET/MR imaging fusion images (*B, E*). The axial (*C*) and coronal (*F*) volumetric noncontrast T1-weighted MR images demonstrate volume loss in the left mesial temporal lobe (*dashed yellow circle*). The combined metabolic and anatomic findings suggest a left mesial temporal lobe seizure focus.

Epilepsy

For patients with epilepsy refractory to medication, evaluation for surgical management includes MR imaging and, in some cases, interictal FDG-PET.[153] Between seizures, the epileptogenic focus and surrounding brain tissue is typically hypometabolic, although in some cases of cortical dysplasia, the FDG uptake may be similar to or greater than normal cortex. FDG-PET typically provides lateralization (eg, left vs right temporal lobe) rather than discrete localization of the seizure focus. In some cases, FDG abnormalities aid in the identification of subtle regions of cortical dysplasia not identified on MR imaging,[154,155] and interpretation of brain FDG-PET in this setting should be performed with a high-quality structural MR imaging study whenever possible.

Initial studies suggest that brain FDG-PET/MR imaging for evaluation of seizure foci has similar to slightly superior performance to PET/CT with separately acquired MR imaging,[156–158] although some of the differences in FDG-PET could be due to uptake time differences related to study design as PET/CT was performed first followed by PET/MR imaging, both after the same FDG administration. As with PET/MR imaging for cognitive impairment, volumetric MR imaging can be used to confirm regional brain volume loss such as hippocampal atrophy in temporal lobe epilepsy[159] and to automatically generate regions of interest for regional brain analysis of PET. An example of FDG-PET/MR imaging for seizure focus localization is shown in **Fig. 9**. A small study in 15 patients with extratemporal nonlesional epilepsy using dynamic FDG-PET/MR imaging with a 60-minute acquisition time suggests that quantitative estimates of regional brain glucose metabolic rate with an image-derived input function using PET and MR angiography data performed better than standard visual analysis of delayed FDG-PET images.[160]

SUMMARY

Significant clinical experience has been gained with integrated PET/MR scanner over the past decade. PET/MRI systems capable of simultaneous acquisition of PET and MRI sequences provide advantages in workflow and accuracy of anatomical coregistration that particularly benefit evaluation of brain, liver, pelvic structures and soft tissues, and otherwise performs at least as well as PET/CT for whole body oncologic imaging. Reduce radiation exposure compared to PET/CT is an important consideration in pediatric applications. Specific MRI sequences are being introduced into clinical practice to improve evaluation of lung parenchyma and identify small pulmonary nodules. With newer PET radiopharmaceuticals receiving regulatory approval and routine reimbursement, there is increasing interest and clinical need in utilizing the diagnostic synergy between multiparametric MRI and PET for better identification of lesions and characterization of pathophysiological processes.

CLINICS CARE POINTS

- PET/MR imaging performs at least as well as PET/CT for whole-body oncologic and dedicated brain imaging.
- Whole-body PET/MR imaging can substantially reduce radiation dose to the patient compared with PET/CT.
- Malignancies involving the liver, pelvic structures, and soft tissues may benefit the most from PET/MR imaging.
- Specific MR imaging sequences are needed to identify small pulmonary nodules.
- PET/MR imaging is well suited to clinical brain PET with diagnostic synergy between PET and MR imaging with expected increases in volume as newer PET agents receive regulatory approval and routine reimbursement.

DISCLOSURE

F. Moradi has nothing to disclose. A. Iagaru disclosed receiving consulting and research support from GE Healthcare, Progenics, and Novartis and consulting fee from ITM. J. McConathy disclosed receiving consulting and research support from GE Healthcare, Blue Earth Diagnostics, and Eli Lilly/Avid Radiopharmaceuticals.

REFERENCES

1. Stortz G, Thiessen JD, Bishop D, et al. Performance of a PET Insert for High-Resolution Small-Animal PET/MRI at 7 Tesla. J Nucl Med 2018;59(3):536–42.
2. Delso G, Furst S, Jakoby B, et al. Performance measurements of the Siemens mMR integrated whole-body PET/MR scanner. Research Support, Non-U.S. Gov't. J Nucl Med 2011;52(12):1914–22.
3. Yamamoto S, Kuroda K, Senda M. Scintillator selection for MR-compatible gamma detectors. IEEE Trans Nucl Sci 2003;50(5):1683–5.

4. Seith F, Gatidis S, Schmidt H, et al. Comparison of Positron Emission Tomography Quantification Using Magnetic Resonance- and Computed Tomography-Based Attenuation Correction in Physiological Tissues and Lesions: A Whole-Body Positron Emission Tomography/Magnetic Resonance Study in 66 Patients. Invest Radiol 2016;51(1):66–71.

5. Su Y, Rubin BB, McConathy J, et al. Impact of MR-Based Attenuation Correction on Neurologic PET Studies. J Nucl Med 2016;57(6):913–7.

6. Liu G, Cao T, Hu L, et al. Validation of MR-Based Attenuation Correction of a Newly Released Whole-Body Simultaneous PET/MR System. Biomed Res Int 2019;2019:8213215.

7. Fraum TJ, Fowler KJ, McConathy J. Conspicuity of FDG-Avid Osseous Lesions on PET/MRI Versus PET/CT: a Quantitative and Visual Analysis. Nucl Med Mol Imaging 2016;50(3):228–39.

8. Yu J, Jian Y, Lindsay S, et al. Attenuation measurement of a new ultra-light surface coil for PET/MR system. J Nucl Med 2017;58(supplement 1):1326.

9. Deller TW, Mathew NK, Hurley SA, et al. PET Image Quality Improvement for Simultaneous PET/MRI with a Lightweight MRI Surface Coil. Radiol 2020; 3:200967.

10. Delso G, Wiesinger F, Sacolick LI, et al. Clinical evaluation of zero-echo-time MR imaging for the segmentation of the skull. J Nucl Med 2015;56(3): 417–22.

11. Baran J, Chen Z, Sforazzini F, et al. Accurate hybrid template-based and MR-based attenuation correction using UTE images for simultaneous PET/MR brain imaging applications. BMC Med Imaging 2018;18(1):41.

12. Leynes AP, Yang J, Wiesinger F, et al. Zero-Echo-Time and Dixon Deep Pseudo-CT (ZeDD CT): Direct Generation of Pseudo-CT Images for Pelvic PET/MRI Attenuation Correction Using Deep Convolutional Neural Networks with Multiparametric MRI. J Nucl Med 2018;59(5):852–8.

13. Mecheter I, Alic L, Abbod M, et al. MR Image-Based Attenuation Correction of Brain PET Imaging: Review of Literature on Machine Learning Approaches for Segmentation. J Digit Imaging 2020;33(5): 1224–41.

14. Hwang D, Kang SK, Kim KY, et al. Generation of PET Attenuation Map for Whole-Body Time-of-Flight (18)F-FDG PET/MRI Using a Deep Neural Network Trained with Simultaneously Reconstructed Activity and Attenuation Maps. J Nucl Med 2019;60(8): 1183–9.

15. Kolbitsch C, Neji R, Fenchel M, et al. Respiratory-resolved MR-based attenuation correction for motion-compensated cardiac PET-MR. Phys Med Biol 2018;63(13):135008.

16. Ahn S, Cheng L, Shanbhag DD, et al. Joint estimation of activity and attenuation for PET using pragmatic MR-based prior: application to clinical TOF PET/MR whole-body data for FDG and non-FDG tracers. Phys Med Biol 2018;63(4):045006.

17. Rezaei A, Schramm G, Willekens SMA, et al. A Quantitative Evaluation of Joint Activity and Attenuation Reconstruction in TOF PET/MR Brain Imaging. J Nucl Med 2019;60(11):1649–55.

18. Riola-Parada C, Garcia-Canamaque L, Perez-Duenas V, et al. Simultaneous PET/MRI vs PET/CT in oncology. A systematic review. Rev Esp Med Nucl Imagen Mol 2016;35(5):306–12.

19. Hope TA, Fayad ZA, Fowler KJ, et al. Summary of the First ISMRM-SNMMI Workshop on PET/MRI: Applications and Limitations. J Nucl Med 2019; 60(10):1340–6.

20. Pareek A, Muehe AM, Theruvath AJ, et al. Whole-body PET/MRI of Pediatric Patients: The Details That Matter. J Vis Exp 2017;130.

21. de Galiza Barbosa F, Geismar JH, Delso G, et al. Pulmonary nodule detection in oncological patients - Value of respiratory-triggered, periodically rotated overlapping parallel T2-weighted imaging evaluated with PET/CT-MR. Eur J Radiol 2018;98:165–70.

22. Fraum TJ, Fowler KJ, McConathy J, et al. PET/MRI for the body imager: abdominal and pelvic oncologic applications. Abdom Imaging 2015;40(6):1387–404.

23. Daou D. Respiratory motion handling is mandatory to accomplish the high-resolution PET destiny. Eur J Nucl Med Mol Imaging 2008;35(11):1961–70.

24. Osman MM, Cohade C, Nakamoto Y, et al. Clinically significant inaccurate localization of lesions with PET/CT: frequency in 300 patients. J Nucl Med 2003;44(2):240–3.

25. Huang T-C, Chou K-T, Wang Y-C, et al. Motion freeze for respiration motion correction in PET/CT: a preliminary investigation with lung cancer patient data. Biomed Research International 2014;2014.

26. Petibon Y, Sun T, Han PK, et al. MR-based cardiac and respiratory motion correction of PET: application to static and dynamic cardiac 18F-FDG imaging. Phys Med Biol 2019;64(19):195009.

27. Sher AC, Seghers V, Paldino MJ, et al. Assessment of Sequential PET/MRI in Comparison With PET/CT of Pediatric Lymphoma: A Prospective Study. AJR Am J Roentgenol 2016;206(3):623–31.

28. Sekine T, Delso G, Zeimpekis KG, et al. Reduction of (18)F-FDG Dose in Clinical PET/MR Imaging by Using Silicon Photomultiplier Detectors. Radiol 2018;286(1):249–59.

29. Muehe AM, Theruvath AJ, Lai L, et al. How to Provide Gadolinium-Free PET/MR Cancer Staging of Children and Young Adults in Less than 1 h: the Stanford Approach. Mol Imaging Biol 2018;20(2): 324–35.

30. Martin O, Schaarschmidt BM, Kirchner J, et al. PET/MRI Versus PET/CT for Whole-Body Staging: Results from a Single-Center Observational Study

on 1,003 Sequential Examinations. J Nucl Med 2020;61(8):1131–6.

31. Pearce MS, Salotti JA, Little MP, et al. Radiation exposure from CT scans in childhood and subsequent risk of leukaemia and brain tumours: a retrospective cohort study. Lancet 2012;380(9840): 499–505.

32. Meulepas JM, Ronckers CM, Smets A, et al. Radiation Exposure From Pediatric CT Scans and Subsequent Cancer Risk in the Netherlands. J Natl Cancer Inst 2019;111(3):256–63.

33. Huellner MW, Appenzeller P, Kuhn FP, et al. Whole-body nonenhanced PET/MR versus PET/CT in the staging and restaging of cancers: preliminary observations. Radiol 2014;273(3):859–69.

34. Metser U, Chan R, Veit-Haibach P, et al. Comparison of MRI Sequences in Whole-Body PET/MRI for Staging of Patients With High-Risk Prostate Cancer. AJR Am J Roentgenol 2019;212(2):377–81.

35. Melsaether AN, Raad RA, Pujara AC, et al. Comparison of Whole-Body (18)F FDG PET/MR Imaging and Whole-Body (18)F FDG PET/CT in Terms of Lesion Detection and Radiation Dose in Patients with Breast Cancer. Radiology 2016;281(1): 193–202.

36. Celebi F, Cindil E, Sarsenov D, et al. Added Value of Contrast Medium in Whole-Body Hybrid Positron Emission Tomography/Magnetic Resonance Imaging: Comparison between Contrast-Enhanced and Non-Contrast-Enhanced Protocols. Med Princ Pract 2020;29(1):54–60.

37. Yoon JH, Lee JM, Chang W, et al. Initial M Staging of Rectal Cancer: FDG PET/MRI with a Hepatocyte-specific Contrast Agent versus Contrast-enhanced CT. Radiol 2020;294(2):310–9.

38. Miles KA, Voo SA, Groves AM. Additional Clinical Value for PET/MRI in Oncology: Moving Beyond Simple Diagnosis. J Nucl Med 2018;59(7):1028–32.

39. Morsing A, Hildebrandt MG, Vilstrup MH, et al. Hybrid PET/MRI in major cancers: a scoping review. Eur J Nucl Med Mol Imaging 2019;46(10): 2138–51.

40. Mayerhoefer ME, Prosch H, Beer L, et al. PET/MRI versus PET/CT in oncology: a prospective single-center study of 330 examinations focusing on implications for patient management and cost considerations. Eur J Nucl Med Mol Imaging 2020;47(1): 51–60.

41. Samolyk-Kogaczewska N, Sierko E, Dziemianczyk-Pakiela D, et al. Usefulness of Hybrid PET/MRI in Clinical Evaluation of Head and Neck Cancer Patients. Cancers (Basel) 2020;(2):12. https://doi.org/10.3390/cancers12020511.

42. Yeh CH, Chan SC, Lin CY, et al. Comparison of (18) F-FDG PET/MRI, MRI, and (18)F-FDG PET/CT for the detection of synchronous cancers and distant metastases in patients with oropharyngeal and hypopharyngeal squamous cell carcinoma. Eur J Nucl Med Mol Imaging 2020;47(1):94–104.

43. Szyszko TA, Cook GJR. PET/CT and PET/MRI in head and neck malignancy. Clin Radiol 2018; 73(1):60–9.

44. Ryan JL, Aaron VD, Sims JB. PET/MRI vs PET/CT in Head and Neck Imaging: When, Why, and How? Semin Ultrasound CT MR 2019;40(5):376–90.

45. Chen WS, Li JJ, Hong L, et al. Comparison of MRI, CT and 18F-FDG PET/CT in the diagnosis of local and metastatic of nasopharyngeal carcinomas: an updated meta analysis of clinical studies. Am J Transl Res 2016;8(11):4532–47.

46. Kuhn FP, Hüllner M, Mader CE, et al. Contrast-enhanced PET/MR imaging versus contrast-enhanced PET/CT in head and neck cancer: how much MR information is needed? J Nucl Med 2014;55(4):551–8.

47. Martens RM, Noij DP, Koopman T, et al. Predictive value of quantitative diffusion-weighted imaging and 18-F-FDG-PET in head and neck squamous cell carcinoma treated by (chemo)radiotherapy. Eur J Radiol 2019;113:39–50.

48. Kirchner J, Schaarschmidt BM, Sauerwein W, et al. (18) F-FDG PET/MRI vs MRI in patients with recurrent adenoid cystic carcinoma. Head Neck 2019; 41(1):170–6.

49. Schaarschmidt BM, Heusch P, Buchbender C, et al. Locoregional tumour evaluation of squamous cell carcinoma in the head and neck area: a comparison between MRI, PET/CT and integrated PET/MRI. Eur J Nucl Med Mol Imaging 2016; 43(1):92–102.

50. Moradi F. Positron Emission Tomography and Molecular Imaging of Head and Neck Malignancies. Curr Radiol Rep 2020;8(11):1–19.

51. Cheng Y, Bai L, Shang J, et al. Preliminary clinical results for PET/MR compared with PET/CT in patients with nasopharyngeal carcinoma. Oncol Rep 2020;43(1):177–87.

52. Pyatigorskaya N, De Laroche R, Bera G, et al. Are Gadolinium-Enhanced MR Sequences Needed in Simultaneous (18)F-FDG-PET/MRI for Tumor Delineation in Head and Neck Cancer? AJNR Am J Neuroradiol 2020;41(10):1888–96.

53. Zheng D, Liu Y, Liu J, et al. Improving MR sequence of 18F-FDG PET/MR for diagnosing and staging gastric Cancer: a comparison study to (18)F-FDG PET/CT. Cancer Imaging 2020; 20(1):39.

54. Dresen RC, De Vuysere S, De Keyzer F, et al. Whole-body diffusion-weighted MRI for operability assessment in patients with colorectal cancer and peritoneal metastases. Cancer Imaging 2019. https://doi.org/10.1186/s40644-018-0187-z.

55. Hope TA, Kassam Z, Loening A, et al. The use of PET/MRI for imaging rectal cancer. Abdom Radiol (NY) 2019;44(11):3559–68.

56. Paspulati RM, Partovi S, Herrmann KA, et al. Comparison of hybrid FDG PET/MRI compared with PET/CT in colorectal cancer staging and restaging: a pilot study. Abdom Imaging 2015;40(6):1415–25.

57. Li Y, Mueller LI, Neuhaus JP, et al. (18)F-FDG PET/MR versus MR Alone in Whole-Body Primary Staging and Restaging of Patients with Rectal Cancer: What Is the Benefit of PET? J Clin Med 2020; 9(10). https://doi.org/10.3390/jcm9103163.

58. Crimì F, Spolverato G, Lacognata C, et al. 18F-FDG PET/MRI for Rectal Cancer TNM Restaging After Preoperative Chemoradiotherapy: Initial Experience. Dis Colon Rectum 2020;63(3):310–8.

59. Plodeck V, Rahbari NN, Weitz J, et al. FDG-PET/MRI in patients with pelvic recurrence of rectal cancer: first clinical experiences. Eur Radiol 2019; 29(1):422–8.

60. Rutegård MK, Båtsman M, Blomqvist L, et al. Rectal cancer: a methodological approach to matching PET/MRI to histopathology. Cancer Imaging 2020;20(1):80.

61. Bailey JJ, Jordan EJ, Burke C, et al. Does Extended PET Acquisition in PET/MRI Rectal Cancer Staging Improve Results? AJR Am J Roentgenol 2018;211(4):896–900.

62. Amorim BJ, Hong TS, Blaszkowsky LS, et al. Clinical impact of PET/MR in treated colorectal cancer patients. Eur J Nucl Med Mol Imaging 2019;46(11): 2260–9.

63. Rutegård MK, Båtsman M, Axelsson J, et al. PET/MRI and PET/CT hybrid imaging of rectal cancer - description and initial observations from the RECTOPET (REctal Cancer trial on PET/MRI/CT) study. Cancer Imaging 2019;19(1):52.

64. Donati OF, Hany TF, Reiner CS, et al. Value of retrospective fusion of PET and MR images in detection of hepatic metastases: comparison with 18F-FDG PET/CT and Gd-EOB-DTPA-enhanced MRI. J Nucl Med 2010;51(5):692–9.

65. Hong SB, Choi SH, Kim KW, et al. Diagnostic performance of [(18)F]FDG-PET/MRI for liver metastasis in patients with primary malignancy: a systematic review and meta-analysis. Eur Radiol 2019;29(7):3553–63.

66. Hope TA, Pampaloni MH, Nakakura E, et al. Simultaneous (68)Ga-DOTA-TOC PET/MRI with gadoxetate disodium in patients with neuroendocrine tumor. Abdom Imaging 2015;40(6):1432–40.

67. Pirasteh A, Riedl C, Mayerhoefer ME, et al. PET/MRI for neuroendocrine tumors: a match made in heaven or just another hype? Clin Transl Imaging 2019;7(6):405–13.

68. Seith F, Schraml C, Reischl G, et al. Fast non-enhanced abdominal examination protocols in PET/MRI for patients with neuroendocrine tumors (NET): comparison to multiphase contrast-enhanced PET/CT. Radiol Med 2018;123(11):860–70.

69. Farchione A, Rufini V, Brizi MG, et al. Evaluation of the Added Value of Diffusion-Weighted Imaging to Conventional Magnetic Resonance Imaging in Pancreatic Neuroendocrine Tumors and Comparison With 68Ga-DOTANOC Positron Emission Tomography/Computed Tomography. Pancreas 2016;45(3):345–54.

70. Gaur S, Harmon S, Gupta RT, et al. A Multireader Exploratory Evaluation of Individual Pulse Sequence Cancer Detection on Prostate Multiparametric Magnetic Resonance Imaging (MRI). Acad Radiol 2019;26(1):5–14.

71. Felker ER, Margolis DJ, Nassiri N, et al. Prostate cancer risk stratification with magnetic resonance imaging. Urol Oncol 2016;34(7):311–9.

72. Kim TH, Woo S, Han S, et al. The Diagnostic Performance of the Length of Tumor Capsular Contact on MRI for Detecting Prostate Cancer Extraprostatic Extension: A Systematic Review and Meta-Analysis. Korean J Radiol 2020;21(6):684–94.

73. Yu KK, Hricak H, Alagappan R, et al. Detection of extracapsular extension of prostate carcinoma with endorectal and phased-array coil MR imaging: multivariate feature analysis. Radiol 1997;202(3): 697–702.

74. Kasivisvanathan V, Rannikko AS, Borghi M, et al. MRI-Targeted or Standard Biopsy for Prostate-Cancer Diagnosis. N Engl J Med 2018;378(19): 1767–77.

75. Brown LC, Ahmed HU, Faria R, et al. Multiparametric MRI to improve detection of prostate cancer compared with transrectal ultrasound-guided prostate biopsy alone: the PROMIS study. Health Technol Assess 2018;22(39):1–176.

76. van der Leest M, Cornel E, Israël B, et al. Head-to-head Comparison of Transrectal Ultrasound-guided Prostate Biopsy Versus Multiparametric Prostate Resonance Imaging with Subsequent Magnetic Resonance-guided Biopsy in Biopsy-naïve Men with Elevated Prostate-specific Antigen: A Large Prospective Multicenter Clinical Study. Eur Urol 2019;75(4):570–8.

77. Schoots IG, Roobol MJ, Nieboer D, et al. Magnetic resonance imaging-targeted biopsy may enhance the diagnostic accuracy of significant prostate cancer detection compared to standard transrectal ultrasound-guided biopsy: a systematic review and meta-analysis. Eur Urol 2015;68(3):438–50.

78. Park SY, Zacharias C, Harrison C, et al. Gallium 68 PSMA-11 PET/MR Imaging in Patients with Intermediate- or High-Risk Prostate Cancer. Radiology 2018;288(2):495–505.

79. Eiber M, Weirich G, Holzapfel K, et al. Simultaneous (68)Ga-PSMA HBED-CC PET/MRI Improves

the Localization of Primary Prostate Cancer. Eur Urol 2016;70(5):829–36.

80. Jena A, Taneja R, Taneja S, et al. Improving Diagnosis of Primary Prostate Cancer With Combined (68)Ga-Prostate-Specific Membrane Antigen-HBED-CC Simultaneous PET and Multiparametric MRI and Clinical Parameters. AJR Am J Roentgenol 2018;211(6):1246–53.

81. Scheltema MJ, Chang JI, Stricker PD, et al. Diagnostic accuracy of (68) Ga-prostate-specific membrane antigen (PSMA) positron-emission tomography (PET) and multiparametric (mp)MRI to detect intermediate-grade intra-prostatic prostate cancer using whole-mount pathology: impact of the addition of (68) Ga-PSMA PET to mpMRI. BJU Int 2019;124(Suppl 1):42–9.

82. Hicks RM, Simko JP, Westphalen AC, et al. Diagnostic Accuracy of (68)Ga-PSMA-11 PET/MRI Compared with Multiparametric MRI in the Detection of Prostate Cancer. Radiology 2018;289(3):730–7.

83. Simopoulos DN, Natarajan S, Jones TA, et al. Targeted Prostate Biopsy Using (68)Gallium PSMA-PET/CT for Image Guidance. Urol Case Rep 2017;14:11–4.

84. Fendler WP, Eiber M, Beheshti M, et al. 68)Ga-PSMA PET/CT: Joint EANM and SNMMI procedure guideline for prostate cancer imaging: version 1.0. Eur J Nucl Med Mol Imaging 2017;44(6):1014–24.

85. Zamboglou C, Klein CM, Thomann B, et al. The dose distribution in dominant intraprostatic tumour lesions defined by multiparametric MRI and PSMA PET/CT correlates with the outcome in patients treated with primary radiation therapy for prostate cancer. Radiat Oncol 2018;13(1):65.

86. Luiting HB, van Leeuwen PJ, Busstra MB, et al. Use of gallium-68 prostate-specific membrane antigen positron-emission tomography for detecting lymph node metastases in primary and recurrent prostate cancer and location of recurrence after radical prostatectomy: an overview of the current literature. BJU Int 2020;125(2):206–14.

87. Jansen BHE, Bodar YJL, Zwezerijnen GJC, et al. Pelvic lymph-node staging with (18)F-DCFPyL PET/CT prior to extended pelvic lymph-node dissection in primary prostate cancer - the SALT trial. Eur J Nucl Med Mol Imaging 2020. https://doi.org/10.1007/s00259-020-04974-w.

88. Scholte M, Barentsz JO, Sedelaar JPM, et al. Modelling Study with an Interactive Model Assessing the Cost-effectiveness of (68)Ga Prostate-specific Membrane Antigen Positron Emission Tomography/Computed Tomography and Nano Magnetic Resonance Imaging for the Detection of Pelvic Lymph Node Metastases in Patients with Primary Prostate Cancer. Eur Urol Focus 2020;6(5):967–74.

89. Hofman MS, Lawrentschuk N, Francis RJ, et al. Prostate-specific membrane antigen PET-CT in patients with high-risk prostate cancer before curative-intent surgery or radiotherapy (proPSMA): a prospective, randomised, multicentre study. Lancet 2020;395(10231):1208–16.

90. Fendler WP, Weber M, Iravani A, et al. Prostate-Specific Membrane Antigen Ligand Positron Emission Tomography in Men with Nonmetastatic Castration-Resistant Prostate Cancer. Clin Cancer Res 2019;25(24):7448–54.

91. Afshar-Oromieh A, Holland-Letz T, Giesel FL, et al. Erratum to: Diagnostic performance of (68)Ga-PSMA-11 (HBED-CC) PET/CT in patients with recurrent prostate cancer: evaluation in 1007 patients. Eur J Nucl Med Mol Imaging 2017;44(10):1781.

92. Wu LM, Gu HY, Zheng J, et al. Diagnostic value of whole-body magnetic resonance imaging for bone metastases: a systematic review and meta-analysis. J Magn Reson Imaging 2011;34(1):128–35.

93. Li B, Li Q, Nie W, et al. Diagnostic value of whole-body diffusion-weighted magnetic resonance imaging for detection of primary and metastatic malignancies: a meta-analysis. Eur J Radiol 2014;83(2):338–44.

94. Shen G, Deng H, Hu S, et al. Comparison of choline-PET/CT, MRI, SPECT, and bone scintigraphy in the diagnosis of bone metastases in patients with prostate cancer: a meta-analysis. Skeletal Radiol 2014;43(11):1503–13.

95. Jambor I, Kuisma A, Ramadan S, et al. Prospective evaluation of planar bone scintigraphy, SPECT, SPECT/CT, 18F-NaF PET/CT and whole body 1.5T MRI, including DWI, for the detection of bone metastases in high risk breast and prostate cancer patients: SKELETA clinical trial. Acta Oncol 2016;55(1):59–67.

96. Zhou J, Gou Z, Wu R, et al. Comparison of PSMA-PET/CT, choline-PET/CT, NaF-PET/CT, MRI, and bone scintigraphy in the diagnosis of bone metastases in patients with prostate cancer: a systematic review and meta-analysis. Skeletal Radiol 2019;48(12):1915–24.

97. Bian LH, Wang M, Gong J, et al. Comparison of integrated PET/MRI with PET/CT in evaluation of endometrial cancer: a retrospective analysis of 81 cases. PeerJ 2019;7:e7081.

98. Tsuyoshi H, Tsujikawa T, Yamada S, et al. Diagnostic value of [(18)F]FDG PET/MRI for staging in patients with ovarian cancer. EJNMMI Res 2020;10(1):117.

99. Tsuboyama T, Tatsumi M, Onishi H, et al. Assessment of combination of contrast-enhanced magnetic resonance imaging and positron emission tomography/computed tomography for evaluation

of ovarian masses. Invest Radiol 2014;49(8): 524–31.

100. Xin J, Ma Q, Guo Q, et al. PET/MRI with diagnostic MR sequences vs PET/CT in the detection of abdominal and pelvic cancer. Eur J Radiol 2016; 85(4):751–9.

101. Liu B, Gao S, Li S. A Comprehensive Comparison of CT, MRI, Positron Emission Tomography or Positron Emission Tomography/CT, and Diffusion Weighted Imaging-MRI for Detecting the Lymph Nodes Metastases in Patients with Cervical Cancer: A Meta-Analysis Based on 67 Studies. Gynecol Obstet Invest 2017;82(3):209–22.

102. Sanli Y, Turkmen C, Bakir B, et al. Diagnostic value of PET/CT is similar to that of conventional MRI and even better for detecting small peritoneal implants in patients with recurrent ovarian cancer. Nucl Med Commun 2012;33(5):509–15.

103. Fraum TJ, Fowler KJ, Crandall JP, et al. Measurement Repeatability of (18)F-FDG PET/CT Versus (18)F-FDG PET/MRI in Solid Tumors of the Pelvis. J Nucl Med 2019;60(8):1080–6.

104. Gao S, Du S, Lu Z, et al. Multiparametric PET/MR (PET and MR-IVIM) for the evaluation of early treatment response and prediction of tumor recurrence in patients with locally advanced cervical cancer. Eur Radiol 2020;30(2):1191–201.

105. Sarabhai T, Tschischka A, Stebner V, et al. Simultaneous multiparametric PET/MRI for the assessment of therapeutic response to chemotherapy or concurrent chemoradiotherapy of cervical cancer patients: Preliminary results. Clin Imaging 2018;49: 163–8.

106. Sawicki LM, Kirchner J, Grueneisen J, et al. Comparison of (18)F-FDG PET/MRI and MRI alone for whole-body staging and potential impact on therapeutic management of women with suspected recurrent pelvic cancer: a follow-up study. Eur J Nucl Med Mol Imaging 2018;45(4):622–9.

107. Virarkar M, Ganeshan D, Devine C, et al. Diagnostic value of PET/CT versus PET/MRI in gynecological malignancies of the pelvis: A meta-analysis. Clin Imaging 2020;60(1):53–61.

108. Eiber M, Takei T, Souvatzoglou M, et al. Performance of whole-body integrated 18F-FDG PET/MR in comparison to PET/CT for evaluation of malignant bone lesions. J Nucl Med 2014;55(2):191–7.

109. Zamagni E, Nanni C, Patriarca F, et al. A prospective comparison of 18F-fluorodeoxyglucose positron emission tomography-computed tomography, magnetic resonance imaging and whole-body planar radiographs in the assessment of bone disease in newly diagnosed multiple myeloma. Haematologica 2007;92(1):50–5.

110. Mesguich C, Hulin C, Latrabe V, et al. Prospective comparison of 18-FDG PET/CT and whole-body diffusion-weighted MRI in the assessment of multiple myeloma. Ann Hematol 2020;99(12):2869–80.

111. Chen J, Li C, Tian Y, et al. Comparison of Whole-Body DWI and (18)F-FDG PET/CT for Detecting Intramedullary and Extramedullary Lesions in Multiple Myeloma. AJR Am J Roentgenol 2019; 213(3):514–23.

112. Albano D, Patti C, Lagalla R, et al. Whole-body MRI, FDG-PET/CT, and bone marrow biopsy, for the assessment of bone marrow involvement in patients with newly diagnosed lymphoma. J Magn Reson Imaging 2017;45(4):1082–9.

113. Lecouvet FE, Boyadzhiev D, Collette L, et al. MRI versus (18)F-FDG-PET/CT for detecting bone marrow involvement in multiple myeloma: diagnostic performance and clinical relevance. Eur Radiol 2020;30(4):1927–37.

114. Stecco A, Buemi F, Iannessi A, et al. Current concepts in tumor imaging with whole-body MRI with diffusion imaging (WB-MRI-DWI) in multiple myeloma and lymphoma. Leuk Lymphoma 2018;59(11):2546–56.

115. Stecco A, Trisoglio A, Soligo E, et al. Whole-Body MRI with Diffusion-Weighted Imaging in Bone Metastases: A Narrative Review. Diagnostics 2018; 8(3). https://doi.org/10.3390/diagnostics8030045.

116. Park HY, Kim KW, Yoon MA, et al. Role of whole-body MRI for treatment response assessment in multiple myeloma: comparison between clinical response and imaging response. Cancer Imaging 2020;20(1):14.

117. Roberts CC, Daffner RH, Weissman BN, et al. ACR appropriateness criteria on metastatic bone disease. J Am Coll Radiol 2010;7(6):400–9.

118. Bäuerle T, Bartling S, Berger M, et al. Imaging antiangiogenic treatment response with DCE-VCT, DCE-MRI and DWI in an animal model of breast cancer bone metastasis. Eur J Radiol 2010;73(2): 280–7.

119. Gatidis S, Schmidt H, Gücke B, et al. Comprehensive Oncologic Imaging in Infants and Preschool Children With Substantially Reduced Radiation Exposure Using Combined Simultaneous ^{18}F-Fluorodeoxyglucose Positron Emission Tomography/Magnetic Resonance Imaging: A Direct Comparison to ^{18}F-Fluorodeoxyglucose Positron Emission Tomography/Computed Tomography. Invest Radiol 2016;51(1):7–14.

120. States LJ, Reid JR. Whole-Body PET/MRI Applications in Pediatric Oncology. AJR Am J Roentgenol 2020;215(3):713–25.

121. Uslu-Beşli L, Atay Kapucu L, Karadeniz C, et al. Comparison of FDG PET/MRI and FDG PET/CT in Pediatric Oncology in Terms of Anatomic Correlation of FDG-positive Lesions. J Pediatr Hematol Oncol 2019;41(7):542–50.

122. Theruvath AJ, Siedek F, Muehe AM, et al. Therapy Response Assessment of Pediatric Tumors with

Whole-Body Diffusion-weighted MRI and FDG PET/MRI. Radiology Jul 2020;296(1):143–51.

123. Kouwe AJW, Benner T, Dale AM. Real-time rigid body motion correction and shimming using cloverleaf navigators. Magn Reson Med 2006;56(5):1019–32.

124. Catana C, Benner T, Kouwe Avd, et al. MRI-Assisted PET Motion Correction for Neurologic Studies in an Integrated MR-PET Scanner. J Nucl Med 2011;52(1):154–61.

125. Inomata T, Watanuki S, Odagiri H, et al. A systematic performance evaluation of head motion correction techniques for 3 commercial PET scanners using a reproducible experimental acquisition protocol. Ann Nucl Med 2019;33(7):459–70.

126. Keller SH, Hansen C, Hansen C, et al. Motion correction in simultaneous PET/MR brain imaging using sparsely sampled MR navigators: a clinically feasible tool. EJNMMI Phys 2015;2(1):14.

127. Ullisch MG, Scheins JJ, Weirich C, et al. MR-Based PET Motion Correction Procedure for Simultaneous MR-PET Neuroimaging of Human Brain. PLoS One 2012;7(11):e48149.

128. Schramm G, Rigie D, Vahle T, et al. Approximating anatomically-guided PET reconstruction in image space using a convolutional neural network. Neuroimage 2021;224:117399.

129. Raman F, Grandhi S, Murchison CF, et al. Biomarker Localization, Analysis, Visualization, Extraction, and Registration (BLAzER) Methodology for Research and Clinical Brain PET Applications. J Alzheimers Dis 2019;70(4):1241–57.

130. Albert NL, Weller M, Suchorska B, et al. Response Assessment in Neuro-Oncology working group and European Association for Neuro-Oncology recommendations for the clinical use of PET imaging in gliomas. Neuro-oncology 2016. https://doi.org/10.1093/neuonc/now058.

131. Law I, Albert NL, Arbizu J, et al. Joint EANM/EANO/RANO practice guidelines/SNMMI procedure standards for imaging of gliomas using PET with radiolabelled amino acids and [(18)F]FDG: version 1.0. Eur J Nucl Med Mol Imaging 2019;46(3):540–57.

132. Quartuccio N, Laudicella R, Vento A, et al. The Additional Value of (18)F-FDG PET and MRI in Patients with Glioma: A Review of the Literature from 2015 to 2020. Diagnostics (Basel) 2020;10(6). https://doi.org/10.3390/diagnostics10060357.

133. Langen KJ, Galldiks N. Update on amino acid PET of brain tumours. Curr Opin Neurol 2018;31(4):354–61.

134. Pyka T, Hiob D, Preibisch C, et al. Diagnosis of glioma recurrence using multiparametric dynamic 18F-fluoroethyl-tyrosine PET-MRI. Eur J Radiol 2018;103:32–7.

135. Deuschl C, Kirchner J, Poeppel TD, et al. 11)C-MET PET/MRI for detection of recurrent glioma. Eur J Nucl Med Mol Imaging 2018;45(4):593–601.

136. Thon N, Kunz M, Lemke L, et al. Dynamic ^{18}F-FET PET in suspected WHO grade II gliomas defines distinct biological subgroups with different clinical courses. Int J Cancer 2015;136(9):2132–45.

137. Jansen NL, Suchorska B, Wenter V, et al. Dynamic 18F-FET PET in newly diagnosed astrocytic low-grade glioma identifies high-risk patients. J Nucl Med 2014;55(2):198–203.

138. Galldiks N, Stoffels G, Filss C, et al. The use of dynamic O-(2-18F-fluoroethyl)-l-tyrosine PET in the diagnosis of patients with progressive and recurrent glioma. Neuro-oncology 2015;17(9):1293–300.

139. Einhellig HC, Siebert E, Bauknecht HC, et al. Comparison of diagnostic value of 68 Ga-DOTATOC PET/MRI and standalone MRI for the detection of intracranial meningiomas. Sci Rep 2021;11(1):9064.

140. Kunz WG, Jungblut LM, Kazmierczak PM, et al. Improved Detection of Transosseous Meningiomas Using ^{68}Ga-DOTATATE PET-CT Compared to Contrast-Enhanced MRI. J Nucl Med 2017. https://doi.org/10.2967/jnumed.117.191932.

141. Galldiks N, Albert NL, Sommerauer M, et al. PET imaging in patients with meningioma-report of the RANO/PET Group. Neurooncol 2017;19(12):1576–87.

142. Maclean J, Fersht N, Sullivan K, et al. Simultaneous (68)Ga DOTATATE Positron Emission Tomography/Magnetic Resonance Imaging in Meningioma Target Contouring: Feasibility and Impact Upon Interobserver Variability Versus Positron Emission Tomography/Computed Tomography and Computed Tomography/Magnetic Resonance Imaging. Clin Oncol (R Coll Radiol 2017;29(7):448–58.

143. Afshar-Oromieh A, Wolf MB, Kratochwil C, et al. Comparison of (6)(8)Ga-DOTATOC-PET/CT and PET/MRI hybrid systems in patients with cranial meningioma: Initial results. Neurooncol 2015;17(2):312–9.

144. Mosconi L. Brain glucose metabolism in the early and specific diagnosis of Alzheimer's disease. FDG-PET studies in MCI and AD. Eur J Nucl Med Mol Imaging 2005;32(4):486–510.

145. Jagust W, Reed B, Mungas D, et al. What does fluorodeoxyglucose PET imaging add to a clinical diagnosis of dementia? Neurology 2007;69(9):871–7.

146. Foster NL, Heidebrink JL, Clark CM, et al. FDG-PET improves accuracy in distinguishing frontotemporal dementia and Alzheimer's disease. Brain 2007;130(Pt 10):2616–35.

147. Jack CR Jr, Bennett DA, Blennow K, et al. NIA-AA Research Framework: Toward a biological definition of Alzheimer's disease. Alzheimers Dement 2018;14(4):535–62.

148. McDade E, Wang G, Gordon BA, et al. Longitudinal cognitive and biomarker changes in dominantly inherited Alzheimer disease. Neurology 2018;91(14):e1295–306.

149. Tanpitukpongse TP, Mazurowski MA, Ikhena J, et al. Alzheimer's Disease Neuroimaging I.

Predictive Utility of Marketed Volumetric Software Tools in Subjects at Risk for Alzheimer Disease: Do Regions Outside the Hippocampus Matter? AJNR Am J neuroradiology 2017;38(3):546–52.

150. Okazawa H, Ikawa M, Jung M, et al. Multimodal analysis using [(11)C]PiB-PET/MRI for functional evaluation of patients with Alzheimer's disease. EJNMMI Res 2020;10(1):30.

151. Raman F, Dean YH, Grandhi S, et al. Dynamic Amyloid PET: Relationships to Flortaucipir Tau PET Measures. J Nucl Med 2021. https://doi.org/10.2967/jnumed.120.254490.

152. Chen KT, Gong E, de Carvalho Macruz FB, et al. Ultra-Low-Dose (18)F-Florbetaben Amyloid PET Imaging Using Deep Learning with Multi-Contrast MRI Inputs. Radiol 2019;290(3):649–56.

153. Ponisio MR, Zempel JM, Day BK, et al. The Role of SPECT and PET in Epilepsy. AJR Am J Roentgenol 2021;216(3):759–68.

154. Salamon N, Kung J, Shaw SJ, et al. FDG-PET/MRI coregistration improves detection of cortical dysplasia in patients with epilepsy. Neurol 2008; 71(20):1594–601.

155. Desarnaud S, Mellerio C, Semah F, et al. (18)F-FDG PET in drug-resistant epilepsy due to focal cortical dysplasia type 2: additional value of electroclinical data and coregistration with MRI. Eur J Nucl Med Mol Imaging 2018;45(8):1449–60.

156. Paldino MJ, Yang E, Jones JY, et al. Comparison of the diagnostic accuracy of PET/MRI to PET/CT-acquired FDG brain exams for seizure focus detection: a prospective study. Pediatr Radiol 2017; 47(11):1500–7.

157. Poirier SE, Kwan BYM, Jurkiewicz MT, et al. An evaluation of the diagnostic equivalence of (18)F-FDG-PET between hybrid PET/MRI and PET/CT in drug-resistant epilepsy: A pilot study. Epilepsy Res 2021;172:106583.

158. Kikuchi K, Togao O, Yamashita K, et al. Diagnostic accuracy for the epileptogenic zone detection in focal epilepsy could be higher in FDG-PET/MRI than in FDG-PET/CT. Eur Radiol 2021;31(5):2915–22.

159. Mettenburg JM, Branstetter BF, Wiley CA, et al. Improved Detection of Subtle Mesial Temporal Sclerosis: Validation of a Commercially Available Software for Automated Segmentation of Hippocampal Volume. AJNR Am J neuroradiology 2019; 40(3):440–5.

160. Traub-Weidinger T, Muzik O, Sundar LKS, et al. Utility of Absolute Quantification in Non-lesional Extratemporal Lobe Epilepsy Using FDG PET/MR Imaging. Front Neurol 2020;11:54.

Immune PET Imaging

Osigbemhe Iyalomhe, MD, PhD, Michael D. Farwell, MD*

KEYWORDS

- Immunotherapy • Immune-related adverse events • FDG • PET/CT • Immune imaging

KEY POINTS

- Immunotherapy causes infiltration of tumors by immune cells and in rare cases is associated with unique response patterns, such as pseudoprogression.
- FDG PET/CT is frequently used to assess response to immunotherapy, and, although it cannot distinguish immune-related activity from tumor growth, it has the potential to provide insight into the immune response.
- New probes for PET imaging of the immune system are likely to be helpful in predicting response to cancer immunotherapy and separating immune-related changes from progressive disease.

INTRODUCTION

To promote their own proliferation and survival, cancer cells are known to escape immune surveillance and suppress the immune response.[1,2] Although the processes by which tumors escape immune surveillance are not understood completely, some of these mechanisms have been elucidated.[3] For example, tumors can express T-cell suppressor proteins, either constitutively or in response to the initial immune response in the tumor microenvironment.[4] As a result, drugs that target suppressors of cytotoxic T cells have been seen as attractive tools in immunotherapy.

Exemplary immunotherapeutic agents that have demonstrated survival benefit include immune checkpoint inhibitors (ICIs), such as ipilimumab, pembrolizumab, and nivolumab, which usually are administered every 2 weeks to 3 weeks.[5–7] Ipilimumab inhibits cytotoxic T-lymphocyte–associated protein 4 (CTLA-4) by preventing CTLA-4 binding to the B7 ligand on antigen-presenting cells or even tumors.[8–11] Nivolumab and pembrolizumab inhibit the membrane protein programmed cell death receptor (PD-1) on cytotoxic T cells, preventing PD-1 binding to PD ligand 1 (PD-L1) or PD ligand 2 (PD-L2) (Fig. 1).[12,13] Similarly, PD-L1 inhibitors, such as atezolizumab, avelumab, and durvalumab, prevent PD-1 binding on cytotoxic T cells. In the absence of therapy, signaling through CTLA-4 or the PD-1 axis leads to suppression of cytotoxic T-cell function and persistence of tumors. Treatment with checkpoint inhibitors blocks these inhibitory signals and leads to activation of the immune response with T-cell activation and expansion.

Immunotherapies have been used to re-engage and augment the immune response against a variety of malignancies, such as melanoma, non–small cell lung cancer, renal cell cancer, urothelial cancer, head and neck squamous cell cancer, Merkel cell carcinoma, and Hodgkin lymphoma, and the role of immunotherapy in the treatment of cancer continues to expand.[5–7,14–19] Although immunotherapy generally is associated with more frequent durable responses compared with chemotherapy or targeted therapy, more than 50% of patients do not respond.[20–22] Given nonredundancy in immune checkpoint pathways, combination immunotherapy has been utilized to increase efficacy, although combination therapies also are associated with greater toxicity.[7,23–27]

Imaging is used routinely for diagnosis, staging, treatment planning and response assessment in

Funding Source: This work was supported by National Institutes of Health grants 5R01EB026892 and NIH 2T32EB004311-16.

Conflicts of interest: None.

Department of Radiology, University of Pennsylvania, 3400 Spruce Street, Philadelphia, PA 19104, USA

* Corresponding author.

E-mail address: Michael.Farwell@pennmedicine.upenn.edu

Radiol Clin N Am 59 (2021) 875–886

https://doi.org/10.1016/j.rcl.2021.05.010

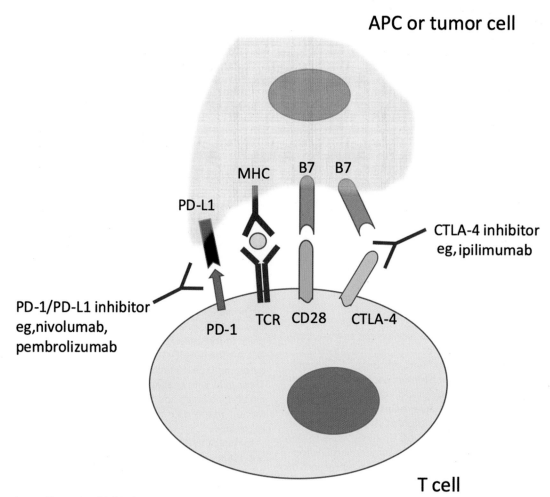

Fig. 1. Illustration highlighting the interaction between CTLA-4 (on a T cell) and B7 (on an APC or tumor), and interaction between PD-1 (on a T cell) and PD-L1 (on an APC or tumor). Inhibitors of CTLA-4 (for example, ipili-mumab) block the interaction between CTLA-4 and B7. Nivolumab and pembrolizumab are examples of immu-notherapy agents that block PD-1, preventing the interaction between PD-1 and PD-L1. These inhibitors enhance antitumor activity through the aforementioned blockades. Yellow circular insert between MHC and TCR indicates processed peptide presented by MHC to TCR/T cell. APC, antigen-presenting cell; TCR, T-cell recep-tor; MHC, major histocompatibility complex, CD28 interacts with B7 to generate a co-stimulatory signal to T cells.

oncology. Ultrasound, computed tomography (CT), and MR imaging can identify potential tumor lesions and assess changes in the size and density of lesions after treatment. In addition, functional imaging using PET with ^{18}F-fluorodeoxyglucose (FDG) is used routinely due to its high sensitivity for detecting malignancy and characterizing tumor metabolism. This article discusses the role of FDG PET/CT in the assessment of treatment response after cancer immunotherapy and identifies a few approaches that utilize FDG PET/CT to evaluate the immune response. New immune-specific PET imaging probes that are just beginning to be explored in early-phase clinical trials also are reviewed.

ATYPICAL RESPONSE PATTERNS IN IMMUNOTHERAPY

The novel mechanism of action of immunother-apies, with immune and T-cell activation, has the potential to lead to unusual patterns of response, such as pseudoprogression or hyper-progression, which are discussed later. These atypical responses are, however, quite rare, and a vast majority of patients treated with cur-rent immunotherapy regimens have typical response patterns. In addition, it is important to be aware of potential immune-related adverse events (irAEs), which can result in misleading findings on imaging.

Pseudoprogression

For some patients on immunotherapy, tumors can transiently increase in size, or new lesions may be seen.[28] If follow-up evaluation shows resolution of the new lesions and decreasing size or resolution of the lesions that had previously grown, this is termed, pseudoprogression (**Fig. 2**), and can be early or delayed.[29] This phenomenon likely occurs as a result of tumor infiltration by immune cells, which has been confirmed by biopsy in a few cases.[30–32] Many of these transiently increased/new lesions also are avid on FDG PET/CT,[33] and, in some patients, pseudoprogression may be associated with clinical symptoms.[34]

Pseudoprogression has been reported mainly in melanoma patients treated with ipilimumab (occurring in up to 15% of cases), and appears much rarer with the use of anti–PD-1/PD-L1 agents.[35–37] Billan and colleagues[28] have compiled frequencies of pseudoprogression in pooled studies and clinical trials where anti–PD-1 axis immunotherapy agents were used to treat different cancers, and frequencies ranged from 1.3% to 9.3%. In the largest analysis to date involving 19 clinical trials and 2400 participants, nivolumab and pembrolizumab were investigated in various advanced solid tumors, and pseudoprogression was observed in 6.3% of patients.[38] Thus, morphologic increase in tumor volume or metabolic activity on FDG PET/CT is much more likely to reflect true progressive disease.

Pseudoprogression also has been seen with chimeric antigen receptor (CAR) T-cell therapy when patients are imaged early; a case report of a patient with relapsed B-cell acute lymphoblastic leukemia noted pseudoprogression of extramedullary disease on MR imaging at 16 days post–CAR T-cell treatment, with subsequent response on day 30.[39] In contrast, when patients with lymphoma were imaged at 1 month post–CAR T-cell therapy via FDG PET/CT, no evidence of pseudoprogression was identified even in patients that had cytokine release syndrome, suggesting that pseudoprogression should not be a confounding factor for routine follow-up scans in patients treated with CAR T-cell therapy.[40]

Hyperprogression

Hyperprogression of cancer after the initiation of ICIs is a recently described response pattern in a subset of patients receiving PD-1/PD-L1 axis inhibitors.[41] Hyperprogression is considered a therapy-induced acceleration of tumor growth kinetics (see **Fig. 2**) and has been defined as treatment failure of less than 2 months, or a 2-fold or greater increase in tumor burden/growth rate during immunotherapy.[42] The existence of hyperprogression continues to be controversial, however, given that it is difficult to establish if rapid progression is due to the natural history of the disease or an immunotherapy-induced process.[42,43]

In several reports, prebaseline, baseline, and post-treatment scans were utilized, so that the tumor growth rate during immunotherapy could be compared with the growth rate prior to immunotherapy. Champiat and colleagues[41] used this approach to show that 12/131 (9%) patients who received anti–PD-1/PD-L1 immunotherapy could be classified as hyperprogressors. In another study where prebaseline, baseline, and post-therapy scans were available, 6/155 (4%) of patients experienced hyperprogression.[44] Additional

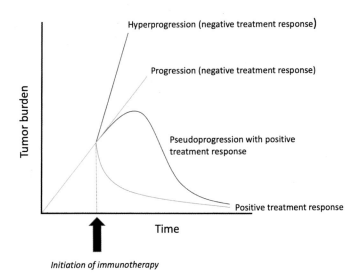

Fig. 2. Schematic comparing response patterns following immunotherapy. Hyperprogression (*red line*) indicates a rapid increase in disease burden following immunotherapy, such that disease progresses at a significantly faster rate compared with the preimmunotherapy period. In routine progression (*yellow line*), tumor growth is grossly unchanged or only slightly diminished after initiation of immunotherapy. In pseudoprogression (*blue line*), tumors initially increase in size; however, subsequent anatomic or metabolic imaging demonstrates a decrease in disease burden. The green curve represents a typical response pattern, with tumor shrinkage following treatment.

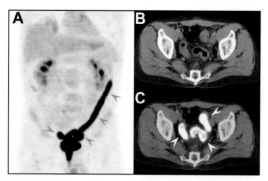
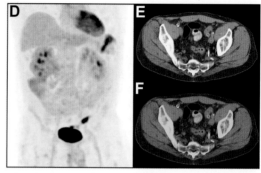

Fig. 3. Colitis in a 53-year-old woman with poorly differentiated adenocarcinoma of the lung treated with durvalumab (anti–PD-L1 therapy). Maximum intensity projection (*A*), CT (*B*), and fused FDG PET/CT images (*C*) acquired 3.5 months after treatment initiation revealed marked FDG uptake in the descending and sigmoid colon (*arrowheads*) with associated wall thickening and fat stranding consistent with colitis. The patient had bloody diarrhea at the time of the scan; sigmoidoscopy performed a week later showed acute colitis. Symptoms resolved following treatment with prednisone. Follow-up maximum intensity projection (*D*), CT (*E*), and fused FDG PET/CT images (*F*) obtained 5 months later demonstrated marked improvement.

studies are needed, however, to understand the biology driving hyperprogression and provide more evidence for this controversial phenomenon.

Immune-related Adverse Events

Immunotherapeutic agents can cause off-target side effects known as irAEs, which result from inflammation of various organs/organ systems. irAEs usually occur within 12 weeks of immunotherapy initiation and commonly occur in the skin and gastrointestinal tract (**Fig. 3**), although the pancreas (**Fig. 4**), thyroid gland (**Fig. 5**), pituitary gland, liver, lung (**Fig. 6**), heart, and joints also may be affected.[45,46] Sarcoid-like reactions also can occur as a manifestation of irAE (**Fig. 7**).[47] Although incidence rates vary by organ system, irAEs may occur in more than 50% of patients and they appear to be more common in patients on anti–CTLA-4 monotherapy and combination immunotherapy.[45,46,48] Fatality is rare and ranges from 0.3% to 1.3% in patients treated with PD-1/

PD-L1 and CTLA-4 inhibitors and is more frequently attributable to colitis-related toxicity in patients treated with ipilimumab, and pneumonitis when patients receive anti–PD-1/PD-L1 therapy.[49]

irAEs can manifest on imaging in a range of organs and organ systems, can precede clinical symptoms, and even may mimic metastatic disease[45,50–52]; therefore, it is important that radiologists are aware of this entity so that is included in the differential diagnoses for patients on immunotherapy. On FDG PET/CT, irAEs manifest as increased FDG uptake in the involved organs, and subsequent decreased uptake suggests resolution of acute inflammation.[53–55] irAEs also may predict response to immunotherapy,[56,57] although this may be organ/system dependent.[46]

RESPONSE EVALUATION

Response criteria in solid tumors (RECIST) and other metrics are used routinely to assess response to cancer therapy.[58–61] The observation

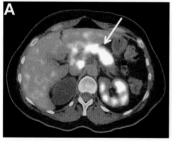
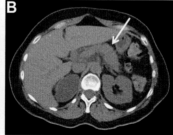
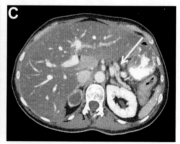

Fig. 4. Pancreatitis in a 57-year-old woman with metastatic anal cancer on nivolumab. Fused FDG PET/CT (*A*) and CT (*B*) images acquired 7.5 months after initiation of treatment demonstrate increased FDG uptake in an edematous pancreas (*arrows*); the patient had diarrhea at the time of the scan. Nivolumab was held for 1 cycle and pancreatic enzyme supplementation was started. A follow-up contrast-enhanced CT (*C*) performed 9 months later showed resolution with interval atrophy of the pancreas. Chronic right-sided hydronephrosis also is seen.

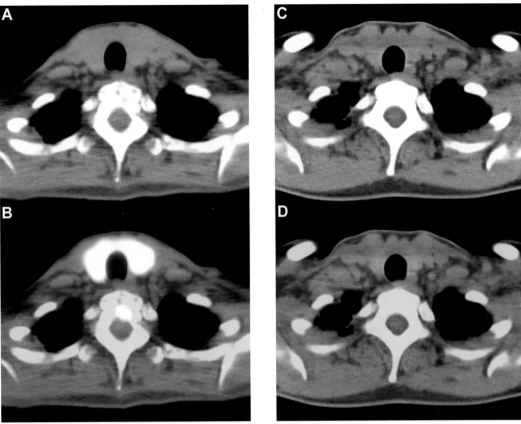

Fig. 5. Thyroiditis in a 56-year-old woman with metastatic melanoma treated with ipilimumab/nivolumab. CT (A) and fused FDG PET/CT images (B) acquired 2.5 months after treatment initiation revealed marked FDG uptake in the thyroid gland consistent with thyroiditis; the patient had thyrotoxicosis at the time of the scan, which was followed by persistent hypothyroidism requiring levothyroxine replacement. Follow-up CT (C) and fused FDG PET/CT images (D) obtained 1 year later demonstrated resolution of the abnormal uptake in the thyroid gland.

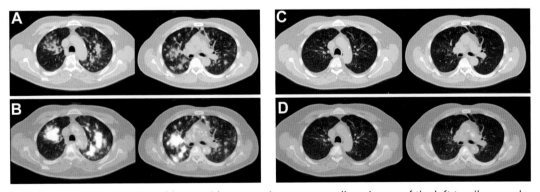

Fig. 6. Pneumonitis in a 61-year-old man with metastatic squamous cell carcinoma of the left tonsil on pembro-lizumab. CT (A) and fused FDG PET/CT images (B) acquired 7.5 months after initiation of treatment demonstrate FDG-avid nodular opacities in the lungs in a peribronchovascular distribution consistent with pneumonitis; at the time of the scan, the patient had shortness of breath and cough. Pembrolizumab was held and steroids were initi-ated, and the patient's symptoms improved. Follow-up CT (C) and fused FDG PET/CT images (D) acquired 4 months later demonstrate resolution of the pneumonitis.

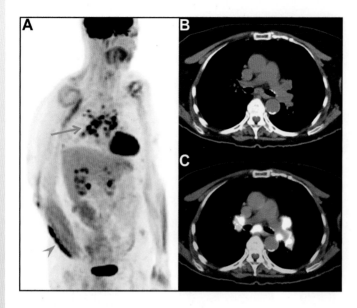

Fig. 7. Sarcoid-like reaction in a 77-year-old woman with metastatic melanoma treated with pembrolizumab. Oblique maximum intensity projection (A), CT (B), and fused FDG PET/CT images (C) acquired 13 months after treatment initiation revealed marked FDG uptake in mediastinal and bilateral hilar lymph nodes (arrow), which were new from the prior study and consistent with a sarcoid-like reaction. At the time of the scan, there also was a new FDG-avid right forearm mass (arrowhead); biopsy of the mass revealed granulomatous inflammation and no tumor. The mass persisted for an additional 12 months (including 5 months of pembrolizumab and 7 months of no therapy) and then resolved spontaneously.

of pseudoprogression, however, in a subgroup of patients treated primarily with ipilimumab motivated the development of new criteria for response assessment in the setting of cancer immunotherapy, in order to distinguish true progressive disease from pseudoprogression. In a majority of these new immune-related response criteria, such as irRC, iRECIST, and iPERCIST,[33,37,62,63] an increase in size of lesions and/or appearance of new sites of disease on the first follow-up (relative to baseline imaging) reflects unconfirmed progressive disease. If follow-up anatomic imaging and/or FDG PET/CT after greater than or equal to 4 weeks demonstrates no improvement or even worsening of disease, patients are classified as confirmed progressive disease. In the modified Lugano criteria for immunotherapy in lymphoma, biopsy or subsequent imaging can be performed.[64] In addition, some investigators have combined anatomic and molecular imaging criteria to characterize response,[65] whereas others have used thresholds of lesion size and number to determine progressive disease.[66,67] Despite this wide variety of new immune-related response criteria, RECIST remains the primary method of response assessment for most clinical trials, including immunotherapy trials, with immune-related response criteria used for exploratory endpoints.

IMMUNE IMAGING WITH FDG PET/CT

FDG is known to be taken up by activated immune cells. In clinical FDG PET/CT scans, this is reflected in inflammatory conditions, such as infection, rheumatoid arthritis, and sarcoidosis, which demonstrate elevated FDG uptake.[68–70] Additionally, in vitro studies have demonstrated markedly increased uptake in activated T cells compared with unstimulated T cells.[71] In the routine clinical setting, FDG activity in immune cells cannot be discriminated from FDG activity in tumor cells. If a baseline FDG PET/CT is compared, however, with an early post-treatment FDG PET/CT over a short interval that minimizes changes in the tumor, any increase in FDG uptake should reflect tumor infiltration by activated immune cells. This metabolic "flare" phenomenon has been demonstrated in a preclinical mouse tumor model and reported in a few clinical cases and potentially is an earlier and more sensitive measure of response to cancer immunotherapy.[72–74] A recent clinical trial demonstrated that a metabolic flare could be detected in 2/16 (13%) patients with melanoma on pembrolizumab as early as 6 days to 7 days post-therapy, with dramatic increases in tumor maximum standardized uptake value that more than doubled and predicted a complete response to therapy; no tumor flare was seen in nonresponders.[75] Future studies need to test this approach in a larger cohort of patients and explore the optimal posttreatment imaging time.

Other approaches to use FDG PET/CT imaging to predict response to immunotherapy also have been explored. For example, 2 studies have reported that an increased ratio of mean standardized uptake value of bone marrow to liver on baseline FDG PET/CT has been associated with decreased survival after anti–PD-1 immunotherapy in the setting of metastatic melanoma.[76,77] This bone marrow hypermetabolism in patients with cancer is hypothesized to reflect a systemic inflammatory response, which leads to immuno-suppression and is associated with cancer progression. Additional support for this hypothesis is provided by a significant positive correlation between FDG uptake in bone marrow and serum inflammatory markers including the white blood cell count and C-reactive protein.[76]

During immunotherapy, activation of the immune system can cause infiltration of lymphoid organs by immune cells. Sarcoid-like reaction, although considered to be an irAE, has been shown to reflect nodal infiltration by immune cells postimmunotherapy, and such nodal infiltration corresponds to associated FDG avidity (see **Fig. 7**).[78] In a recent study, all patients with FDG-avid sarcoid-like reactions following immunotherapy demonstrated positive response.[79] Pseudoprogression also appears to indicate infiltration of tumors by immune cells which are FDG avid.[31,80]

FDG PET/CT also has been used to visualize the immune response following vaccination. Increased FDG uptake has been seen in ipsilateral axillary lymph nodes following the influenza vaccine for up to 2 weeks to 4 weeks, with the highest uptake seen within the first week after the vaccine.[81,82] In 1 case report, transiently increased FDG activity also was seen in the spleen at 2 days to 3 days post-vaccination, which resolved 12 days later.[83] A similar pattern of increased FDG uptake in the deltoid muscle and ipsilateral axillary lymph nodes has been seen for up to several weeks following COVID-19 vaccination (**Fig. 8**).[84] These cases underscore the need for an accurate patient history, to ensure that FDG avid reactive axillary lymph nodes are not mistaken for metastatic disease.

NEW IMMUNE-SPECIFIC PET IMAGING PROBES

Because FDG accumulates in both tumor cells and activated immune cells, FDG uptake can be nonspecific. In order to overcome this limitation, PET probes with higher specificity for immune-related targets are needed, which can be grouped into 2 different categories: (1) imaging probes that target general immune-related markers or (2) probes designed to target markers that are expressed more uniquely in the setting of immune activation.

Given that tumor-infiltrating CD8+ T cells are predictive of response to immunotherapy,[80] whole-body CD8 PET/CT imaging is of interest, because it has the potential to allow noninvasive assessment of temporal changes in CD8+ T-cell concentration in tumors, both before and after immunotherapy. Although a majority of immune-specific probes are in preclinical development, a few are in early-phase clinical trials. For example,

an [89]Zr-labeled anti-CD8 minibody ([89]Zr-Df-IAB22M2C) currently is in a phase 2 trial (NCT03802123) as a PET probe for imaging CD8+ T cells in patients with metastatic solid tumors, with the goal of correlating CD8 signal on PET/CT imaging to CD8+ T-cell infiltration from biopsy samples and response to cancer immunotherapy. Results from the phase 1 trial of [89]Zr-Df-IAB22M2C demonstrated tracer uptake in tumors (**Fig. 9**) and CD8-rich tissues (eg, spleen, bone marrow, and lymph nodes) with maximum uptake at 24 hours to 48 hours postinjection and low background activity in non–T-cell-rich tissues (eg, muscle and heart).[85] In preclinical models of cancer immunotherapy, CD8-specific and CD3-specific imaging agents both have demonstrated greater trafficking and/or a more central distribution of tumor-infiltrating T cells in responders versus nonresponders, which supports the potential utility of these agents as an early measure of response to immunotherapy.[86–89] In addition, imaging agents that target immune cells have the potential to serve as noninvasive predictive biomarkers by differentiating patients with hot versus cold tumors and their likelihood of responding to immunotherapy.[90] CD8 PET/CT imaging also could be helpful in distinguishing pseudoprogression from treatment failure and may complement FDG PET/CT as a problem-solving tool when immune-related changes need to be isolated from tumor growth.

Other immune-specific imaging agents that are in clinical trials include probes that target PD-L1 ([89]Zr-atezolizumab and ^{18}F-BMS-986192) and PD-1 ([89]Zr-nivolumab).[91–93] Given that PD-L1 expression levels have been shown to be a positive (albeit imperfect) predictive biomarker for patients undergoing immune checkpoint blockade therapy, these agents have the potential to serve as a noninvasive measure of PD-L1 expression, which would have particular utility in patients with lung cancer where assessment of PD-L1 expression is required prior to first-line treatment with anti–PD-1 therapy.[94] A wide variety of other imaging probes that target immune-related markers, such as CD4, CTLA-4, CD11b, CD47, VLA-4, and CXCR4 (and other chemokine receptors and ligands), are in preclinical development and also may prove to have utility in the setting of cancer immunotherapy in the future.[95,96]

Imaging agents that target immune activation also are being developed, which will be helpful in distinguishing activated immune cells present in the tumor microenvironment from quiescent immune cells. These include agents that are specific for key enzymes involved in T-lymphocyte and other immune cell activation and proliferation

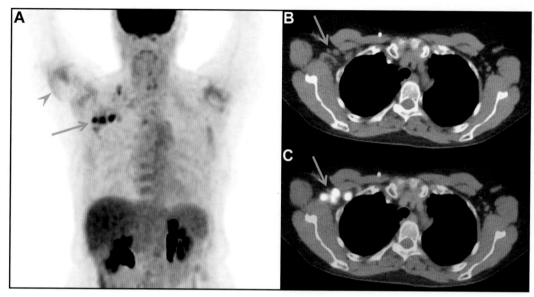

Fig. 8. Imaging findings of COVID-19 vaccination. Maximum intensity projection (*A*), CT (*B*), and fused FDG PET/CT images (*C*) acquired 2 days after COVID-19 vaccination in the right arm revealed increased FDG uptake in the right deltoid muscle (*arrowhead*) and markedly increased uptake in right axillary lymph nodes (*arrows*) and a supraclavicular lymph node, which were normal in size. These findings were consistent with reactive changes from COVID-19 vaccination in a 70-year-old woman with a history of treated lung cancer and no evidence of recurrent disease for 4+ years.

(^{18}F-FAC, ^{18}F-CFA, and ^{18}F-AraG), which are in early-phase clinical trials and have been used preclinically for detecting the location of activated T cells, monitoring graft-versus-host disease, and evaluating autoimmune disorders.[95,96] Clinical data on the utility of these imaging agents in the setting of cancer immunotherapy, however, have not yet been published. Other probes that are specific for activated immune cells include agents that target granzyme B (^{68}Ga-NOTA-GZP), interleukin-2 (^{18}F-FB-IL2), OX40 (^{64}Cu-DOTA-AbOX40), and ICOS (^{89}Zr-DFO-ICOS mAb).[96] PET imaging probes that target granzyme B, OX40, and ICOS have been tested in preclinical models of cancer immunotherapy and demonstrated increased tumor uptake in responders

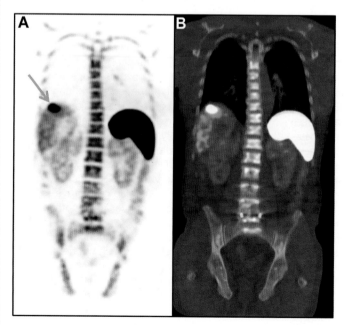

Fig. 9. A 67-year-old man with metastatic hepatocellular carcinoma (HCC) treated with nivolumab. A CD8 PET/CT scan acquired 14 days after starting immunotherapy demonstrated increased tracer activity in the primary tumor (*arrow*) (maximum standardized uptake value = 22.9) on the coronal PET (*A*) and fused PET/CT (*B*) images, suggestive of tumor infiltration by CD8$^+$ T cells and a productive antitumor immune response; physiologic tracer activity is seen in the spleen, liver, bone marrow, and kidneys. Follow-up imaging demonstrated a partial response to therapy, which has lasted 3+ years, with an associated drop in alpha-fetoprotein from 33.2 ng/mL at baseline to 1.4 ng/mL at 3 years.

versus nonresponders, suggesting that they could serve as an early measure of response.[97–99] In addition, granzyme B PET/CT imaging using ^{68}Ga-NOTA-hGZP is currently in a phase 1 clinical trial (NCT04169321).

The aforementioned studies indicate that the immune-specific PET imaging toolbox is likely to expand and will provide information that supplements FDG PET/CT and anatomic imaging.[100] These new imaging tools have the potential to have a major impact on patient management in the setting of cancer immunotherapy and likely will have applications outside of oncology for other conditions in which the immune system plays a role, such as autoimmune and inflammatory diseases, transplant rejection, and infection.

CLINICS CARE POINTS

- Signal on FDG PET/CT can be due to viable tumor cells as well as activated immune cells.
- FDG PET/CT scans should be assessed for potential immune-related adverse events.
- In the setting of immunotherapy, an increase in tumor size or metabolic activity should be interpreted as progressive disease, since pseudoprogression is rare.

REFERENCES

1. Butt AQ, Mills KH. Immunosuppressive networks and checkpoints controlling antitumor immunity and their blockade in the development of cancer immunotherapeutics and vaccines. Oncogene 2014;33(38):4623–31.
2. Liu Y, Cao X. Immunosuppressive cells in tumor immune escape and metastasis. J Mol Med (Berl) 2016;94(5):509–22.
3. Leach DR, Krummel MF, Allison JP. Enhancement of antitumor immunity by CTLA-4 blockade. Science 1996;271(5256):1734–6.
4. Jiang X, Wang J, Deng X, et al. Role of the tumor microenvironment in PD-L1/PD-1-mediated tumor immune escape. Mol Cancer 2019;18(1):10.
5. Hodi FS, O'Day SJ, McDermott DF, et al. Improved survival with ipilimumab in patients with metastatic melanoma. N Engl J Med 2010;363(8):711–23.
6. Topalian SL, Hodi FS, Brahmer JR, et al. Safety, activity, and immune correlates of anti-PD-1 antibody in cancer. N Engl J Med 2012;366(26):2443–54.
7. Wolchok JD, Kluger H, Callahan MK, et al. Nivolumab plus ipilimumab in advanced melanoma. N Engl J Med 2013;369(2):122–33.

8. Ni L, Dong C. New B7 family checkpoints in human cancers. Mol Cancer Ther 2017;16(7):1203–11.
9. Rowshanravan B, Halliday N, Sansom DM. CTLA-4: a moving target in immunotherapy. Blood 2018; 131(1):58–67.
10. Tirapu I, Huarte E, Guiducci C, et al. Low surface expression of B7-1 (CD80) is an immunoescape mechanism of colon carcinoma. Cancer Res 2006;66(4):2442–50.
11. Walunas TL, Bakker CY, Bluestone JA. CTLA-4 ligation blocks CD28-dependent T cell activation. J Exp Med 1996;183(6):2541–50.
12. Freeman GJ, Long AJ, Iwai Y, et al. Engagement of the PD-1 immunoinhibitory receptor by a novel B7 family member leads to negative regulation of lymphocyte activation. J Exp Med 2000;192(7): 1027–34.
13. Latchman Y, Wood CR, Chernova T, et al. PD-L2 is a second ligand for PD-1 and inhibits T cell activation. Nat Immunol 2001;2(3):261–8.
14. Ansell SM, Lesokhin AM, Borrello I, et al. PD-1 blockade with nivolumab in relapsed or refractory Hodgkin's lymphoma. N Engl J Med 2015;372(4): 311–9.
15. Armand P, Engert A, Younes A, et al. Nivolumab for relapsed/refractory classic Hodgkin lymphoma after failure of autologous hematopoietic cell transplantation: extended follow-up of the multicohort single-arm phase II CheckMate 205 trial. J Clin Oncol 2018;36(14):1428–39.
16. Brahmer J, Reckamp KL, Baas P, et al. Nivolumab versus docetaxel in advanced squamous-cell non-small-cell lung cancer. N Engl J Med 2015;373(2): 123–35.
17. Motzer RJ, Rini BI, McDermott DF, et al. Nivolumab for metastatic renal cell carcinoma: results of a randomized phase II trial. J Clin Oncol 2015;33(13): 1430–7.
18. Nghiem PT, Bhatia S, Lipson EJ, et al. PD-1 blockade with pembrolizumab in advanced Merkel-cell carcinoma. N Engl J Med 2016; 374(26):2542–52.
19. van den Bulk J, Verdegaal EM, de Miranda NF. Cancer immunotherapy: broadening the scope of targetable tumours. Open Biol 2018;8(6):180037.
20. Darvin P, Toor SM, Sasidharan Nair V, et al. Immune checkpoint inhibitors: recent progress and potential biomarkers. Exp Mol Med 2018;50(12):1–11.
21. Pons-Tostivint E, Latouche A, Vaflard P, et al. Comparative analysis of durable responses on immune checkpoint inhibitors versus other systemic therapies: a pooled analysis of phase III trials. JCO Precision Oncol 2019;3(3):1–10.
22. Rotte A. Combination of CTLA-4 and PD-1 blockers for treatment of cancer. J Exp Clin Cancer Res 2019;38(1):255.

23. Gao J, Navai N, Alhalabi O, et al. Neoadjuvant PD-L1 plus CTLA-4 blockade in patients with cisplatin-ineligible operable high-risk urothelial carcinoma. Nat Med 2020;26(12):1845–51.

24. Larkin J, Chiarion-Sileni V, Gonzalez R, et al. Combined nivolumab and ipilimumab or monotherapy in untreated melanoma. N Engl J Med 2015; 373(1):23–34.

25. Long GV, Atkinson V, Lo S, et al. Combination nivolumab and ipilimumab or nivolumab alone in melanoma brain metastases: a multicentre randomised phase 2 study. Lancet Oncol 2018;19(5):672–81.

26. Rozeman EA, Menzies AM, van Akkooi ACJ, et al. Identification of the optimal combination dosing schedule of neoadjuvant ipilimumab plus nivolumab in macroscopic stage III melanoma (OpA-CIN-neo): a multicentre, phase 2, randomised, controlled trial. Lancet Oncol 2019;20(7):948–60.

27. van Dijk N, Gil-Jimenez A, Silina K, et al. Preoperative ipilimumab plus nivolumab in locoregionally advanced urothelial cancer: the NABUCCO trial. Nat Med 2020;26(12):1839–44.

28. Billan S, Kaidar-Person O, Gil Z. Treatment after progression in the era of immunotherapy. Lancet Oncol 2020;21(10):e463–76.

29. Hodi FS, Hwu WJ, Kefford R, et al. Evaluation of immune-related response criteria and RECIST v1.1 in patients with advanced melanoma treated with pembrolizumab. J Clin Oncol 2016;34(13): 1510–7.

30. Di Giacomo AM, Danielli R, Guiboni M, et al. Therapeutic efficacy of ipilimumab, an anti-CTLA-4 monoclonal antibody, in patients with metastatic melanoma unresponsive to prior systemic treatments: clinical and immunological evidence from three patient cases. Cancer Immunol Immunother 2009;58(8):1297–306.

31. Kong BY, Menzies AM, Saunders CA, et al. Residual FDG-PET metabolic activity in metastatic melanoma patients with prolonged response to anti-PD-1 therapy. Pigment Cell Melanoma Res 2016;29(5):572–7.

32. Ledezma B, Binder S, Hamid O. Atypical clinical response patterns to ipilimumab. Clin J Oncol Nurs 2011;15(4):393–403.

33. Goldfarb L, Duchemann B, Chouahnia K, et al. Monitoring anti-PD-1-based immunotherapy in non-small cell lung cancer with FDG PET: introduction of iPERCIST. EJNMMI Res 2019;9(1):8.

34. Sarfaty M, Moore A, Dudnik E, et al. Not only for melanoma. Subcutaneous pseudoprogression in lung squamous-cell carcinoma treated with nivolumab: a case report. Medicine (Baltimore) 2017; 96(4):e5951.

35. Aide N, Hicks RJ, Le Tourneau C, et al. FDG PET/CT for assessing tumour response to immunotherapy: report on the EANM symposium on immune modulation and recent review of the literature. Eur J Nucl Med Mol Imaging 2019;46(1): 238–50.

36. Wong ANM, McArthur GA, Hofman MS, et al. The advantages and challenges of using FDG PET/CT for response assessment in melanoma in the era of targeted agents and immunotherapy. Eur J Nucl Med Mol Imaging 2017;44(Suppl 1):67–77.

37. Wolchok JD, Hoos A, O'Day S, et al. Guidelines for the evaluation of immune therapy activity in solid tumors: immune-related response criteria. Clin Cancer Res 2009;15(23):7412–20.

38. Queirolo P, Spagnolo F. Atypical responses in patients with advanced melanoma, lung cancer, renal-cell carcinoma and other solid tumors treated with anti-PD-1 drugs: a systematic review. Cancer Treat Rev 2017;59:71–8.

39. Huang J, Rong L, Wang E, et al. Pseudoprogression of extramedullary disease in relapsed acute lymphoblastic leukemia after CAR T-cell therapy. Immunotherapy 2021;13(1):5–10.

40. Shah NN, Nagle SJ, Torigian DA, et al. Early positron emission tomography/computed tomography as a predictor of response after CTL019 chimeric antigen receptor -T-cell therapy in B-cell non-Hodgkin lymphomas. Cytotherapy 2018;20(12):1415–8.

41. Champiat S, Dercle L, Ammari S, et al. Hyperprogressive disease is a new pattern of progression in cancer patients treated by anti-PD-1/PD-L1. Clin Cancer Res 2017;23(8):1920–8.

42. Understanding hyperprogression in cancer. Cancer Discov 2019;9(7):821.

43. Adashek JJ, Kato S, Ferrara R, et al. Hyperprogression and immune checkpoint inhibitors: hype or progress? Oncologist 2020;25(2):94–8.

44. Kato S, Goodman A, Walavalkar V, et al. Hyperprogressors after immunotherapy: analysis of genomic alterations associated with accelerated growth rate. Clin Cancer Res 2017;23(15): 4242–50.

45. Martins F, Sofiya L, Sykiotis GP, et al. Adverse effects of immune-checkpoint inhibitors: epidemiology, management and surveillance. Nat Rev Clin Oncol 2019;16(9):563–80.

46. Xing P, Zhang F, Wang G, et al. Incidence rates of immune-related adverse events and their correlation with response in advanced solid tumours treated with NIVO or NIVO+IPI: a systematic review and meta-analysis. J Immunother Cancer 2019;7(1):341.

47. Tirumani SH, Ramaiya NH, Keraliya A, et al. Radiographic profiling of immune-related adverse events in advanced melanoma patients treated with ipilimumab. Cancer Immunol Res 2015;3(10):1185–92.

48. Bertrand A, Kostine M, Barnetche T, et al. Immune related adverse events associated with anti-CTLA-

4 antibodies: systematic review and meta-analysis. BMC Med 2015;13:211.

49. Wang DY, Salem JE, Cohen JV, et al. Fatal toxic effects associated with immune checkpoint inhibitors: a systematic review and meta-analysis. JAMA Oncol 2018;4(12):1721–8.

50. Kwak JJ, Tirumani SH, Van den Abbeele AD, et al. Cancer immunotherapy: imaging assessment of novel treatment response patterns and immune-related adverse events. Radiographics 2015; 35(2):424–37.

51. Das JP, Postow MA, Friedman CF, et al. Imaging findings of immune checkpoint inhibitor associated pancreatitis. Eur J Radiol 2020;131:109250.

52. Das JP, Halpenny D, Do RK, et al. Focal immunotherapy-induced pancreatitis mimicking metastasis on FDG PET/CT. Clin Nucl Med 2019; 44(10):836–7.

53. Mekki A, Dercle L, Lichtenstein P, et al. Detection of immune-related adverse events by medical imaging in patients treated with anti-programmed cell death 1. Eur J Cancer 2018;96:91–104.

54. Nawwar AA, Searle J, Lyburn ID. Pembrolizumab-induced thyroiditis and colitis-presentation and resolution on serial FDG PET/CT. Clin Nucl Med 2021;46(2):e121–2.

55. Razzouk-Cadet M, Picard A, Grangeon-Chapon C, et al. Nivolumab-induced pneumonitis in patient with metastatic melanoma showing complete remission on 18F-FDG PET/CT. Clin Nucl Med 2019;44(10):806–7.

56. Ayati N, Sadeghi R, Kiamanesh Z, et al. The value of (18)F-FDG PET/CT for predicting or monitoring immunotherapy response in patients with metastatic melanoma: a systematic review and meta-analysis. Eur J Nucl Med Mol Imaging 2021;48(2): 428–48.

57. Nobashi T, Baratto L, Reddy SA, et al. Predicting response to immunotherapy by evaluating tumors, lymphoid cell-rich organs, and immune-related adverse events using FDG-PET/CT. Clin Nucl Med 2019;44(4):e272–9.

58. Eisenhauer EA, Therasse P, Bogaerts J, et al. New response evaluation criteria in solid tumours: revised RECIST guideline (version 1.1). Eur J Cancer 2009;45(2):228–47.

59. Miller AB, Hoogstraten B, Staquet M, et al. Reporting results of cancer treatment. Cancer 1981;47(1): 207–14.

60. Wahl RL, Jacene H, Kasamon Y, et al. From RECIST to PERCIST: evolving considerations for PET response criteria in solid tumors. J Nucl Med 2009;50(Suppl 1):122S–50S.

61. Young H, Baum R, Cremerius U, et al. Measurement of clinical and subclinical tumour response using [18F]-fluorodeoxyglucose and positron emission tomography: review and 1999 EORTC recommendations. European Organization for Research and Treatment of Cancer (EORTC) PET Study Group. Eur J Cancer 1999;35(13):1773–82.

62. Nishino M, Giobbie-Hurder A, Gargano M, et al. Developing a common language for tumor response to immunotherapy: immune-related response criteria using unidimensional measurements. Clin Cancer Res 2013;19(14):3936–43.

63. Seymour L, Bogaerts J, Perrone A, et al. iRECIST: guidelines for response criteria for use in trials testing immunotherapeutics. Lancet Oncol 2017; 18(3):e143–52.

64. Cheson BD, Ansell S, Schwartz L, et al. Refinement of the Lugano Classification lymphoma response criteria in the era of immunomodulatory therapy. Blood 2016;128(21):2489–96.

65. Cho SY, Lipson EJ, Im HJ, et al. Prediction of response to immune checkpoint inhibitor therapy using early-time-point (18)F-FDG PET/CT imaging in patients with advanced melanoma. J Nucl Med 2017;58(9):1421–8.

66. Anwar H, Sachpekidis C, Winkler J, et al. Absolute number of new lesions on (18)F-FDG PET/CT is more predictive of clinical response than SUV changes in metastatic melanoma patients receiving ipilimumab. Eur J Nucl Med Mol Imaging 2018;45(3):376–83.

67. Sachpekidis C, Anwar H, Winkler J, et al. The role of interim (18)F-FDG PET/CT in prediction of response to ipilimumab treatment in metastatic melanoma. Eur J Nucl Med Mol Imaging 2018; 45(8):1289–96.

68. Hess S, Hansson SH, Pedersen KT, et al. FDG-PET/CT in infectious and inflammatory diseases. PET Clin 2014;9(4):497–519. vi-vii.

69. Huber H, Hodolic M, Stelzmuller I, et al. Malignant disease as an incidental finding at (1)(8)F-FDG-PET/CT scanning in patients with granulomatous lung disease. Nucl Med Commun 2015;36(5):430–7.

70. Meller J, Sahlmann CO, Scheel AK. 18F-FDG PET and PET/CT in fever of unknown origin. J Nucl Med 2007;48(1):35–45.

71. Patsoukis N, Bardhan K, Chatterjee P, et al. PD-1 alters T-cell metabolic reprogramming by inhibiting glycolysis and promoting lipolysis and fatty acid oxidation. Nat Commun 2015;6:6692.

72. Chargari C, Le Moulec S, Bonardel G, et al. Ipilimumab in cancer patients: the issue of early metabolic response. Anticancer Drugs 2013;24(3):324–6.

73. Escuin-Ordinas H, Elliott MW, Atefi M, et al. PET imaging to non-invasively study immune activation leading to antitumor responses with a 4-1BB agonistic antibody. J Immunother Cancer 2013;1:14.

74. Sachpekidis C, Larribere L, Pan L, et al. Predictive value of early 18F-FDG PET/CT studies for treatment response evaluation to ipilimumab in metastatic melanoma: preliminary results of an

ongoing study. Eur J Nucl Med Mol Imaging 2015; 42(3):386–96.

75. Chang B, Huang A, Shang C, et al. Evaluation of the anti-PD-1 flare response in patients with advanced melanoma using FDG PET/CT imaging and hematologic biomarkers. J Nucl Med 2019; 60:1270.

76. Nakamoto R, Zaba LC, Liang T, et al. Prognostic value of bone marrow metabolism on pretreatment (18)F-FDG PET/CT in patients with metastatic melanoma treated with anti-PD-1 therapy. J Nucl Med 2021. doi: 10.2967/jnumed.120.254482.

77. Seban RD, Nemer JS, Marabelle A, et al. Prognostic and theranostic 18F-FDG PET biomarkers for anti-PD1 immunotherapy in metastatic melanoma: association with outcome and transcriptomics. Eur J Nucl Med Mol Imaging 2019;46(11): 2298–310.

78. Cheshire SC, Board RE, Lewis AR, et al. Pembrolizumab-induced sarcoid-like reactions during treatment of metastatic melanoma. Radiology 2018; 289(2):564–7.

79. Sachpekidis C, Larribere L, Kopp-Schneider A, et al. Can benign lymphoid tissue changes in (18) F-FDG PET/CT predict response to immunotherapy in metastatic melanoma? Cancer Immunol Immunother 2019;68(2):297–303.

80. Tumeh PC, Harview CL, Yearley JH, et al. PD-1 blockade induces responses by inhibiting adaptive immune resistance. Nature 2014;515(7528): 568–71.

81. Burger IA, Husmann L, Hany TF, et al. Incidence and intensity of F-18 FDG uptake after vaccination with H1N1 vaccine. Clin Nucl Med 2011;36(10): 848–53.

82. Thomassen A, Lerberg Nielsen A, Gerke O, et al. Duration of 18F-FDG avidity in lymph nodes after pandemic H1N1v and seasonal influenza vaccination. Eur J Nucl Med Mol Imaging 2011;38(5): 894–8.

83. Mingos M, Howard S, Giacalone N, et al. Systemic immune response to vaccination on FDG-PET/CT. Nucl Med Mol Imaging 2016;50(4):358–61.

84. Eifer M, Eshet Y. Imaging of COVID-19 vaccination at FDG PET/CT. Radiology 2021;299(2):E248.

85. Pandit-Taskar N, Postow MA, Hellmann MD, et al. First-in-humans imaging with (89)Zr-Df-IAB22M2C anti-CD8 minibody in patients with solid malignancies: preliminary pharmacokinetics, biodistribution, and lesion targeting. J Nucl Med 2020;61(4):512–9.

86. Kristensen LK, Christensen C, Alfsen MZ, et al. Monitoring CD8a(+) T cell responses to radiotherapy and CTLA-4 blockade using [(64)Cu] NOTA-CD8a PET imaging. Mol Imaging Biol 2020; 22(4):1021–30.

87. Kristensen LK, Frohlich C, Christensen C, et al. CD4(+) and CD8a(+) PET imaging predicts response to novel PD-1 checkpoint inhibitor: studies of Sym021 in syngeneic mouse cancer models. Theranostics 2019;9(26):8221–38.

88. Larimer BM, Wehrenberg-Klee E, Caraballo A, et al. Quantitative CD3 PET imaging predicts tumor growth response to anti-CTLA-4 therapy. J Nucl Med 2016;57(10):1607–11.

89. Tavare R, Escuin-Ordinas H, Mok S, et al. An effective immuno-PET imaging method to monitor CD8-dependent responses to immunotherapy. Cancer Res 2016;76(1):73–82.

90. Vonderheide RH, Domchek SM, Clark AS. Immunotherapy for breast cancer: what are we missing? Clin Cancer Res 2017;23(11):2640–6.

91. Bensch F, van der Veen EL, Lub-de Hooge MN, et al. (89)Zr-atezolizumab imaging as a noninvasive approach to assess clinical response to PD-L1 blockade in cancer. Nat Med 2018;24(12): 1852–8.

92. Huisman MC, Niemeijer AN, Windhorst AD, et al. Quantification of PD-L1 expression with (18)F-BMS-986192 PET/CT in patients with advanced-stage non-small cell lung cancer. J Nucl Med 2020;61(10):1455–60.

93. Niemeijer AN, Leung D, Huisman MC, et al. Whole body PD-1 and PD-L1 positron emission tomography in patients with non-small-cell lung cancer. Nat Commun 2018;9(1):4664.

94. Buttner R, Gosney JR, Skov BG, et al. Programmed death-ligand 1 immunohistochemistry testing: a review of analytical assays and clinical implementation in non-small-cell lung cancer. J Clin Oncol 2017;35(34):3867–76.

95. Ponomarev V. Advancing immune and cell-based therapies through imaging. Mol Imaging Biol 2017;19(3):379–84.

96. Wei W, Jiang D, Ehlerding EB, et al. Noninvasive PET imaging of T cells. Trends Cancer 2018;4(5): 359–73.

97. Alam IS, Mayer AT, Sagiv-Barfi I, et al. Imaging activated T cells predicts response to cancer vaccines. J Clin Invest 2018;128(6):2569–80.

98. Larimer BM, Wehrenberg-Klee E, Dubois F, et al. Granzyme B PET imaging as a predictive biomarker of immunotherapy response. Cancer Res 2017;77(9):2318–27.

99. Xiao Z, Mayer AT, Nobashi TW, et al. ICOS is an indicator of T-cell-mediated response to cancer immunotherapy. Cancer Res 2020;80(14):3023–32.

100. Iravani A, Hicks RJ. Imaging the cancer immune environment and its response to pharmacologic intervention, part 2: the role of novel PET agents. J Nucl Med 2020;61(11):1553–9.

Novel Tracers and Radionuclides in PET Imaging

Christian Mason, PhD[a], Grayson R. Gimblet, BS[b,1], Suzanne E. Lapi, PhD[c,d,1], Jason S. Lewis, PhD[a,e,f],*

KEYWORDS

- PET imaging • Oncology • Cardiology • Neurodegenerative disease • Personalized medicine
- Novel PET tracers

KEY POINTS

- New radiopharmaceuticals can enable imaging strategies for the better understanding of disease states in oncology, neurology, and cardiovascular disease.
- Oncologic PET imaging agents are intended to probe the biological characteristics of cancers to improve diagnostics and the efficacy of therapeutic strategies.
- Nononcology neurologic PET imaging focuses on a range of neurologic disorders with an emphasis placed on neurodegenerative diseases such as Parkinson disease and Alzheimer disease.
- Most cardiac PET imaging has focused on blood flow and metabolism and is complemented by additional compounds for imaging of atherosclerosis.

PROMINENT PET TRACERS IN ONCOLOGY

This article first discusses many of the most prominent PET imaging agents in late preclinical and early clinical development in oncology. These agents are intended to take advantage of the unique biological and physiologic characteristics of tumors to delineate malignant from normal tissues as a means of improving current methods of diagnosis. In addition, numerous PET imaging agents focus on probing the biological characteristics of cancers and other cell populations of interest in tumors to monitor and predict the efficacy of various therapeutic strategies.

Fibroblast Activation Protein Inhibitors

Cancer-associated fibroblasts and extracellular fibroblasts are among the most abundant cell types in solid cancers.[1] These cells, which dominate the tumor stoma, have been found to play a significant role in regulating the antitumor immune response and thus have been a noteworthy target of interest for both diagnostic and therapeutic applications.[1,2] Cancer-associated fibroblasts overexpress the fibroblast activation protein (FAP), which has led to the development of fibroblast-activating protein inhibitors (FAPIs), as a means of selectively targeting these cells to improve therapeutic outcomes.[3] Although therapeutic radionuclides attach via

[a] Department of Radiology, Memorial Sloan Kettering Cancer Center, 417 East 68th Street, New York, NY 10065, USA; [b] School of Medicine, University of Alabama at Birmingham, Birmingham, AL 35233, USA; [c] Department of Radiology, University of Alabama at Birmingham, Birmingham, AL 35233, USA; [d] Department of Chemistry, University of Alabama at Birmingham, Birmingham, AL 35205, USA; [e] Molecular Pharmacology Program, Memorial Sloan Kettering Cancer Center, New York, NY 10065, USA; [f] Weill Cornell Medical College, New York, NY 10065, USA

[1] Present address: 1824 6th Avenue South, Birmingham, AL 35294.
* Corresponding author. 417 East 68th Street, New York, NY 10065.
E-mail address: lewisj2@mskcc.org

Radiol Clin N Am 59 (2021) 887–918
https://doi.org/10.1016/j.rcl.2021.05.012

chelators to FAPI and have been evaluated in numerous types of cancer, the focus here is on PET imaging applications. An extensive amount of research has focused on the preclinical and clinical evaluation of variations of the [68Ga]Ga-FAPI PET tracer, including [68Ga]Ga-FAPI-2, [68Ga]Ga-FAPI-4, [68Ga]Ga-FAPI-46, and [68Ga]Ga-FAPI-74 in various types of cancers.[4–14]

One such prominent study extensively assessed the use of [68Ga]Ga-FAPI-04 as an imaging agent in 28 different types of cancers. Images generated from this study are shown in **Fig. 1**.[4] The standard uptake value (SUV) varied depending on the type of cancer, but the investigators reported tumor to background ratios greater than 3 for the moderate uptake groups and more than 6 for the high-intensity uptake groups.[4] In addition, studies have been performed directly comparing the imaging capabilities of [68Ga]FAPI and [18F]-fluoro-deoxyglucose (FDG),[9,11,12] and some physicians argue that this tracer could replace [18F]FDG, especially in cancers where surrounding tissues show high rates of metabolism resulting in high background signal.[15] More recent work has explored the capabilities of an [18F]-labeled FAPI imaging agent as a means of extending the radioactive half-life of the tracer to improve its availability to more remote locations.[14] The results of these studies have shown the potential of these tracers in numerous types of cancer for both diagnostic and staging applications. There are currently 20 active clinical trials exploring the use of FAPI PET imaging agents in various cancers and diseases. There is significant optimism that these tracers could play a prominent role in addressing pitfalls in current standard of care techniques and improve patient outcomes.

Imaging Increased Rates of Cellular Proliferation

The [18F]-labeled nucleoside analogue 3′-fluoro-3′deoxythymidine (FLT) is a PET imaging agent that has seen significant interest for its ability to quantify cellular proliferation. The capabilities of this tracer were initially reported in 1998, and have since sparked a large number of preclinical and clinical evaluations for its potential in overcoming the challenges associated with [18F]FDG.[16] [18F]FLT has the potential to better delineate malignant tissues in areas with high metabolic rates, such as muscle, lymphocytes, brain tissue, as well as in head and neck cancers.[17–19] In a clinical evaluation performed by Buck and colleagues,[20] the uptake of [18F]FLT better correlated with staging than [18F]FDG in soft tissue tumors, with mean SUVs of 0.7, 1.3, 4.1, and 6.1 in benign lesions, low-grade sarcoma, grade 2 tumors, and grade 3 tumors respectively.

In addition, the ability to monitor cell proliferation has made [18F]FLT PET a promising tool to noninvasively monitor therapeutic response and predict outcomes in patients with a variety of cancers.[21] Numerous studies have been performed to evaluate the potential of [18F]FLT to predict patient response to several treatment strategies. A recent study explored the use of [18F]FLT PET imaging to determine response to neoadjuvant chemotherapy targeting the c-met pathway in soft tissue sarcomas.[19] Researchers observed, in a small subset of 15 patients, that 12 had observable changes in [18F]FLT accumulation, 8 patients showed response, and 4 progressed. The results of this pilot study support the potential of this tracer to monitor response, and further evaluation of this tracer is currently being explored.[19] [18F]FLT has been evaluated in numerous types of cancer.[21] In some studies in head and neck cancer and non–small cell lung cancer, [18F]FLT performs worse or about the same as [18F]FDG in monitoring therapeutic response.[22,23] In other studies in patients with ovarian cancer and lymphoma, [18F]FLT has better performance in determining therapeutic outcomes.[24,25] Although results can vary depending on the type of cancer and treatment strategy, [18F]FLT is a prominent imaging agent that has significant potential in improving detection and monitoring therapeutic outcomes.

Prostate-Specific Membrane Antigen

The development of PET imaging agents targeting the prostate-specific membrane antigen (PSMA) has been an extensive area of research over the past decade, generating close to 1000 research articles in the past 2 years alone. PSMA PET imaging has been implemented in the clinic as an improved method of staging and restaging patients as well as to monitor for recurrence and metastatic dissemination after therapy.[26–28] More recent work has been designed to evaluate [68Ga]PSMA PET imaging for initial diagnosis that could potentially improve detection of early-stage recurrence in patients with only moderately increased levels of prostate-specific antigen.[29] In addition, there is significant interest in using PSMA PET imaging to guide therapeutic strategies, such as radiotherapy and radioimmunotherapy, as well as predict patient outcomes.[30–32]

One of the most widely used PSMA targeted tracers is [68Ga]PSMA-11, which is the focus of numerous preclinical and clinical studies and has recently been approved by the US Food and Drug Administration (FDA) in patients with

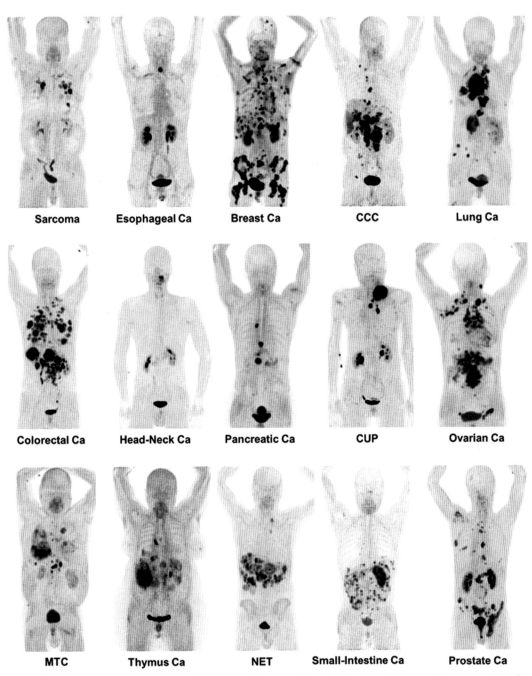

Fig. 1. [^{68}Ga] fibroblast-activating protein inhibitor-4 imaging in multiple types of cancer. Ca, cancer; CCC, circulating cancer cell; CUP, cancer of unknown primary; MTC, medullary thyroid cancer; NET, neuroendocrine tumor. (*From* Kratochwil C, Flechsig P, Lindner T, et al. (68)Ga-FAPI PET/CT: Tracer Uptake in 28 Different Kinds of Cancer. *J Nucl Med.* 2019;60(6):801-805.)

suspected metastatic and recurrent prostate cancer. A more novel tracer, [^{18}F]PSMA-1007, is also being evaluated in the clinic and has the advantage of a longer physical half-life compared with [^{68}Ga]PSMA-11.[33] Another PSMA imaging agent in late phase development is [^{18}F]F-2-(3-{1-carboxy-5-[(6-[^{18}F]fluoro-pyridine-3-carbonyl)-amino]-pentyl}-ureido)-pentanedioic acid (DCFPyL). In a study of 262 patients with biochemically recurrent prostate cancer, 91.4% of lesions with an SUV$_{peak}$ greater than 3.5 and 95.5% of lesions with an SUV$_{peak}$ greater than

4.0 were considered malignant on [^{18}F]F-DCFPyL PET.[34]

Although prostate cancer has been the main area of focus in most of the studies performed to date, more recent work has begun to elucidate the significance of PSMA expression in other types of cancers. PSMA expression in the neovasculature of many different cancers has been shown to be increased, and thus recent research has aimed to take advantage of this increased expression in cancers such as breast cancer, non–small cell lung cancer, colorectal cancer, renal cell carcinoma, pancreatic cancer, and highly vascularized gliomas, such as glioblastoma multiforme.[28,35,36] One such example includes a recent study evaluating the use of [^{68}Ga]PSMA-11 to detect and stage primary and metastatic breast cancer lesions.[37] The researchers reported promising detection rates in lesions identified by [^{18}F]FDG.[37] These results along with numerous preclinical and clinical evaluations support the prominent role PSMA targeted PET tracers may have on the diagnosis and therapeutic outcomes in patients with prostate cancer and other cancers with PSMA expression in their neovasculature.

Deltalike Protein 3

The deltalike protein 3 (DLL3) is an inhibitory ligand of the Notch pathway and is upregulated in 85% of small cell lung cancers and other neuroendocrine cancers, whereas nonneuroendocrine cancers and normal tissues do not express DLL3.[38] Castration-resistant neuroendocrine prostate cancers also show increased expression of DLL3 and thus this ligand has received attention in recent years for its potential as a target in immunotherapies such as rovalpituzumab teserine (SC16LD6.5),[39] and radioimmunotherapies including ^{225}Ac and ^{177}Lu labeled anti-DLL3 monoclonal antibodies.[40] Several multicenter clinical trials have been performed exploring the use of rovalpituzumab teserine as a therapy in small cell lung cancer.

The use of PET imaging to guide therapies is of significant interest in these indications because conventional methods of analyzing DLL3 expression are limited. These limitations include insufficient contemporaneous analysis of DLL3 expression, sampling bias resulting from intratumoral and intertumoral heterogeneity, and the inherently high false-negative rate for histopathologic assessment of DLL3 expression.[41] The implementation of PET imaging can overcome many of these limitations and thus has been of significant interest in this field. Sharma and colleagues[41] reported the preclinical evaluation of

an [^{89}Zr]Zr-DFO-SC16 PET imaging agent in small cell lung cancer xenografts as a means of noninvasively quantifying DLL3 expression. In this work, statistically significant differences in tumor accumulation were observed between the high and low DLL3-expressing small cell lung cancer xenograft models. In addition, uptake of the [^{89}Zr]Zr-DFO-SC16 correlated with therapeutic response, highlighting the potential of these tracers to predict patient outcome.[41] With the promising results of this preclinical analysis, a clinical trial (NCT04199741) was initiated to evaluate the use of [^{89}Zr]Zr-DFO-SC16.56 to noninvasively monitor DLL3 expression in patients, and is currently ongoing.

Poly(ADP-ribose) Polymerase 1

Poly(ADP-ribose) polymerase 1 (PARP1) is part of a family of proteins tasked with repairing single-strand DNA breaks as part of the base excision repair pathway.[42] With increased rates of metabolism and proliferation, cancer cells are more prone to developing single-strand breaks and thus show increased expression and activity of PARP1.[43,44] The increased reliance on DNA repair pathways is a prominent characteristic of many types of cancer, and thus a significant amount of research has been aimed at targeting these pathways to prevent DNA repair, ultimately leading to cell death.[42,45–47] There are currently 4 FDA-approved inhibitors of PARP1: olaparib, niraparib, rucaparib, and talazoparib.[46]

A significant volume of research is focused on the development of imaging agents that are based on these PARP inhibitor (PARPi) scaffolds for their potential applications in cancer diagnosis, patient stratification, and monitoring therapy.[48] As a diagnostic, these imaging agents are particularly focused on improving current standard-of-care modalities such as [^{18}F]FDG, which has limitations in certain areas of the body because of high background signal in normal tissues. Several PARP-selective tracers have been developed and evaluated in preclinical and/or clinical studies, including [^{18}F]FluorThanatrace and [^{18}F]PARPi.[49–53] The [^{18}F]PARPi tracer was developed based on the FDA-approved olaparib scaffold, and the [^{18}F]PARPi tracer was evaluated extensively in preclinical settings as a diagnostic and a means of monitoring the accumulation and retention of PARPi in the tumor.[54,55] This tracer has since been used in clinical trials (NCT04173104 and NCT03631017) for multiple types of cancer and has shown promising results, as shown in **Fig. 2**. Continued development of these tracers will likely lead to multiple novel

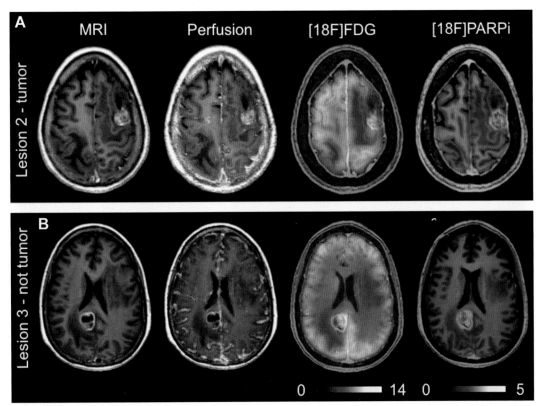

Fig. 2. [^{18}F]-PARPi imaging in a patient with benign and malignant lesions within the brain. (*A*) Lesion from patient confirmed to be cancerous (*B*) Lesion from patient confirmed to be non-cancerous. (*From* Young RJ, Demétrio De Souza França P, Pirovano G, et al. Preclinical and first-in-human-brain-cancer applications of [18F]poly-(ADP-ribose) polymerase inhibitor PET/MR. *Neuro-Oncology Advances*. 2020.)

radiotracers that can provide improved contrast in PET images, stratify patients, and identify tumors that are likely to respond to therapies targeting the PARP enzyme.

Immune Checkpoint Inhibitors

Immune checkpoint inhibitors such as programmed cell death protein 1 (PD-1)/programmed death-ligand 1 (PD-L1) and cytotoxic T lymphocyte–associated protein 4 (CTLA-4) have received significant attention for their impressive results in some patients.[56,57] However, one of the major limitations of these therapies is the lack of a marker that can be used to stratify patients who are likely to respond to immune checkpoint blockade.[58,59] There are several possible explanations as to why traditional immunohistochemistry quantification of expression for the ligands that play a role in immune activity does not correlate with patient outcomes. Many in the field believe that heterogeneous expression and the dynamic nature of the ligand expression are the leading factors preventing clinicians from determining

whether a patient is likely to respond.[60,61] PET imaging has the potential of overcoming these 2 limitations and thus has led to a significant effort to develop an effective PET tracer that can noninvasively monitor expression and correlate well with patient outcomes.[62]

One strategy is to prepare ^{89}Zr-labeled monoclonal antibodies that selectively bind with the particular immune checkpoint ligand. There are several monoclonal antibodies to date that have been approved by the FDA for use in immune checkpoint therapies.[63] One such monoclonal antibody is pembrolizumab, one of the earliest FDA-approved and widely implemented immune checkpoint inhibitors.[63] There are several researchers who have prepared ^{89}Zr-labeled versions of the pembrolizumab antibody to evaluate its potential in quantifying PD-1 expression using varying approaches.[64–66] Several clinical trials (NCT02760225, NCT04605614, and NCT03065764) have also been initiated to evaluate PET tracers based on the pembrolizumab antibody in the clinic. Additional clinical trials are also underway for PET tracers based on other

FDA-approved antibodies, including ipilimumab, atezolizumab, and avelumab.

Another prominent approach that has seen success in preclinical settings attempts to monitor T-cell activation as a consequence of immune checkpoint therapies using PET/computed tomography (CT) by administering the 18-fluoro-9-(β-D-arabinofuranosyl) guanine ([18F]F-AraG) imaging agent. [18F]F-AraG has been established as selective for activated T lymphocytes,[67] and accumulation of [18F]F-AraG paralleled the course of adaptive immune response in a preclinical colorectal cancer model.[68] Multiple clinical trials are currently investigating the ability of this tracer to monitor T-cell activation in response to immune checkpoint blockade in several types of cancer.

Imaging Extracellular Acidic and Hypoxic Conditions

There are several distinct characteristics of cancer that allow researchers and clinicians to develop novel therapeutic and diagnostic agents that specifically target tumors. One such characteristic is the reduced pH and hypoxic conditions within the extracellular environment of most tumors as a result of the poorly formed vasculature as well as aberrant and increased rates of metabolism and cell proliferation.[69,70] This characteristic has led to a significant research effort to devise unique and clever ways to take advantage of this phenomenon. These efforts have brought to fruition numerous pH-sensitive cleavable linkers that can improve the selectivity and efficacy of drug molecules, peptides that can alter their structure as a result of pH and insert themselves into the membrane of cells, and radiolabeled molecules that are metabolized by cells that have altered metabolic pathways as a result of environmental stimuli.[70–76]

The evaluation of the family of pH (low) insertion peptides has produced promising results and has shown the capabilities of targeting the acidic microenvironment within tumors. These peptides alter their structures in a low-pH environment, forming a transmembrane alpha helix that inserts itself into the cell membrane.[72,73,77] These peptides have been labeled with several different isotopes for PET imaging, including 18F and 64Cu.[73,77] The research performed to date evaluating these peptides has focused on their potential as diagnostic agents as well as discerning which patients or tumors are likely to respond to pH low insertion peptide (pHLIP) variants designed for delivery of therapeutic payloads.[78] At present, a clinical trial has been initiated for an 18F-labeled version of the pHLIP peptide to evaluate its efficacy for imaging the low-pH environments in patients with breast cancer (NCT04054986).

Another strategy for imaging tumor microenvironment focuses on the hypoxic conditions in the extracellular matrix and the variations in cell metabolism that result.[74,79] The tracer [18F]fluoro-misonidazole ([18F]FMISO) is reduced by hypoxic cells and accumulates in regions of the body where these conditions exist. Imaging hypoxia has several clinically relevant applications. These agents can act as a companion diagnostic in regions of the body where imaging metabolism using [18F]FDG is insufficient in diagnosing cancer and/or the presence of hypoxia could alter the therapeutic plan.[80] Imaging hypoxia can act as a prognostic indicator and guide therapeutic strategy, and also has a significant impact on radiotherapy where hypoxic cells are much more radiation resistant than normoxic cells, thus requiring increased radiation dose to obtain sufficient therapeutic efficacy.[74] Although [18F]FMISO seems to be the most prominent tracer currently being explored, many other tracers are also in development, including [18F]fluoroazomycin arabinoside ([18F]FAZA),[80–82] with numerous ongoing clinical trials such as NCT03418818, NCT04395469, and NCT02701699, and [64Cu]Cu-diacetyl-bis(N4-methylthiosemicarbazone) ([64Cu]Cu-ATSM)[83–85] also with ongoing clinical trials NCT03951337.

Radiolabeled Analogues of Bioactive Molecules

As researchers continue to elucidate the complex mechanisms involved in cancer biology and metabolism, many novel radiotracers have been developed based on bioactive molecules such as amino acids, hormones, and antibodies that target or interact with processes more specifically associated with cancer. Many of the tracers mentioned previously would be considered among this class of tracers. Although a complete list of novel and promising PET tracers is beyond the scope of this article, briefly, the following tracers are examples of this diverse and powerful field and will likely make their way into clinical settings in the very near future if they have not already.

The PET tracers 3,4-dihydroxy-6[18F]fluoro-L-phenylalanine ([18F]FDOPA), L-[11C]methionine ([11C]MET), and O-(2-[18F]fluoroethyl)-L-tyrosine ([18F]F-FET) are amino acid analogues of particular interest for their potential in improving diagnosis of primary brain tumors, including glioblastoma.[86–90] These tracers improve on current standard of care because they are capable of passing through an intact blood-brain barrier and have much improved tumor/normal brain uptake ratio compared with [^{18}F]FDG. Each of these tracers is currently under investigation in ongoing clinical trials. Another example of radiolabeled amino acids is the (4S)-4-(3[^{18}F]fluoropropyl)-L-glutamic acid ([^{18}F]F-FSPG) PET tracer. This tracer is of particular interest for its ability to determine drug resistance because the tumor uptake can indicate the upregulation of antioxidant pathways. This tracer has been shown to provide an early indicator for tumor response in preclinical studies, preceding other standard methods such as tumor size regression or reduced glucose metabolism.[91] These results have led to several clinical trials that are evaluating the ability of these tracers to act as a diagnostic and monitor therapeutic response in patients.

A tracer that uses a radiolabeled hormone analogue is the 16α-[^{18}F]fluoroestradiol ([^{18}F]F-FES), which is capable of providing a method of noninvasively assessing estrogen expression within a tumor and was approved by the FDA in June of 2020. This tracer has been studied as a diagnostic for recurrent and metastatic breast cancer in patients with a history of estrogen-positive primary cancer.[92,93] Ongoing clinical trials, such as NCT02398773, are evaluating the ability of [^{18}F]FES to improve current diagnostic techniques for assessing recurrent and metastatic breast cancer as well as predict patient response to endocrine therapies. Additional hormone analogues currently under study include 21-[^{18}F]fluoro-furanyl-norprogesterone ([^{18}F]FFNP) as a means of evaluating progesterone expression in breast cancers (NCT03212170), as well as the 16β-[^{18}F]fluoro-5α-dihydrotestosterone ([^{18}F]F-FDHT) to diagnose recurrent and metastatic prostate cancer and evaluate androgen receptor expression to guide therapeutic strategies.[93–95] These tracers have provided promising results with high selectivity and sensitivity, noninvasive quantitation of receptor expression to inform therapeutic strategies, and the capability of monitoring changes in hormone receptor expression as a result of endocrine therapies.

Antibodies and the various fragments that can be engineered from portions of the antibody is an expansive and invaluable area of research that has generated an extensive and ever-growing library of highly specific therapeutic and diagnostic agents that have seen tremendous success in preclinical and clinical studies.[96] The investigators of the Antibodies to Watch series presented an excellent breakdown of the current field of antibody-based therapeutics for treatment in multiple diseases from academic and industrial laboratories that are at varying stages of clinical development.[96] As antibodies are evaluated and confirmed to be effective

therapeutics, novel PET imaging agents can readily be prepared by labeling these antibodies with chelators capable of incorporating radioactive isotopes. Thus, as the number of viable and effective therapeutic antibodies continues to grow, so does the library of imaging agents with the potential of improving diagnostic capabilities, stratifying patients who are more likely to respond to therapy, and more quickly and accurately monitoring patient response. Some examples of approved antibodies that have been adapted as PET imaging agents include [^{89}Zr]Zr-durvalumab for imaging PD-L1 expression in head and neck cancers as well as lymphoma (NCT03610061, NCT03829007), [^{89}Zr]Zr-ramucirumab for imaging VEGFR-2 expression in prostate cancer,[97] and [^{64}Cu]Cu-Bn-NOTA-hu14.18K322A, a humanized version of the chimeric antibody dinutuximab, used to image disialoganglioside GD2 expression in neuroblastoma and osteosarcoma.[98] In addition, some of the previously discussed imaging agents were developed from approved antibodies such as [^{89}Zr]Zr-atezolizumab (NCT04564482, NCT03850028, NCT04222426), [^{89}Zr]Zr-avelumab (NCT03514719), and [^{89}Zr]Zr-ipilimumab (NCT04029181, NCT03313323).

RADIOPHARMACEUTICALS FOR PET IMAGING IN NEUROLOGY

Highlighted here are the radiopharmaceuticals, for nononcology neurologic PET imaging, that are either FDA approved or in late-stage clinical trials. Nononcology neurologic PET imaging focuses on a range of neurologic disorders,[99,100] with an emphasis placed on neurodegenerative diseases such as Parkinson disease (PD) and Alzheimer disease (AD). Such neurodegenerative disorders are notable for the accumulation of protein inclusions in the brain and their impact on neurotransmission.

To illustrate this point, patients with PD experience a degeneration of the nigrostriatal pathway that results in the loss of dopaminergic neurons. This neuronal loss has been shown to correlate with the aggregation of protein α-synuclein in the neuronal perikarya, forming the characteristic Lewy body.[101] In addition, the primary pathology features of AD is the aggregate burden of 2 proteins: β-amyloid, the principal component of neurotic plaques, and tau protein, a component of neurofibrillary tangles.[102] Impairment of the cholinergic system is also thought to play a significant role in the cognitive decline experienced by patients with AD.[103]

These unique disease indications, in combination with the chronic inflammation they produce, are used as potential targets in the development and use of radiopharmaceuticals for the PET imaging of neurologic disorders.

Protein-Targeted Imaging

One of the primary pathology features in neurodegenerative diseases such as PD and AD is protein aggregation. Thus, protein-targeted imaging is an especially notable modality in AD, which has a significant aggregate burden of amyloid-beta (Aβ) plaques and tau protein. Note that preclinical targeting of the PD aggregate protein α-synuclein has met with limited success to date, with recent efforts showing promise.[104]

The clinical relevance of imaging agents targeting Aβ plaques and tau protein in AD are discussed next.

β-Amyloid imaging agents

The accumulation of β-amyloid into Aβ plaques is one of the hallmarks of AD. The first widely used PET imaging agent for detecting these plaques, [11C]PiB (2-[4-([11C]methylamino)phenyl]-1,3-benzothiazol-6-ol; Pittsburgh compound B), continues to have widespread use in research ever since its first use in human studies in the early 2000s.[105] Although this tracer is not approved for clinical use by the FDA, it is notable for its high specificity for Aβ plaques and ability to differentiate AD from other types of neurodegeneration that do not involve Aβ deposition, such as frontotemporal lobar degeneration (FTLD).[106] For this reason, [11C]PiB has been used as a comparative standard in the development of new β-amyloid imaging agents. There is also increasing evidence for the presence of comorbidities in neurodegenerative disorders, such as the presence of Aβ plaques in some patients with PD.[107,108] [11C]PiB is being used in clinical trials to measure the amyloid burden in PD (NCT03555292), to evaluate the potential presence of comorbid AD. The results of this trial could provide unique clinical insight into the disease burden of Aβ plaques in PD and other types of neurodegeneration.

Beyond [11C]C-PiB, 3 18F-labeled amyloid imaging agents have been approved for use by the FDA, within the last decade, for the detection of Aβ plaques in patients undergoing evaluation for cognitive impairment with AD as a potential cause. These 3 tracers are [18F]florbetapir (4-[(E)-2-[6-[2-[2-(2-[18F]fluoranylethoxy)ethoxy]ethoxy]pyridin-3-yl]ethenyl]-N-methylaniline; Amyvid), [18F]florbetaben (4-[(E)-2-[4-[2-[2-(2-[18F]fluoranylethoxy)ethoxy]ethoxy]phenyl]ethenyl]-N-methylaniline; NeuraCeq), and [18F]flutemetamol (2-[3-[18F]fluoranyl-4-(methylamino)phenyl]-1,3-benzothiazol-6-ol; Vizamyl), and have proven efficacy in several clinical trials.[109–111] The tracers can be used to estimate the Aβ plaque density in patients with suspected AD but are not indicated to diagnose AD or other neurodegenerative disorders based on imaging alone. These 3 tracers continue to undergo clinical development and are commonly used as a standard with which to compare novel tracers. For example, florbetaben is being examined, similarly to [11C]C-PiB, as a means to quantify the comorbid Aβ plaque burden experienced by patients with other neurodegenerative diseases, such as PD.[112]

There are 2 next-generation radiopharmaceuticals for imaging β-amyloid that have potential for clinical impact in the coming years: [18F]FIBT (2-(p-methylaminophenyl)-7-(2-[18F]fluoroethoxy)imidazo-[2,1-b]benzothiazole) and [18F]NAV4694 (2-[2-[18F]fluoro-6-(methylamino)-3-pyridinyl]-1-benzofuran-5-ol). In a human study involving 6 patients with AD, [18F]FIBT showed imaging quality comparable with [11C]PiB.[113] [18F]FIBT was also shown to have a higher binding affinity and specificity for Aβ plaques. This study followed the first human study for [18F]FIBT in 2015, which involved 2 patients: 1 patient with AD and 1 control. In this preliminary study, [18F]FIBT was able to successfully differentiate the patient with AD from the control and showed a strong pattern of tracer uptake consistent with AD.[114] Because of the small number of subjects in these studies, larger clinical trials are required to further understand the utility of these agents.

The second radiopharmaceutical, [18F]NAV4694 (also known as [18F]AZD4694), has been shown to have imaging characteristics nearly identical to those of [11C]PiB[115] and has recently undergone phase 2 and phase 3 trials (NCT01886820, NCT01680588). Despite its demonstrated efficacy, a recently conducted human trial showed low uptake of the tracer in the preclinical phase of AD, suggesting a limit for its clinical use.[116] However, this tracer remains promising for future clinical use because of its favorable imaging characteristics.

Tau imaging agents

Tau protein is most associated with cognitive decline in neurodegenerative diseases such as AD. Note that tau protein accumulation is not a specific biomarker for AD; the protein is also present during acute brain conditions such as stroke.[117] In addition, different forms of tau accumulate in different neurodegenerative diseases, and PET tracers targeting tau typically bind preferentially to certain forms of tau.[118] However, research has shown that measuring the buildup of tau, which can occur before the formation of Aβ plaques, may be important in detecting AD in early stages.[119] Studies such as these suggest the important complementary role nonspecific protein imaging can play in disease-targeted imaging.

There are 3 radiopharmaceuticals that have been widely studied in the targeting of tau protein: [18F]THK5351 ((2S)-1-[18F]fluoranyl-3-[2-[6-(methylamino)pyridin-3-yl]quinolin-6-yl]oxypropan-2-ol), [18F]AV1451 (7-(6-fluoropyridine-3-yl)-5H-pyrido[4,3-b]indole), [11C]PBB3 (2-((1E,3E)-4-(6-(11C-methylamino)pyridine-3-yl)buta-1,3-dienyl)benzo[d]thiazol-6-ol). In general, these 3 tracers were found to have excellent selectivity for tau protein compared with Aβ plaques with some off-target binding.[120] For example, [18F]THK5351 binds to monoamine oxidase B and [11C]PBB3 has been shown to bind to α-synuclein.[121] A study with [18F]AV1451 involving 8 patients with AD and 8 healthy controls showed some age-related uptake of the compound among the healthy controls, indicating some off-target uptake.[122]

Beyond these 3 compounds, a new generation of tau tracers were designed to reduce off-target binding. Among these new radiopharmaceuticals, [18F]MK-6240 (6-[18F]fluoranyl-3-pyrrolo[2,3-c]pyridin-1-ylisoquinolin-5-amine) and [18F]RO-6958948 (2-(6-[18F]fluoro-pyridin-3-yl)-9H-1,6,9-triaza-fluorene) have shown promising results. The safety and efficacy of [18F]MK-6240 has been shown preclinically[123] and is currently the subject of several active clinical trials (NCT04104659, NCT03706261). Large clinical trials have shown that [18F]MK-6240 is able to identify individuals with AD with high fidelity and accuracy.[121] The tracer has also been an important tool in developing a better understanding of the role the tau protein plays in AD progression.

A human trial comparing [11C]PiB and [18F]MK-6240 showed patients with increased Aβ burden experience cognitive decline largely accounted for by the level of tau protein.[124] This trial highlights a potentially important role for future tau imaging to monitor disease progression. In addition, the short half-life of [11C]PiB could allow the imaging of Aβ plaques and tau protein in the same patient on the same day (Fig. 3).

The tracer [18F]RO-6958948 has undergone preclinical testing in mice, which showed its highly specific binding to tau and rapid kinetics.[125] The tracer has also recently completed several phase 1 trials testing for safety and efficiency in humans (NCT02792179, NCT02187627). Future clinical trials showing its clinical relevance in targeting tau protein are expected in the future.

Neurotransmission-Targeted Imaging

Dopaminergic system imaging
Patients with PD are known to experience a neurodegeneration affecting the nigrostriatal system, one of the 4 dopaminergic pathways in the brain. A well-established tracer for dopamine metabolism is [18F]FDOPA.[126] This tracer is a substrate for aromatic acid decarboxylase (AADC), an enzyme necessary for the conversion of aromatic amino acids into neurotransmitters such as dopamine. This tracer was approved by the FDA in 2019 for the evaluation of adult patients with suspected parkinsonian syndromes, including PD, through the visualization dopaminergic nerve terminals. Human trials have shown that this tracer is both highly sensitive and highly specific.[127]

The design of the next generation of radiopharmaceuticals in this area is primarily focused on targeting 2 additional proteins: dopamine transporter (DAT) and vesicular monoamine transporter 2 (VMAT2). There are 2 novel tracers of interest related to these protein targets: [18F]FP-CIT (methyl(1R,2S,3S,5S)-8-(3-fluoropropyl)-3-(4-[18F]fluorophenyl)-8-azabicyclo[3.2.1]octane2-carboxylate) and [18F]FE-PE2I ((E)-N-(3-iodoprop-2-enyl)-2β-carbo[18F]fluoroethoxy-3β-(4'-methyl-phenyl)nortropane). In the case of FP-CIT, its 123I-labeled form, ioflupane, is used clinically for single-photon emission computed tomography (SPECT) imaging in patients with suspected PD. An analysis of 6 PET clinical studies showed that [18F]FP-CIT is a potential biomarker for early PD diagnosis.[128] In addition, a study with 9 patients with early PD was conducted using [18F]FE-PE2I, which was successful in differentiating healthy controls and patients with early PD.[129] This same compound also showed good repeatability and reliability and is a possible marker to monitor the progress of DAT decline.[130] There has also been interest in imaging vesicular acetylcholine transporter, which has been associated with PD, using the PET ligand (2R,3R)-5-[18F]fluoroethoxybenzovesamicol.[131]

Inflammation-Targeted Imaging and Synaptic Density

There is considerable evidence that both chronic inflammation[132] and reduced synaptic density[133] are associated with neurodegenerative disorders. As a result, there is interest in identifying markers for these two conditions associated with neurodegeneration. Of particular interest for inflammation is the translocator protein (TSPO) that is upregulated with high density in many neurologic disorders.[134] Markers of interest for synaptic density include high-density neural synapse proteins, one of which is synaptic vesicle protein 2A (SV2A).[135] The loss or decrease in density of these synaptic proteins indicates disease progression.

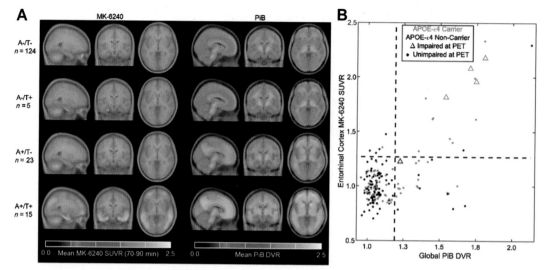

Fig. 3. MK-6240 and PiB PET/CT images, and biomarker group stratification. (*A*) PET/CT images of the [11C]PiB and [18F]MK6240 tracers in different patient groups. (*B*) Quantrant plots representing the relationship between global PiB distribution volume ratio (DVR) and MK6240 standard uptake value ratio (SUVR) in entorhinal cortex. Results suggest that changes in PiB precede detectable changes in MK-6240 in most cases. Individuals with mild cognitive impairment at PET (*triangles*) were more likely to be both amyloid (A) and tau (T) positive than any other group. (*From* Betthauser TJ, Koscik RL, Jonaitis EM, et al. Amyloid and tau imaging biomarkers explain cognitive decline from late middle-age. *Brain.* Jan 1 2020;143(1):320-335. https://doi.org/10.1093/brain/awz378.)

Translocator protein imaging

TSPO is a transmembrane protein upregulated during periods of neuroinflammation, following the activation of microglial cells.[134] One of the first radiopharmaceuticals targeting this protein was [11C]PK-11195 (*N-sec*-butyl-1-(2-chlorophenyl)-*N*-[11C]methyl-3-isoquinolinecarboxamide), which was widely used in research for several decades. However, clinical use of this compound was limited by nonspecific binding, low brain uptake, and the short half-life of [11C].[136]

A second generation of TSPO-targeting radiopharmaceuticals was developed to address these limitations. Compounds in this second generation include [11C]DAA1106 (*N*-(5-fluoro-2-phenoxy-phenyl)-*N*-[(5-methoxy-2-[11C]methoxyphenyl) methyl]acetamide), [11C]PBR28 (*N*-[(2-[11C] methoxyphenyl)methyl]-*N*-(6-phenoxypyridin-3-yl) acetamide), [18F]FEPPA (*N*-[[2-(2-[18F]fluoranyle-thoxy)phenyl]methyl]-*N*-(4-phenoxypyridin-3-yl) acetamide), [18F]PBR06 (*N*-[(2,5-dimethoxyphenyl) methyl]-2-[18F]fluoranyl-*N*-(2-phenoxyphenyl) acetamide), [18F]PBR11 (2-(6-chloro-2-(4-(3-[18F] fluoropropoxy)phenyl)imidazo[1,2-a]pyridin-3-yl)-*N,N*-diethylacetamide), and [18F]DPA714 ([*N,N*-diethyl-2-(2-(4-(2[18F]fluoroethoxy)phenyl) 5,7dimethylpyrazolo[1,5a]pyrimidin-3-yl)acet-amide]). Many of these new compounds showed higher brain uptake and greater specificity for the TSPO target compared with [11C]PK-11195.[137] However, additional studies also revealed that

genetic variation in the TSPO gene among participants resulted in TSPO expression with varied the binding affinity for the tracer, leading to the classification of so-called high-affinity, low-affinity, and mixed-affinity binding groups.[138] Patients with low-affinity TSPO binding present a significant clinical contraindication for TSPO-targeted imaging and have been excluded from some clinical trials. Despite this limitation, the largest improvement in TSPO-targeted imaging with second-generation radiopharmaceuticals was the development of [18F]-labeled compounds, which benefit from a longer half-life compared with their [11C]-labeled counterparts to allow more widespread use.

TSPO-targeted imaging studies of neurodegenerative disorders with second-generation DPA-714 modeled acute inflammation in rats and showed that [18F]DPA-714 is a selective and reliable biomarker[139] with a more favorable signal/noise ratio than [11C]PK-11195.[140] However, one of the first human trials, involving 10 patients with AD and 6 healthy controls, showed no significant difference in [18F]DPA-714 uptake between the two groups.[141] Note that no information on the binding status of the participants of this trial was available for this study. A subsequent human trial, involving 64 patients with AD and 32 controls, specifically studied high-affinity and mixed-affinity binders. The results of the trial showed greater TSPO uptake among high-affinity and mixed-affinity binders compared with healthy controls and also showed that participants with a greater uptake of TSPO had a slower disease progression over a period of 2 years, indicating a possible protective effect provided by TSPO.[142] The results of these 2 clinical trials introduce new questions regarding the use of [18F]DPA-714 in identifying neurodegeneration and the potential importance of binding status on TSPO-targeted imaging. Further exploration of this compound continues, including current clinical trials to determine whether patients who experience higher neuroinflammation have more symptoms from neuroinflammatory diseases (NCT03759522). Overall, the development of second-generation TSPO imaging agents has shown promise regarding binding specificity and brain uptake, but continued developments may improve image quality and diagnostic utility.[143]

Synaptic vesicle protein 2A

SV2A is a membrane protein localized to the synapse in neural cells.[135] Many neurodegenerative diseases are known to reduce the density of these synapses, thereby reducing the amount of SV2A.[144] As a result, SV2A has been investigated as a clinical marker for neurodegeneration.

Among the first-generation SV2A tracers, 3 have been identified with potential clinical relevance: [18F]UCB-H, [11C]UCB-A, and [11C]UCB-J (4R)-1-(3-([11C]methylpyridin-4-yl)methyl)-4-(3,4,5-trifluorophenyl)pyrrolidin-2-one. A preclinical analysis of these 3 compounds found [11C]UCB-J to have superior imaging characteristics, including rapid brain uptake, and fast, reversible binding with high specificity to SV2A.[144] Compared with [11C]UCB-J, [11C]UCB-A was found to have a slower kinetics, whereas [18F]UCB-H had less specific binding.

To date, there have been several clinical trials that have shown the efficacy of these 3 compounds as a diagnostic measure in neurodegenerative disorders (NCT03577262, NCT04243304). The safety and efficacy of [18F]UCB-H as a means of studying synaptic density was first shown in a small human study involving 4 healthy subjects.[145] Similar efficacy was shown in a clinical trial of [11C]UCB-J involving 10 patients with AD and 11 healthy controls, which found a significant reduction of SV2A in areas of the brain associated with the progression of AD disease.[146] A larger clinical trial of [18F]UCB-H involving 24 patients with AD and 19 healthy controls also showed a significantly reduced uptake of the tracer in areas of the brain related to cognitive decline in patients with AD.[147]

Out of the 3 first-generation SV2A tracers, [11C]UCB-J, is considered the best in its class because of its rapid uptake, fast kinetics, and specific binding. However, the short half-life of ^{11}C presents a limitation for widespread use, similar to the first-generation TSPO-targeting compound [11C]PK-11195. Independent attempts to synthesize a longer-lived [18F] derivative were met with success by 2 research groups, who synthesized a compound that was jointly named [18F]SynVesT-1 (4R)-1-(3-([18F]methylpyridin-4-yl)methyl)-4-(3,4,5-trifluorophenyl)pyrrolidin-2-one.[148] In a preliminary study comparing the efficacy of [18F]FSDM-8 and [11C]UCB-J, the former was found to have imaging properties comparable with the first-generation compound with the added benefit of a longer half-life.[149] Current clinical trials with this second generation of SV2A tracers are ongoing or recently completed (NCT03587649).

RADIOPHARMACEUTICALS FOR CARDIOVASCULAR PET IMAGING

Most cardiac PET imaging has focused on blood flow ([82]Rb and [13N]NH$_3$) and metabolism ([18F] FDG). Research into newer agents for both of these areas continues and is complemented by additional compounds in imaging of atherosclerosis and angiogenesis.

PET Agents for Myocardial Perfusion Imaging

Although the approval of [82]Rb and [13N]NH$_3$ has enabled widespread cardiac PET imaging, the very short half-lives of [82]Rb and ^{13}N make these studies accessible only at sites with access to an [82]Sr/[82]Rb generator or an on-site cyclotron. Thus, there has been significant research into longer-lived imaging agents for this purpose.

[18F]Flurpiridaz (2-tert-butyl-4-chloro-5-[4-(2-[18F]fluoroethoxymethyl)-benzyloxy]-2H-pyridazin-3-1) is under investigation for myocardial perfusion imaging in late-stage clinical trials.[150] A phase III clinical trial recently reported that, although the imaging study was not as specific as other available agents, the sensitivity was significantly higher than SPECT agents, as shown in Fig. 4. Studies comparing imaging characteristics of [18F]flurpiridaz with those of [13N]NH$_3$ showed no significant differences between parameters derived from images with either agent.[151] Other agents labeled with [18F] and ^{68}Ga are also under investigation in preclinical studies.[152,153]

PET Agents for Imaging of Cardiac Metabolism

[18F]FDG is widely available and has been used for cardiac metabolism and sarcoidosis. However, complementary agents have provided additional insight into cardiac function.

[11C]Acetate has long been used for imaging of metabolism in a variety of disease states. In the

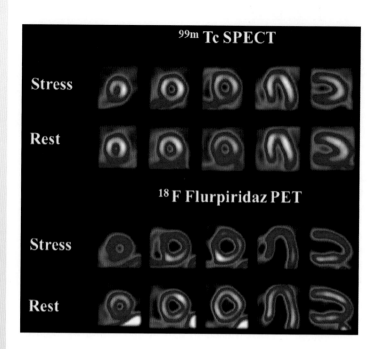

Fig. 4. Rest and pharmacological stress SPECT and [18F]flurpiridaz PET images. This 82-year-old male patient without a history of myocardial infarction had 100% proximal obtuse marginal occlusion as well as 56% proximal and 80% distal left circumflex stenoses. Both studies are true-positive, but stress and rest perfusion defects in the lateral wall are more prominent and larger on PET than on SPECT images. (*From* Maddahi J, Lazewatsky J, Udelson JE, et al. Phase-III Clinical Trial of Fluorine-18 Flurpiridaz Positron Emission Tomography for Evaluation of Coronary Artery Disease. *Journal of the American College of Cardiology.* 2020/07/28/ 2020;76(4):391-401.)

research setting, this imaging strategy has been used to study cardiac metabolism in several investigations. For example, in a study of asymptomatic men with chromic alcohol consumption, investigators showed that [11C]acetate PET/CT could be used to detect metabolic changes in the myocardium.[154] Newer imaging analysis techniques combined with dynamic imaging have also shown the feasibility of oxygen consumption, myocardial external efficiency, and blood flow in a single scan.[155,156]

Imaging of fatty acid metabolism has also been an ongoing area of study in cardiac research. In particular, [11C]palmitate has been used for many years in basic metabolism studies.[157] In a multiple tracer study involving [15O]water and [1-11C] glucose, palmitate, and leucine, investigators were able to image myocardial metabolic changes associated with Barth syndrome.[158] Newer fatty acid agents such as [18F]fluoro-4-thiapalmitate (FTP) are also being studied in ongoing clinical trials in cardiac metabolism. In a paired study with lean controls and diabetic glycemically controlled volunteers, investigators found fatty acid oxidation was higher in the diabetic group and could be altered in both groups by the administration of insulin.[159]

PET Agents for Imaging of Cardiovascular Disease

As mentioned earlier, there are several agents that have shown utility in assessment of amyloid burden in patients with cognitive impairment. Atherosclerosis has also been shown to contain amyloid proteins. Thus, imaging using previously developed agents for β-amyloid has been investigated in atherosclerosis and cardiac amyloidosis. Other biomarkers, including CCR2, are also currently being studied.

Amyloid imaging

Preliminary human imaging studies using [18F]flutemetamol showed visible uptake in carotid arteries, with male gender associated with enhanced uptake.[160] In a recent study in patients with suspected cardiac amyloidosis, imaging with [18F]florbetaben at delayed timepoints allowed the differentiation of immunoglobulin light chain–derived amyloidosis from transthyretin-related amyloidosis.[161] Similar results were also reported using [11C]PiB in multiple studies.[162,163] However, in several recent [18F]flutemetamol studies in patients with cardiac amyloidosis, results were mixed, with 1 group reporting that PET/CT could be used to differentiate between patients with transthyretin amyloidosis and another reporting that the diagnostic yield from images acquired was low.[164,165] Additional clinical trials in this area are ongoing (NCT01683825, NCT04105634, NCT02641145, NCT04392960).

Other targets in atherosclerosis

Macrophages and other inflammatory cells are known to be associated with atherosclerotic processes.[166] Existing agents targeting TSPO and somatostatin receptors have been investigated for

Table 1
Prominent and novel tracers and their current status

Imaging Agent	Clinical Application	Biological Target	Current Status	Example Clinical Trials
[68Ga]Ga-FAPI	Oncology;[4] Head and neck cancer[168] Esophageal cancer Breast cancer Metastatic Breast cancer[9] Sarcoma Lung cancer[169] Colorectal cancer[170] Pancreatic cancer[171] Prostate cancer[172] Ovarian cancer Cardiology: myocardial infarction[173]	Fibroblast activation protein expressed on fibroblasts	Phase I/II clinical trials	NCT04588064, NCT04457258, NCT04504110, NCT04147494, NCT04441606, NCT04457232, NCT04459273, NCT04571086, NCT04499365, NCT04554719, NCT04416165, NCT04367948
[18F]F-FLT	Oncology; Glioblastoma multiforme[174] Head and neck cancer[22] Breast cancer[175] Metastatic Breast cancer[176] Small cell lung cancer[177] Non–small cell lung cancer[178] Lymphoma[18,25180] Sarcoma[19]	Internalized and phosphorylated by proliferating cells	Phase II/III clinical trials	NCT03318497, NCT04221438, NCT04271436, NCT01244737, NCT02392429, NCT03276676, NCT04037462
[68Ga]Ga-PSMA	Oncology: Glioblastoma[179] Breast cancer[35,37] Metastatic Breast cancer[37] Triple-negative breast cancer[180] Prostate cancer[29,31,33]	PSMA expression	Phase II/III clinical trials	NCT04614363, NCT03689582, NCT03903419, NCT04147494, NCT04402151
[89Zr]Zr-SC16	Oncology; Small cell lung cancer[38,41] Neuroendocrine prostate cancer[181,182]	DLL3 expression	Preclinical: Phase I clinical trials	NCT04199741

(continued on next page)

Table 1
(continued)

Imaging Agent	Clinical Application	Biological Target	Current Status	Example Clinical Trials
[18F]F-PARPi	Oncology: Head and neck cancer[51] Brain cancer[183,184] Prostate cancer[50]	PARP1 enzyme in nucleus	Preclinical: Phase I clinical trials	NCT04173104, NCT03631017
[18F]F-FluorThanatrace	Oncology: Glioblastoma Breast cancer[185] Pancreatic cancer[49] Ovarian cancer Prostate cancer	PARP1 enzyme in nucleus	Preclinical: Phase I clinical trials	NCT03492164, NCT03334500, NCT04221061, NCT03604315, NCT03083288
[89Zr]Zr-pembrolizumab	Oncology:[64,65] Non-small cell lung cancer Melanoma	PD-1 expression	Preclinical: Phase I/II clinical trials	NCT02760225, NCT03065764
[89Zr]Zr-ipilimumab	Oncology:[186] Metastatic melanoma	CTLA-4 expression	Preclinical: Phase I clinical trials	NCT03313323
[89Zr]Zr-atezolizumab	Oncology:[187] Metastatic breast cancer Rectal cancer Diffuse large B-cell lymphoma	PD-L1 expression	Preclinical: Phase I clinical trials	NCT04222426, NCT03850028, NCT04564482
[89Zr]Zr-avelumab	Oncology: Breast cancer[188,189] Non-small cell lung cancer	PD-L1 expression	Preclinical: Phase I clinical trials	NCT03514719
[18F]F-AraG	Oncology: Head and neck cancers Triple-negative breast cancer Non-small cell lung cancer Rhabdomyosarcoma[68]	Activated T cells	Preclinical: Phase I clinical trials	NCT04052412, NCT03071757
[18F]F-pHLIP	Oncology: Breast cancer[73] Prostate cancer[190]	Acidic conditions of interstitial space in tumors	Preclinical: Phase I clinical trials	NCT04054986
[18F]FMISO	Oncology: Head and neck cancer[191] brain cancer Breast cancer[192] Non-small cell lung cancer[193]	Hypoxic conditions within tumor microenvironment	Preclinical: Phase I/II clinical trials	NCT02016872, NCT03730077, NCT01967927, NCT03649880, NCT00606294, NCT03865277,

Tracer	Indications	Target/Mechanism	Phase	Clinical trials
	Pancreatic adenocarcinoma[194] Sarcoma Cardiology: Cardiac ischemia[195]			NCT04309552, NCT02498613, NCT01507428
[18F]F-FAZA	Oncology: Head and neck cancer[196] Glioma[82] Neuroendocrine cancer Breast cancer[197] Lung cancer[80] Pancreatic cancer[198,199] Cervical cancer Prostate cancer[200] Colorectal cancer[201] Renal cell carcinoma[202] Sarcoma Rhabdomyosarcoma	Hypoxic conditions within tumor microenvironment	Preclinical: Phase I/II clinical trials	NCT03955393, NCT02701699, NCT01542177, NCT03054792, NCT01567800, NCT03168737, NCT04395469, NCT01549730, NCT02394652, NCT03513042
[64Cu]Cu-ATSM	Oncology: Glioblastoma[203,204] Prostate cancer[205] Rectal cancer Cardiology: Cardiac ischemia[206]	Hypoxic conditions within tumor microenvironment	Preclinical: Phase I clinical trials	NCT03951337
[11C]C-MET	Oncology:[207] Head and neck cancer[208] Glioblastoma[209] Glioma[210] Breast cancer[207] Mesothelioma Prostate cancer[211] Multiple myeloma[212] Melanoma	Increased amino acid transport and protein incorporation in cancer cells	Preclinical: Phase I/II clinical trials	NCT03977896, NCT03739333, NCT03009318, NCT00840047, NCT00002981, NCT02519049
[18F]F-FET	Oncology: Glioblastoma multiforme[213] Glioma[214] Brain neoplasms[90]	LAT-1–based amino acid transport	Preclinical: Phase I/II clinical trials	NCT01756352, NCT03402425, NCT01756352, NCT04001257, NCT04044937
[18F]F-FES	Oncology: Breast cancer[215,216] Metastatic breast cancer	Estrogen receptor expression	Preclinical: Phase I/II/III clinical trials	NCT03544762, NCT03703492, NCT02409316, NCT01986569, NCT04150731

(continued on next page)

Table 1
(continued)

Imaging Agent	Clinical Application	Biological Target	Current Status	Example Clinical Trials
[18F]F-FFNP	Oncology: Breast cancer[93]	Progesterone receptor expression	Preclinical: Phase I/II clinical trials	NCT03212170, NCT02455453, NCT00968409, NCT03212170
[18F]FDOPA	Oncology: Glioblastoma[217] Glioma[88] Neurology: Parkinson disease[218] Schizophrenia[219]	LAT-1 expression in amino acid transport and aromatic acid decarboxylase–mediated conversion to dopamine	Preclinical: Phase I/II clinical trials	NCT03903419, NCT03778294, NCT02104310, NCT03042416 NCT03648905, NCT04459052, NCT04038957
[11C]C-PiB	Neurology: Alzheimer disease[220] Parkinson disease[221] Dementia Cerebral amyloid angiopathy[222] Cardiology: Cardiac amyloidosis[223]	Amyloid-β plaques	Preclinical: Phase I/II/III clinical trials	NCT03555292, NCT03981380, NCT03958630, NCT03172117, NCT03969732
[18F]F-florbetapir	Neurology: Alzheimer disease[224] Parkinson disease[225] Dementia	Amyloid-β plaques	Preclinical: Phase I/II/III clinical trials	NCT03019029, NCT04305210, NCT04248270, NCT02813434, NCT03282916
[18F]F-florbetaben	Neurology: Alzheimer disease[226] Parkinson disease[227] Dementia Cardiology: Atherosclerosis[160]	Amyloid-β plaques	Preclinical: Phase I/II/III clinical trials	NCT03706261, NCT02831283, NCT04576793, NCT03019536
[18F]F-flutemetamol	Neurology: Alzheimer disease[228] PD Dementia Cardiology: Atherosclerosis[229]	Amyloid-β plaques	Preclinical: Phase I clinical trials	NCT03291093, NCT02685969, NCT03174938, NCT01979419, NCT03466177

Tracer	Neurology	Target	Status	NCT numbers
[18F]FIBT	Neurology:[230,231] AD, PD, Dementia	Amyloid-β plaques	Preclinical	—
[18F]NAV4694	Neurology:[232] Alzheimer disease[233], PD, Dementia	Amyloid-β plaques	Preclinical: Phase I clinical trials	NCT00838877, NCT00991419, NCT01325402
[18F]F-THK5351	Neurology: Alzheimer disease[234], Parkinson disease[235], Dementia	Tau protein	Preclinical: Phase I/II clinical trials	NCT02686216, NCT04318626, NCT03430869, NCT04588649
[18F]F-AV-1451	Neurology: Alzheimer disease[236], PD, Dementia[237]	Tau protein	Preclinical: Phase I/II/III clinical trials	NCT02350634, NCT02958670, NCT03189485, NCT03816228, NCT03143374, NCT00950430, NCT01687153, NCT02854033
[11C]C-PBB3	Neurology: Alzheimer disease[238], Parkinson disease[239], Dementia	Tau protein	Preclinical: Phase I clinical trials	NCT04101968
[18F]F-MK-6240	Neurology: Alzheimer disease[120,240], PD, Dementia	Tau protein	Preclinical: Phase I/II clinical trials	NCT03373604, NCT03372317, NCT03706261, NCT04576793, NCT04098666, NCT03053908
[18F]F-Ro-6958948	Neurology: Alzheimer disease[241,242], PD, Dementia	Tau protein	Preclinical: Phase I clinical trials	NCT04482660
[18F]F-FP-CIT	Neurology: Alzheimer disease[243], Parkinson disease[244,245], Dementia	Dopamine transporter	Preclinical: Phase I clinical trials	NCT04334902
[18F]F-FE-PE2I	Neurology: Parkinson disease[131,246]	Dopamine transporter	Preclinical: Phase I clinical trials	NCT04243304

(continued on next page)

Table 1
(continued)

Imaging Agent	Clinical Application	Biological Target	Current Status	Example Clinical Trials
[18F]F-FEOBV	Neurology: Alzheimer disease[247] Parkinson disease[248] Dementia	Vesicular acetylcholine transporter	Preclinical: Phase I clinical trials	NCT03554551, NCT04291144, NCT03647137
[11C]C-PK-11195	Neurology:[249] AD PD Multiple sclerosis[250]	Translocator protein	Preclinical: Phase I clinical trials	NCT04239820, NCT03368677, NCT04171882, NCT04126772, NCT03134716
[11C]C-DAA1106	Neurology:[251] Alzheimer disease[252]	Translocator protein	Preclinical	
[11C]C-PBR28	Neurology: Alzheimer disease[253] Parkinson disease[254] Multiple sclerosis[255] Oncology:[256] Lung cancer Melanoma	Translocator protein	Preclinical: Phase I/II clinical trials	NCT04230174, NCT02831283, NCT04274998, NCT03787446, NCT02702102
[18F]F-FEPPA	Neurology: Alzheimer disease[257] Parkinson disease[257,258] Multiple sclerosis[259] Major depression disorders Oncology: Breast cancer[260]	Translocator protein	Preclinical: Phase I clinical trials	NCT00970333, NCT02983318
[18F]F-PBR06	Neurology: Alzheimer disease[261] PD Multiple sclerosis[262,263] Oncology: Lung cancer[264]	Translocator protein	Preclinical: Phase I clinical trials	NCT04510220, NCT04144257, NCT03983252, NCT01028209

Tracer	Target/Application	Development stage	Clinical trial identifiers
[18F]F-PBR111	Neurology: Alzheimer disease[265] Parkinson disease[266] Multiple sclerosis[267] Schizophrenia[268]	Translocator protein	Preclinical: Phase I/II clinical trials	NCT01209156, NCT02009826, NCT01428505
[18F]F-DPA714	Neurology: Alzheimer disease[141,269] PD Multiple sclerosis Amyotrophic lateral sclerosis[270]	Translocator protein	Preclinical: Phase I/II clinical trials	NCT03691077, NCT04171882, NCT03230526, NCT02305264
[18F]F-UCB-H	Neurology: Alzheimer disease[271] Epilepsy[272]	SV2A	Preclinical	
[11C]C-UCB-A	Neurology: AD Epilepsy[273]	SV2A	Preclinical	
[11C]C-UCB-J	Neurology: AD PD Multiple Sclerosis Epilepsy[274] Schizophrenia	SV2A	Preclinical: Phase I/II clinical trials	NCT03577262, NCT03493282, NCT04038840, NCT04243304, NCT03134716
[18F]F-SynVesT-1	Neurology:[275] AD PD Multiple sclerosis Epilepsy[276]	SV2A	Preclinical: Phase I clinical trials	NCT04634994
[18F]F-flurpiridaz	Cardiology:[151] Coronary artery disease Ischemic heart disease	Myocardial perfusion imaging	Preclinical: Phase I clinical trials	NCT04594941, NCT03354273

(continued on next page)

Table 1
(continued)

Imaging Agent	Clinical Application	Biological Target	Current Status	Example Clinical Trials
[68Ga]Ga-DOTATATE	Cardiology: Atherosclerosis[277] Cardiac sarcoidosis[278] Oncology: Neuroendocrine tumors[279] Breast cancer[280] Pancreatic cancer Prostate cancer	Somatostatin receptor 2	Preclinical: Phase I/II clinical trials	NCT04043377, NCT04073810, NCT04032197, NCT02840149, NCT03145857, NCT04041882
[64Cu]Cu-DOTA-ECL1i	Cardiology: Atherosclerosis Oncology: Head and neck cancer Pancreatic cancer	Somatostatin receptor 2	Preclinical: Phase I clinical trials	NCT04537403, NCT03851237, NCT04217057

The preclinical and clinical research examples provided in this table are not an exhaustive representation of all the work being performed with these PET tracers.

Abbreviation	Chemical Name
FAPI	Fibroblast activation protein inhibitor
FLT	3′-Fluoro-3′ deoxythymidine
FDG	Fluorodeoxyglucose
PSMA	Prostate-specific membrane antigen
[^{18}F]DCFPyL	2-(3-{1-carboxy-5-[(6-[^{18}F]fluoro-pyridine-3-carbonyl)-amino]-pentyl}-ureido)-pentanedioic acid
DFO	Deferoxamine
DLL3	Deltalike protein 3
PARP1	Poly(ADP-ribose) polymerase 1
[^{18}F]F-AraG	[^{18}F]fluoro-9-(β-D-arabinofuranosyl) guanine
pHLIP	pH low insertion peptide
[^{18}F]FMISO	[^{18}F]fluoro-misonidazole
[^{18}F]FAZA	[^{18}F]fluoroazomycin arabinoside
[^{64}Cu]Cu-ATSM	[^{64}Cu]Cu-diacetyl-bis(N^4-methylthiosemicarbazone)
[^{11}C]MET	L-[^{11}C]methionine
[^{18}F]FET	O-(2-[^{18}F]fluoroethyl)-L-tyrosine
[^{18}F]FSPG	(4S)-4-(3[^{18}F]fluoropropyl)-L-glutamic acid
[^{18}F]FES	16α-[^{18}F]fluoroestradiol
[^{18}F]FFNP	21-[^{18}F]F-fluoro-furanyl-norprogesterone
[^{18}F]FDHT	16β-[^{18}F]F-fluoro-5α-dihydrotestosterone
[^{11}C]PiB	2-[4-([^{11}C]methylamino)phenyl]-1,3-benzothiazol-6-ol
[^{18}F]Florbetapir	4-[(E)-2-[6-[2-[2-(2-[^{18}F]fluoranylethoxy)ethoxy]ethoxy]pyridin-3-yl]ethenyl]-N-methylaniline
[^{18}F]Florbetaben	4-[(E)-2-[4-[2-[2-(2-[^{18}F]fluoranylethoxy)ethoxy]ethoxy]phenyl]ethenyl]-N-methylaniline
[^{18}F]Flutemetamol	2-[3-[^{18}F]fluoranyl-4-(methylamino)phenyl]-1,3-benzothiazol-6-ol
[^{18}F]FIBT	2-(p-Methylaminophenyl)-7-(2-[^{18}F]fluoroethoxy)imidazo-[2,1-b]benzothiazole
[^{18}F]NAV4694	2-[2-^{18}F-fluoro-6-(methylamino)-3-pyridinyl]-1-benzofuran-5-ol
[^{18}F]THK5351	(2S)-1-[^{18}F]fluoranyl-3-[2-[6-(methylamino)pyridin-3-yl]quinolin-6-yl]oxypropan-2-ol
	7-(6-fluoropyridine-3-yl)-5H-pyrido[4,3-b]indole
[^{11}C]PBB3	2-((1E,3E)-4-(6-(^{11}C-methylamino)pyridine-3-yl)buta-1,3-dienyl)benzo[d]thiazol-6-ol
[^{18}F]MK-6240	6-[^{18}F]fluoranyl-3-pyrrolo[2,3-c]pyridin-1-ylisoquinolin-5-amine
[^{18}F]Ro-6958948	2-(6-[^{18}F]fluoro-pyridin-3-yl)-9H-1,6,9-triaza-fluorene
[^{18}F]FDOPA	(2S)-2-amino-3-(2-[^{18}F]fluoro-4,5-dihydroxyphenyl)propanoic acid
[^{18}F]FP-CIT	Methyl(1R,2S,3S,5S)-8-(3-fluoropropyl)-3-(4-[^{18}F]fluorophenyl)-8-azabicyclo[3.2.1]octane2-carboxylate
[^{18}F]FE-PE2I	(E)-N-(3-iodoprop-2-enyl)-2β-carbo[^{18}F]fluoroethoxy-3β-(4′-methyl-phenyl)nortropane).
[^{18}F]FEOBV	(2R,3R)-5-[^{18}F]fluoroethoxybenzovesamicol
[^{11}C]CPK-11195	N-sec-Butyl-1-(2-chlorophenyl)-N-[^{11}C]methyl-3-isoquinolinecarboxamide
[^{11}C]DAA1106	N-(5-Fluoro-2-phenoxyphenyl)-N-[(5-methoxy-2-[^{11}C]methoxyphenyl)methyl]acetamide
[^{11}C]PBR28	N-[(2-[^{11}C]methoxyphenyl)methyl]-N-(6-phenoxypyridin-3-yl)acetamide
[^{18}F]FEPPA	N-[[2-(2-[^{18}F]fluoranylethoxy)phenyl]methyl]-N-(4-phenoxypyridin-3-yl)acetamide
[^{18}F]PBR06	N-[(2,5-Dimethoxyphenyl)methyl]-2-[^{18}F]fluoranyl-N-(2-phenoxyphenyl)acetamide
[^{18}F]PBR11	2-(6-Chloro-2-(4-(3-[^{18}F]fluoropropoxy)phenyl)imidazo[1,2-a]pyridin-3-yl)-N,N-diethylacetamide
[^{18}F]DPA714	[N,N-diethyl-2-(2-(4-(2[18F]fluoroethoxy)phenyl)5,7dimethylpyrazolo[1,5a]pyrimidin-3-yl)acetamide]
[^{11}C]UCB-J	(4R)-1-((3-([11C]methylpyridin-4-yl)methyl)-4-(3,4,5-trifluorophenyl)pyrrolidin-2-one
[^{18}F]SynVesT-1	(4R)-1-((3-([18F]methylpyridin-4-yl)methyl)-4-(3,4,5-trifluorophenyl)pyrrolidin-2-one

imaging of inflammatory processes with some success in preclinical models and several clinical trials.[166] For example, in a study involving 42 patients with atherosclerosis [68Ga]DOTATATE outperformed [18F]FDG for the evaluation of high-risk versus low-risk coronary lesions (NCT02021188).[167] Newer agents such as [64Cu] DOTA-ECL1i, which targets CCR2, are currently in clinical trials (NCT04537403) in patients with carotid and femoral artery disease.

Prominent and novel tracers, along with their current status, are listed in **Table 1**.

DISCLOSURE

With regard to the information presented in this article the authors have no potential conflicts of interest to disclose.

REFERENCES

1. Liu T, Han C, Wang S, et al. Cancer-associated fibroblasts: an emerging target of anti-cancer immunotherapy. J Hematol Oncol 2019;12(1):86.
2. Ziani L, Chouaib S, Thiery J. Alteration of the anti-tumor immune response by cancer-associated fibroblasts. Front Immunol 2018;9:414.
3. Lindner T, Loktev A, Giesel F, et al. Targeting of activated fibroblasts for imaging and therapy. EJNMMI Radiopharmacy Chem 2019;4(1):16.
4. Kratochwil C, Flechsig P, Lindner T, et al. 68Ga-FAPI PET/CT: Tracer Uptake in 28 Different Kinds of Cancer. J Nucl Med 2019;60(6):801–5.
5. Giesel FL, Kratochwil C, Lindner T, et al. 68)Ga-FAPI PET/CT: Biodistribution and Preliminary Dosimetry Estimate of 2 DOTA-Containing FAP-Targeting Agents in Patients with Various Cancers. J Nucl Med 2019;60(3):386–92.
6. Koerber SA, Staudinger F, Kratochwil C, et al. The Role of (68)Ga-FAPI PET/CT for Patients with Malignancies of the Lower Gastrointestinal Tract: First Clinical Experience. J Nucl Med 2020;61(9): 1331–6.
7. Ballal S, Yadav MP, Kramer V, et al. A theranostic approach of [(68)Ga]Ga-DOTA.SA.FAPi PET/CT-guided [(177)Lu]Lu-DOTA.SA.FAPi radionuclide therapy in an end-stage breast cancer patient: new frontier in targeted radionuclide therapy. Eur J Nucl Med Mol Imaging 2020. https://doi.org/10.1007/s00259-020-04990-w.
8. Luo Y, Pan Q, Yang H, et al. Fibroblast activation protein targeted PET/CT with (68)Ga-FAPI for imaging IgG4-related disease: comparison to (18)F-FDG PET/CT. J Nucl Med 2020. https://doi.org/10.2967/jnumed.120.244723.
9. Pang Y, Zhao L, Chen H. 68Ga-FAPI Outperforms 18F-FDG PET/CT in identifying bone metastasis and peritoneal carcinomatosis in a patient with metastatic breast cancer. Clin Nucl Med 2020; 45(11):913–5.
10. Shi X, Xing H, Yang X, et al. Comparison of PET imaging of activated fibroblasts and 18F-FDG for diagnosis of primary hepatic tumours: a prospective pilot study. Eur J Nucl Med Mol Imaging 2020. https://doi.org/10.1007/s00259-020-05070-9.
11. Pang Y, Hao B, Shang Q, et al. Comparison of 68Ga-FAPI and 18F-FDG PET/CT in a Patient With Cholangiocellular Carcinoma: A Case Report. Clin Nucl Med 2020;45(7):566–7.
12. Chen H, Pang Y, Wu J, et al. Comparison of [(68) Ga]Ga-DOTA-FAPI-04 and [(18)F] FDG PET/CT for the diagnosis of primary and metastatic lesions in patients with various types of cancer. Eur J Nucl Med Mol Imaging 2020;47(8):1820–32.
13. Meyer C, Dahlbom M, Lindner T, et al. Radiation Dosimetry and Biodistribution of (68)Ga-FAPI-46 PET Imaging in Cancer Patients. J Nucl Med 2020;61(8):1171–7.
14. Giesel F, Adeberg S, Syed M, et al. FAPI-74 PET/CT Using Either (18)F-AlF or Cold-kit (68)Ga-labeling: Biodistribution, Radiation Dosimetry and Tumor Delineation in Lung Cancer Patients. J Nucl Med 2020. https://doi.org/10.2967/jnumed.120.245084.
15. Calais J, Mona CE. Will FAPI PET/CT Replace FDG PET/CT in the Next Decade?—Point: An Important Diagnostic, Phenotypic and Biomarker Role. AJR Am J Roentgenol 2020. https://doi.org/10.2214/AJR.20.24302.
16. Shields AF, Grierson JR, Dohmen BM, et al. Imaging proliferation in vivo with [F-18]FLT and positron emission tomography. Research Support, U.S. Gov't, P.H.S. Nat Med 1998;4(11):1334–6.
17. Bashir A, Vestergaard MB, Marner L, et al. PET imaging of meningioma with 18F-FLT: a predictor of tumour progression. Brain 2020. https://doi.org/10.1093/brain/awaa267.
18. Rybka J, Małkowski B, Olejniczak M, et al. Comparing radioactive tracers 18F-FDG and 18F-FLT in the staging of diffuse large B-cell lymphoma by PET/CT examination: A single-center prospective study. Adv Clin Exp Med 2019;28(8):1095–9.
19. Kairemo K, Santos EB, Macapinlac HA, et al. Molecular Imaging with 3'-deoxy-3'[(18)F]-Fluorothymidine ((18)F-FLT) PET/CT for Early Response to Targeted Therapies in Sarcomas: A Pilot Study. Diagnostics (Basel) 2020;10(3). https://doi.org/10.3390/diagnostics10030125.
20. Buck AK, Herrmann K, Büschenfelde CMz, et al. Imaging Bone and Soft Tissue Tumors with the Proliferation Marker [18F]Fluorodeoxythymidine. Clin Cancer Res 2008;14(10):2970.
21. Peck M, Pollack HA, Friesen A, et al. Applications of PET imaging with the proliferation marker [18F]-FLT. Q J Nucl Med 2015;59(1):95–104.

22. Hoshikawa H, Kishino T, Mori T, et al. The value of 18F-FLT PET for detecting second primary cancers and distant metastases in head and neck cancer patients. Clin Nucl Med 2013;38(8): e318-23.

23. Bhoil A, Singh B, Singh N, et al. Can 3'-deoxy-3'-(18)F-fluorothymidine or 2'-deoxy-2'-(18)F-fluoro-d-glucose PET/CT better assess response after 3-weeks treatment by epidermal growth factor receptor kinase inhibitor, in non-small lung cancer patients? Preliminary results. Hell J Nucl Med 2014; 17(2):90-6.

24. Tsuyoshi H, Morishita F, Orisaka M, et al. 18F-fluorothymidine PET is a potential predictive imaging biomarker of the response to gemcitabine-based chemotherapeutic treatment for recurrent ovarian cancer: preliminary results in three patients. Clin Nucl Med 2013;38(7):560-3.

25. Lee H, Kim SK, Kim YI, et al. Early determination of prognosis by interim 3'-deoxy-3'-18F-fluorothymidine PET in patients with non-Hodgkin lymphoma. J Nucl Med 2014;55(2):216-22.

26. Afshar-Oromieh A, Haberkorn U, Hadaschik B, et al. PET/MRI with a 68Ga-PSMA ligand for the detection of prostate cancer. Eur J Nucl Med Mol Imaging 2013;40(10):1629-30.

27. Barakat A, Yacoub B, Homsi ME, et al. Role of Early PET/CT Imaging with 68Ga-PSMA in Staging and Restaging of Prostate Cancer. Sci Rep 2020; 10(1):2705.

28. Sasikumar A. Specificity of (68)Ga-PSMA PET/CT for Prostate Cancer - Myths and Reality. Indian J Nucl Med 2017;32(1):11-2.

29. Plouznikoff N, Artigas C, Sideris S, et al. Early Detection of Metastatic Prostate Cancer Relapse on 68Ga-PSMA-11 PET/CT in a Patient Still Exhibiting Biochemical Response. Clin Nucl Med 2020; 45(1):81-2.

30. Emmett L, van Leeuwen PJ, Nandurkar R, et al. Treatment Outcomes from (68)Ga-PSMA PET/CT-Informed Salvage Radiation Treatment in Men with Rising PSA after radical prostatectomy: prognostic value of a negative PSMA PET. J Nucl Med 2017;58(12):1972-6.

31. Roberts MJ, Morton A, Donato P, et al. 68)Ga-PSMA PET/CT tumour intensity pre-operatively predicts adverse pathological outcomes and progression-free survival in localised prostate cancer. Eur J Nucl Med Mol Imaging 2020. https://doi.org/10.1007/s00259-020-04944-2.

32. Michalski K, Mix M, Meyer PT, et al. Determination of whole-body tumour burden on [68Ga]PSMA-11 PET/CT for response assessment of [177Lu] PSMA-617 radioligand therapy: a retrospective analysis of serum PSA level and imaging derived parameters before and after two cycles of therapy. Nuklearmedizin 2019;58(6):443-50. Bestimmung der mittels [68Ga]PSMA-11 PET/CT bestimmten Ganzkörper-Tumorlast zur Abschätzung des Therapieansprechens: Eine retrospektive Analyse des Serum-PSA-Wertes und bildgebender Parameter vor und nach 2 Zyklen [177Lu]PSMA-617-Radioligandentherapie.

33. Witkowska-Patena E, Giżewska A, Dziuk M, et al. Diagnostic performance of 18F-PSMA-1007 PET/CT in biochemically relapsed patients with prostate cancer with PSA levels ≤ 2.0 ng/ml. Prostate Cancer Prostatic Dis 2020;23(2):343-8.

34. Meijer D, Jansen BHE, Wondergem M, et al. Clinical verification of 18F-DCFPyL PET-detected lesions in patients with biochemically recurrent prostate cancer. PLoS One 2020;15(10):e0239414.

35. Tolkach Y, Gevensleben H, Bundschuh R, et al. Prostate-specific membrane antigen in breast cancer: a comprehensive evaluation of expression and a case report of radionuclide therapy. Breast Cancer Res Treat 2018;169(3):447-55.

36. Salas Fragomeni RA, Amir T, Sheikhbahaei S, et al. Imaging of nonprostate cancers using PSMA-Targeted Radiotracers: Rationale, Current State of the Field, and a Call to Arms. J Nucl Med 2018; 59(6):871-7.

37. Medina-Ornelas S, García-Perez F, Estrada-Lobato E, et al. (68)Ga-PSMA PET/CT in the evaluation of locally advanced and metastatic breast cancer, a single center experience. Am J Nucl Med Mol Imaging 2020;10(3):135-42.

38. Chen B, Li H, Liu C, et al. Potential prognostic value of delta-like protein 3 in small cell lung cancer: a meta-analysis. World J Surg Oncol 2020;18(1):226.

39. Rudin CM, Pietanza MC, Bauer TM, et al. Rovalpituzumab tesirine, a DLL3-targeted antibody-drug conjugate, in recurrent small-cell lung cancer: a first-in-human, first-in-class, open-label, phase 1 study. Lancet Oncol 2017;18(1):42-51.

40. Lakes AL, An DD, Gauny SS, et al. Evaluating (225) Ac and (177)Lu Radioimmunoconjugates against Antibody-Drug Conjugates for Small-Cell Lung Cancer. Mol Pharm 2020;17(11):4270-9.

41. Sharma SK, Pourat J, Abdel-Atti D, et al. Noninvasive Interrogation of DLL3 Expression in Metastatic Small Cell Lung Cancer. Cancer Res 2017;77(14):3931-41.

42. Chan CY, Tan KV, Cornelissen B. PARP Inhibitors in Cancer Diagnosis and Therapy. Clin Cancer Res 2020. https://doi.org/10.1158/1078-0432.Ccr-20-2766.

43. Liu Y, Zhang Y, Zhao Y, et al. High PARP-1 expression is associated with tumor invasion and poor prognosis in gastric cancer. Oncol Lett 2016; 12(5):3825-35.

44. Ossovskaya V, Koo IC, Kaldjian EP, et al. Upregulation of Poly (ADP-Ribose) Polymerase-1 (PARP1) in Triple-Negative Breast Cancer and Other Primary Human Tumor Types. Genes Cancer 2010;1(8):812-21.

45. Slade D. PARP and PARG inhibitors in cancer treatment. Genes Dev 2020;34(5–6):360–94.

46. Sachdev E, Tabatabai R, Roy V, et al. PARP Inhibition in Cancer: An Update on Clinical Development. Target Oncol 2019;14(6):657–79.

47. Ellisen LW. PARP inhibitors in cancer therapy: promise, progress, and puzzles. Cancer Cell 2011;19(2):165–7.

48. Carney B, Kossatz S, Reiner T. Molecular Imaging of PARP. J Nucl Med 2017;58(7):1025–30.

49. Michel LS, Dyroff S, Brooks FJ, et al. PET of Poly (ADP-Ribose) Polymerase Activity in Cancer: Preclinical Assessment and First In-Human Studies. Radiology 2017;282(2):453–63.

50. Zhou D, Xu J, Mpoy C, et al. Preliminary evaluation of a novel (18)F-labeled PARP-1 ligand for PET imaging of PARP-1 expression in prostate cancer. Nucl Med Biol 2018;66:26–31.

51. Demétrio de Souza França P, Roberts S, Kossatz S, et al. Fluorine-18 labeled poly (ADP-ribose) polymerase1 inhibitor as a potential alternative to 2-deoxy-2-[(18)F]fluoro-d-glucose positron emission tomography in oral cancer imaging. Nucl Med Biol 2020;84-85:80–7.

52. Salinas B, Irwin CP, Kossatz S, et al. Radioiodinated PARP1 tracers for glioblastoma imaging. EJNMMI Res 2015;5(1):123.

53. Sander Effron S, Makvandi M, Lin L, et al. PARP-1 Expression Quantified by [(18)F]FluorThanatrace: A Biomarker of Response to PARP Inhibition Adjuvant to Radiation Therapy. Cancer Biother Radiopharm 2017;32(1):9–15.

54. Carney B, Kossatz S, Lok BH, et al. Target engagement imaging of PARP inhibitors in small-cell lung cancer. Nat Commun 2018;9(1):176.

55. Laird J, Lok BH, Carney B, et al. Positron-Emission Tomographic Imaging of a Fluorine 18-Radiolabeled Poly(ADP-Ribose) Polymerase 1 Inhibitor Monitors the Therapeutic Efficacy of Talazoparib in SCLC Patient-Derived Xenografts. J Thorac Oncol 2019;14(10):1743–52.

56. Kalbasi A, Ribas A. Tumour-intrinsic resistance to immune checkpoint blockade. Nat Rev Immunol 2020;20(1):25–39.

57. Wieder T, Eigentler T, Brenner E, et al. Immune checkpoint blockade therapy. J Allergy Clin Immunol 2018;142(5):1403–14.

58. Zappasodi R, Wolchok JD, Merghoub T. Strategies for Predicting Response to Checkpoint Inhibitors. Curr Hematol Malig Rep 2018;13(5):383–95.

59. Lang D, Wahl G, Poier N, et al. Impact of PET/CT for Assessing Response to Immunotherapy-A Clinical Perspective. J Clin Med 2020;9(11). https://doi.org/10.3390/jcm9113483.

60. Nimmagadda S. Quantifying PD-L1 expression to monitor immune checkpoint therapy: opportunities and challenges. Cancers (Basel) 2020;12(11).

61. Franzin R, Netti GS, Spadaccino F, et al. The use of immune checkpoint inhibitors in oncology and the occurrence of AKI: where do we stand? Review. Front Immunol 2020;11(2619). https://doi.org/10.3389/fimmu.2020.574271.

62. Miao Y, Lv G, Chen Y, et al. One-step radiosynthesis and initial evaluation of a small molecule PET tracer for PD-L1 imaging. Bioorg Med Chem Lett 2020;30(24):127572.

63. Marhelava K, Pilch Z, Bajor M, et al. Targeting Negative and Positive Immune Checkpoints with Monoclonal Antibodies in Therapy of Cancer. Cancers 2019;11(11):1756.

64. Li W, Wang Y, Rubins D, et al. PET/CT Imaging of (89)Zr-N-sucDf-Pembrolizumab in Healthy Cynomolgus Monkeys. Mol Imaging Biol 2020. https://doi.org/10.1007/s11307-020-01558-w.

65. England CG, Ehlerding EB, Hernandez R, et al. Preclinical Pharmacokinetics and Biodistribution Studies of 89Zr-Labeled Pembrolizumab. J Nucl Med 2017;58(1):162–8.

66. van der Veen EL, Giesen D, Pot-de Jong L, et al. 89Zr-pembrolizumab biodistribution is influenced by PD-1-mediated uptake in lymphoid organs. J Immunother Cancer 2020;8(2). https://doi.org/10.1136/jitc-2020-000938.

67. Namavari M, Chang YF, Kusler B, et al. Synthesis of 2'-deoxy-2'-[18F]fluoro-9-β-D-arabinofuranosyl-guanine: a novel agent for imaging T-cell activation with PET. Mol Imaging Biol 2011;13(5):812–8.

68. Levi J, Lam T, Goth SR, et al. Imaging of Activated T Cells as an Early Predictor of Immune Response to Anti-PD-1 Therapy. Cancer Res 2019;79(13):3455–65.

69. Kato Y, Ozawa S, Miyamoto C, et al. Acidic extracellular microenvironment and cancer. Cancer Cell Int 2013;13(1):89.

70. Boedtkjer E, Pedersen SF. The Acidic Tumor Microenvironment as a Driver of Cancer. Annu Rev Physiol 2020;82:103–26.

71. Reshetnyak YK, Moshnikova A, Andreev OA, et al. Targeting Acidic Diseased Tissues by pH-Triggered Membrane-Associated Peptide Folding. Review. Front Bioeng Biotechnol 2020;8:335.

72. Weerakkody D, Moshnikova A, Thakur MS, et al. Family of pH (low) insertion peptides for tumor targeting. Proc Natl Acad Sci U S A 2013;110(15):5834–9.

73. Demoin DW, Wyatt LC, Edwards KJ, et al. PET Imaging of Extracellular pH in Tumors with (64)Cu- and (18)F-Labeled pHLIP Peptides: A Structure-Activity Optimization Study. Bioconjug Chem 2016;27(9):2014–23.

74. Rajendran JG, Krohn KA. F-18 fluoromisonidazole for imaging tumor hypoxia: imaging the microenvironment for personalized cancer therapy. Semin Nucl Med 2015;45(2):151–62.

75. Zhao G, Long L, Zhang L, et al. Smart pH-sensitive nanoassemblies with cleavable PEGylation for tumor targeted drug delivery. Sci Rep 2017;7(1):3383.

76. Wang J, Wen Y, Zheng L, et al. Characterization of chemical profiles of pH-sensitive cleavable D-gluconhydroximo-1, 5-lactam hydrolysates by LC–MS: A potential agent for promoting tumor-targeted drug delivery. J Pharm Biomed Anal 2020;185:113244.

77. Shan L. (64)Cu-1,4,7,10-Tetraazacyclododecane-1,4,7-Tris-acetic acid-10-maleimidoethylacetamide-ACEQNPIYWARYADWLFTTP LLLLLDLALLVDADEGTG. Molecular imaging and contrast agent Database (MICAD). National Center for Biotechnology Information (US); 2004.

78. Wyatt LC, Lewis JS, Andreev OA, et al. Applications of pHLIP Technology for Cancer Imaging and Therapy. Trends Biotechnol 2017;35(7):653–64.

79. Lee ST, Scott AM. Hypoxia positron emission tomography imaging with 18F-fluoromisonidazole. Semin Nucl Med 2007;37(6):451–61.

80. Theodoropoulos AS, Gkiozos I, Kontopyrgias G, et al. Modern radiopharmaceuticals for lung cancer imaging with positron emission tomography/computed tomography scan: A systematic review. SAGE Open Med 2020;8. 2050312120961594.

81. Melsens E, De Vlieghere E, Descamps B, et al. Hypoxia imaging with (18)F-FAZA PET/CT predicts radiotherapy response in esophageal adenocarcinoma xenografts. Radiat Oncol 2018;13(1):39.

82. Mapelli P, Picchio M. 18F-FAZA PET imaging in tumor hypoxia: A focus on high-grade glioma. Int J Biol Markers 2020;35(1_suppl):42–6.

83. Vavere AL, Lewis JS. Cu-ATSM: a radiopharmaceutical for the PET imaging of hypoxia. Dalton Trans 2007;(43):4893–902.

84. Bourgeois M, Rajerison H, Guerard F, et al. Contribution of [64Cu]-ATSM PET in molecular imaging of tumour hypoxia compared to classical [18F]-MISO–a selected review. Nucl Med Rev Cent East Eur 2011;14(2):90–5.

85. Kalinauskaite G, Senger C, Kluge A, et al. 68Ga-PSMA-PET/CT-based radiosurgery and stereotactic body radiotherapy for oligometastatic prostate cancer. PLoS One 2020;15(10):e0240892.

86. Xiao J, Jin Y, Nie J, et al. Diagnostic and grading accuracy of (18)F-FDOPA PET and PET/CT in patients with gliomas: a systematic review and meta-analysis. BMC Cancer 2019;19(1):767.

87. Cicone F, Carideo L, Scaringi C, et al. Long-term metabolic evolution of brain metastases with suspected radiation necrosis following stereotactic radiosurgery: longitudinal assessment by F-DOPA PET. Neuro Oncol 2020. https://doi.org/10.1093/neuonc/noaa239.

88. Zaragori T, Ginet M, Marie P-Y, et al. Use of static and dynamic [(18)F]-F-DOPA PET parameters for detecting patients with glioma recurrence or progression. EJNMMI Res 2020;10(1):56.

89. Cai L, Gao S, Li DC, et al. [Value of 18F-FDG and 11C-MET PET-CT in differentiation of brain ringlike-enhanced neoplastic and non-neoplastic lesions on MRI imaging]. Zhonghua Zhong Liu Za Zhi 2009;31(2):134–8.

90. Muoio B, Giovanella L, Treglia G. Recent Developments of 18F-FET PET in Neuro-oncology. Curr Med Chem 2018;25(26):3061–73.

91. Park SY, Mosci C, Kumar M, et al. Initial evaluation of (4S)-4-(3-[(18)F]fluoropropyl)-L-glutamate (FSPG) PET/CT imaging in patients with head and neck cancer, colorectal cancer, or non-Hodgkin lymphoma. EJNMMI Res 2020;10(1):100.

92. Peterson LM, Kurland BF, Yan F, et al. 18)F-Fluoroestradiol ((18)F-FES)-PET imaging in a Phase II trial of vorinostat to restore endocrine sensitivity in ER+/HER2- metastatic breast cancer. J Nucl Med 2020. https://doi.org/10.2967/jnumed.120.244459.

93. Katzenellenbogen JA. PET Imaging Agents (FES, FFNP, and FDHT) for Estrogen, Androgen, and Progesterone Receptors to Improve Management of Breast and Prostate Cancers by Functional Imaging. Cancers 2020;12(8):2020.

94. Salem K, Kumar M, Yan Y, et al. Sensitivity and Isoform Specificity of (18)F-Fluorofuranylnorprogesterone for Measuring Progesterone Receptor Protein Response to Estradiol Challenge in Breast Cancer. J Nucl Med 2018. https://doi.org/10.2967/jnumed.118.211516.

95. McHugh DJ, Chudow J, DeNunzio M, et al. A Phase I Trial of IGF-1R Inhibitor Cixutumumab and mTOR inhibitor temsirolimus in metastatic castration-resistant prostate cancer. Clin Genitourin Cancer 2020;18(3):171–8.e2.

96. Kaplon H, Muralidharan M, Schneider Z, et al. Antibodies to watch in 2020. mAbs 2020;12(1):1703531.

97. Li M, Jiang D, Barnhart TE, et al. Immuno-PET imaging of VEGFR-2 expression in prostate cancer with (89)Zr-labeled ramucirumab. Am J Cancer Res 2019;9(9):2037–46.

98. Butch ER, Mead PE, Amador Diaz V, et al. Positron Emission Tomography Detects In Vivo Expression of Disialoganglioside GD2 in Mouse Models of Primary and Metastatic Osteosarcoma. Cancer Res 2019;79(12):3112–24.

99. Holland N, Jones PS, Savulich G, et al. Synaptic Loss in Primary Tauopathies Revealed by [(11) C] UCB-J Positron Emission Tomography. Mov Disord 2020;35(10):1834–42.

100. Cybulska K, Perk L, Booij J, et al. Huntington's Disease: A Review of the Known PET Imaging Biomarkers and Targeting Radiotracers. Molecules 2020;25(3). https://doi.org/10.3390/molecules25030482.

101. Kovacs GG, Milenkovic IJ, Preusser M, et al. Nigral burden of alpha-synuclein correlates with striatal dopamine deficit. Mov Disord 2008;23(11):1608–12.

102. Bondi MW, Edmonds EC, Salmon DP. Alzheimer's Disease: Past, Present, and Future. J Int Neuropsychol Soc 2017;23(9–10):818–31.

103. Ferreira-Vieira TH, Guimaraes IM, Silva FR, et al. Alzheimer's disease: Targeting the Cholinergic System. Curr Neuropharmacol 2016;14(1):101–15.

104. Maurer A, Leonov A, Ryazanov S, et al. (11) C Radiolabeling of anle253b: a Putative PET Tracer for Parkinson's Disease That Binds to α-Synuclein Fibrils in vitro and Crosses the Blood-Brain Barrier. ChemMedChem 2020;15(5):411–5.

105. Klunk WE, Engler H, Nordberg A, et al. Imaging brain amyloid in Alzheimer's disease with Pittsburgh Compound-B. Ann Neurol 2004;55(3):306–19.

106. Rabinovici GD, Furst AJ, O'Neil JP, et al. 11C-PIB PET imaging in Alzheimer disease and frontotemporal lobar degeneration. Neurology 2007;68(15):1205–12.

107. Lashley T, Holton JL, Gray E, et al. Cortical alpha-synuclein load is associated with amyloid-beta plaque burden in a subset of Parkinson's disease patients. Acta Neuropathol 2008;115(4):417–25.

108. Colom-Cadena M, Grau-Rivera O, Planellas L, et al. Regional Overlap of Pathologies in Lewy Body Disorders. J Neuropathol Exp Neurol 2017;76(3):216–24.

109. Clark CM, Pontecorvo MJ, Beach TG, et al. Cerebral PET with florbetapir compared with neuropathology at autopsy for detection of neuritic amyloid-β plaques: a prospective cohort study. Lancet Neurol 2012;11(8):669–78.

110. Leinonen V, Rinne JO, Wong DF, et al. Diagnostic effectiveness of quantitative [18F]flutemetamol PET imaging for detection of fibrillar amyloid β using cortical biopsy histopathology as the standard of truth in subjects with idiopathic normal pressure hydrocephalus. Acta Neuropathol Commun 2014;2:46.

111. Sabri O, Sabbagh MN, Seibyl J, et al. Florbetaben PET imaging to detect amyloid beta plaques in Alzheimer's disease: phase 3 study. Alzheimers Dement 2015;11(8):964–74.

112. Yoo HS, Lee S, Chung SJ, et al. Dopaminergic Depletion, β-Amyloid Burden, and Cognition in Lewy Body Disease. Ann Neurol 2020;87(5):739–50.

113. Grimmer T, Shi K, Diehl-Schmid J, et al. (18)F-FIBT may expand PET for β-amyloid imaging in neurodegenerative diseases. Mol Psychiatry 2018. https://doi.org/10.1038/s41380-018-0203-5.

114. Yousefi BH, Manook A, Grimmer T, et al. Characterization and first human investigation of FIBT, a novel fluorinated Aβ plaque neuroimaging PET radioligand. ACS Chem Neurosci 2015;6(3):428–37.

115. Rowe CC, Pejoska S, Mulligan RS, et al. Head-to-head comparison of 11C-PiB and 18F-AZD4694 (NAV4694) for β-amyloid imaging in aging and dementia. J Nucl Med 2013;54(6):880–6.

116. McSweeney M, Pichet Binette A, Meyer PF, et al. Intermediate flortaucipir uptake is associated with Aβ-PET and CSF tau in asymptomatic adults. Neurology 2020;94(11):e1190–200.

117. Lee JC, Kim SJ, Hong S, et al. Diagnosis of Alzheimer's disease utilizing amyloid and tau as fluid biomarkers. Exp Mol Med 2019;51(5):1–10.

118. Robertson JS, Rowe CC, Villemagne VL. Tau imaging with PET: an overview of challenges, current progress, and future applications. Q J Nucl Med Mol Imaging 2017;61(4):405–13.

119. Ritchie C, Smailagic N, Noel-Storr AH, et al. CSF tau and the CSF tau/ABeta ratio for the diagnosis of Alzheimer's disease dementia and other dementias in people with mild cognitive impairment (MCI). Cochrane Database Syst Rev 2017;3(3):Cd010803.

120. Hall B, Mak E, Cervenka S, et al. In vivo tau PET imaging in dementia: Pathophysiology, radiotracer quantification, and a systematic review of clinical findings. Ageing Res Rev 2017;36:50–63.

121. Pascoal TA, Therriault J, Benedet AL, et al. 18F-MK-6240 PET for early and late detection of neurofibrillary tangles. Brain 2020;143(9):2818–30.

122. Barret O, Alagille D, Sanabria S, et al. Kinetic Modeling of the Tau PET Tracer (18)F-AV-1451 in Human Healthy Volunteers and Alzheimer Disease Subjects. J Nucl Med 2017;58(7):1124–31.

123. Koole M, Lohith TG, Valentine JL, et al. Preclinical Safety Evaluation and Human Dosimetry of [(18)F]MK-6240, a Novel PET Tracer for Imaging Neurofibrillary Tangles. Mol Imaging Biol 2020;22(1):173–80.

124. Betthauser TJ, Koscik RL, Jonaitis EM, et al. Amyloid and tau imaging biomarkers explain cognitive decline from late middle-age. Brain 2020;143(1):320–35.

125. Gobbi LC, Knust H, Körner M, et al. Identification of Three Novel Radiotracers for Imaging Aggregated Tau in Alzheimer's Disease with Positron Emission Tomography. J Med Chem 2017;60(17):7350–70.

126. Loane C, Politis M. Positron emission tomography neuroimaging in Parkinson's disease. Am J Transl Res 2011;3(4):323–41.

127. Ibrahim N, Kusmirek J, Struck AF, et al. The sensitivity and specificity of F-DOPA PET in a movement disorder clinic. Am J Nucl Med Mol Imaging 2016; 6(1):102–9.

128. Kong Y, Zhang C, Liu K, et al. Imaging of dopamine transporters in Parkinson disease: a meta-analysis of (18) F/(123) I-FP-CIT studies. Ann Clin Transl Neurol 2020. https://doi.org/10.1002/acn3.51122.

129. Delva A, Van Weehaeghe D, van Aalst J, et al. Quantification and discriminative power of (18)F-FE-PE2I PET in patients with Parkinson's disease. Eur J Nucl Med Mol Imaging 2020;47(8):1913–26.

130. Kerstens VS, Fazio P, Sundgren M, et al. Reliability of dopamine transporter PET measurements with [(18)F]FE-PE2I in patients with Parkinson's disease. EJNMMI Res 2020;10(1):95.

131. Bohnen NI, Kanel P, Zhou Z, et al. Cholinergic system changes of falls and freezing of gait in Parkinson's disease. Ann Neurol 2019;85(4):538–49.

132. DeLegge MH. Smoke A. Neurodegeneration and inflammation. Nutr Clin Pract 2008;23(1):35–41.

133. Jackson J, Jambrina E, Li J, et al. Targeting the Synapse in Alzheimer's Disease. Front Neurosci 2019;13:735.

134. Schain M, Kreisl WC. Neuroinflammation in Neurodegenerative Disorders-a Review. Curr Neurol Neurosci Rep 2017;17(3):25.

135. Madeo M, Kovács AD, Pearce DA. The human synaptic vesicle protein, SV2A, functions as a galactose transporter in Saccharomyces cerevisiae. J Biol Chem 2014;289(48):33066–71.

136. Best L, Ghadery C, Pavese N, et al. New and Old TSPO PET Radioligands for Imaging Brain Microglial Activation in Neurodegenerative Disease. Curr Neurol Neurosci Rep 2019;19(5):24.

137. Knezevic D, Mizrahi R. Molecular imaging of neuroinflammation in Alzheimer's disease and mild cognitive impairment. Prog Neuropsychopharmacol Biol Psychiatry 2018;80(Pt B):123–31.

138. Guo Q, Owen DR, Rabiner EA, et al. Identifying improved TSPO PET imaging probes through biomathematics: the impact of multiple TSPO binding sites in vivo. Neuroimage 2012;60(2): 902–10.

139. Rodríguez-Chinchilla T, Quiroga-Varela A, Molinet-Dronda F, et al. [(18)F]-DPA-714 PET as a specific in vivo marker of early microglial activation in a rat model of progressive dopaminergic degeneration. Eur J Nucl Med Mol Imaging 2020. https://doi.org/10.1007/s00259-020-04772-4.

140. Chauveau F, Van Camp N, Dollé F, et al. Comparative evaluation of the translocator protein radioligands 11C-DPA-713, 18F-DPA-714, and 11C-PK11195 in a rat model of acute neuroinflammation. J Nucl Med 2009;50(3):468–76.

141. Golla SS, Boellaard R, Oikonen V, et al. Quantification of [18F]DPA-714 binding in the human brain:

142. Hamelin L, Lagarde J, Dorothée G, et al. Early and protective microglial activation in Alzheimer's disease: a prospective study using 18F-DPA-714 PET imaging. Brain 2016;139(Pt 4):1252–64.

143. Dimitrova-Shumkovska J, Krstanoski L, Veenman L. Diagnostic and Therapeutic Potential of TSPO Studies Regarding Neurodegenerative Diseases, Psychiatric Disorders, Alcohol Use Disorders, Traumatic Brain Injury, and Stroke: An Update. Cells 2020;9(4). https://doi.org/10.3390/cells9040870.

144. Cai Z, Li S, Matuskey D, et al. PET imaging of synaptic density: A new tool for investigation of neuropsychiatric diseases. Neurosci Lett 2019;691:44–50.

145. Bahri MA, Plenevaux A, Aerts J, et al. Measuring brain synaptic vesicle protein 2A with positron emission tomography and [(18)F]UCB-H. Alzheimers Dement (N Y) 2017;3(4):481–6.

146. Chen MK, Mecca AP, Naganawa M, et al. Assessing Synaptic Density in Alzheimer Disease With Synaptic Vesicle Glycoprotein 2A Positron Emission Tomographic Imaging. JAMA Neurol 2018; 75(10):1215–24.

147. Bastin C, Bahri MA, Meyer F, et al. In vivo imaging of synaptic loss in Alzheimer's disease with [18F] UCB-H positron emission tomography. Eur J Nucl Med Mol Imaging 2020;47(2):390–402.

148. Nabulsi NB, Mercier J, Holden D, et al. Synthesis and Preclinical Evaluation of 11C-UCB-J as a PET Tracer for Imaging the Synaptic Vesicle Glycoprotein 2A in the Brain. J Nucl Med 2016;57(5):777–84.

149. Li S, Cai Z, Wu X, et al. Synthesis and in Vivo Evaluation of a Novel PET Radiotracer for Imaging of Synaptic Vesicle Glycoprotein 2A (SV2A) in Nonhuman Primates. ACS Chem Neurosci 2019;10(3):1544–54.

150. Packard RRS, Cooke CD, Van Train KF, et al. Development, diagnostic performance, and interobserver agreement of a (18)F-flurpiridaz PET automated perfusion quantitation system. J Nucl Cardiol 2020. https://doi.org/10.1007/s12350-020-02335-6.

151. Wang J, Mpharm SL, Liu TW, et al. Preliminary and Comparative Experiment Study Between (18)F-Flurpiridaz and (13)N-NH(3·)H(2)O Myocardial Perfusion Imaging With PET/CT in Miniature Pigs. Mol Imaging 2020;19. 1536012120947506.

152. Jammaz IA, Al-Otaibi B, Al-Hokbani N, et al. Synthesis of novel gallium-68 labeled rhodamine: A potential PET myocardial perfusion agent. Appl Radiat Isot 2019;144:29–33.

153. Sivapackiam J, Laforest R, Sharma V. (68)Ga[Ga]-Galmydar: Biodistribution and radiation dosimetry studies in rodents. Nucl Med Biol 2018;59:29–35.

154. Liu S, Lin X, Shi X, et al. Myocardial tissue and metabolism characterization in men with alcohol

consumption by cardiovascular magnetic resonance and 11C-acetate PET/CT. J Cardiovasc Magn Reson 2020;22(1):23.

155. Wu KY, Dinculescu V, Renaud JM, et al. Repeatable and reproducible measurements of myocardial oxidative metabolism, blood flow and external efficiency using (11)C-acetate PET. J Nucl Cardiol 2018;25(6):1912–25.

156. Harms HJ, Hansson NHS, Kero T, et al. Automatic calculation of myocardial external efficiency using a single (11)C-acetate PET scan. J Nucl Cardiol 2018;25(6):1937–44.

157. Christensen NL, Jakobsen S, Schacht AC, et al. Whole-Body Biodistribution, Dosimetry, and Metabolite Correction of [(11)C]Palmitate: A PET Tracer for Imaging of Fatty Acid Metabolism. Mol Imaging 2017;16. 1536012117734485.

158. Cade WT, Laforest R, Bohnert KL, et al. Myocardial glucose and fatty acid metabolism is altered and associated with lower cardiac function in young adults with Barth syndrome. J Nucl Cardiol 2019. https://doi.org/10.1007/s12350-019-01933-3.

159. Mather KJ, Hutchins GD, Perry K, et al. Assessment of myocardial metabolic flexibility and work efficiency in human type 2 diabetes using 16-[18F]fluoro-4-thiapalmitate, a novel PET fatty acid tracer. Am J Physiol Endocrinol Metab 2016; 310(6):E452–60.

160. Bucerius J, Barthel H, Tiepolt S, et al. Feasibility of in vivo (18)F-florbetaben PET/MR imaging of human carotid amyloid-β. Eur J Nucl Med Mol Imaging 2017;44(7):1119–28.

161. Genovesi D, Vergaro G, Giorgetti A, et al. [18F]-Florbetaben PET/CT for Differential Diagnosis Among Cardiac Immunoglobulin Light Chain, Transthyretin Amyloidosis, and Mimicking Conditions. JACC Cardiovasc Imaging 2020. https://doi.org/10.1016/j.jcmg.2020.05.031.

162. Takasone K, Katoh N, Takahashi Y, et al. Non-invasive detection and differentiation of cardiac amyloidosis using (99m)Tc-pyrophosphate scintigraphy and (11)C-Pittsburgh compound B PET imaging. Amyloid 2020;1–9. https://doi.org/10.1080/13506129.2020.1798223.

163. Rosengren S, Skibsted Clemmensen T, Tolbod L, et al. Diagnostic Accuracy of [(11)C]PIB positron emission tomography for detection of cardiac amyloidosis. JACC Cardiovasc Imaging 2020; 13(6):1337–47.

164. Papathanasiou M, Kessler L, Carpinteiro A, et al. (18)F-flutemetamol positron emission tomography in cardiac amyloidosis. J Nucl Cardiol 2020. https://doi.org/10.1007/s12350-020-02363-2.

165. Möckelind S, Axelsson J, Pilebro B, et al. Quantification of cardiac amyloid with [(18)F]Flutemetamol in patients with V30M hereditary transthyretin amyloidosis. Amyloid 2020;27(3):191–9.

166. Ćorović A, Wall C, Mason JC, et al. Novel Positron Emission Tomography Tracers for Imaging Vascular Inflammation. Curr Cardiol Rep 2020; 22(10):119.

167. Tarkin JM, Joshi FR, Evans NR, et al. Detection of Atherosclerotic Inflammation by (68)Ga-DOTATATE PET Compared to [(18)F]FDG PET Imaging. J Am Coll Cardiol 2017;69(14):1774–91.

168. Syed M, Flechsig P, Liermann J, et al. Fibroblast activation protein inhibitor (FAPI) PET for diagnostics and advanced targeted radiotherapy in head and neck cancers. Eur J Nucl Med Mol Imaging 2020;47(12):2836–45.

169. Giesel FL, Heussel CP, Lindner T, et al. FAPI-PET/CT improves staging in a lung cancer patient with cerebral metastasis. Eur J Nucl Med Mol Imaging 2019;46(8):1754–5.

170. Chen H, Zhao L, Ruan D, et al. 68Ga-FAPI PET/CT improves therapeutic strategy by detecting a second primary malignancy in a patient with rectal cancer. Clin Nucl Med 2020;45(6):468–70.

171. Luo Y, Pan Q, Zhang W, et al. Intense FAPI uptake in inflammation may mask the tumor activity of pancreatic cancer in 68Ga-FAPI PET/CT. Clin Nucl Med 2020;45(4):310–1.

172. Pang Y, Huang H, Fu L, et al. 68Ga-FAPI PET/CT detects gastric signet-ring cell carcinoma in a patient previously treated for prostate cancer. Clin Nucl Med 2020;45(8):632–5.

173. Varasteh Z, Mohanta S, Robu S, et al. Molecular imaging of fibroblast activity after myocardial infarction using a (68)Ga-labeled fibroblast activation protein inhibitor, FAPI-04. J Nucl Med 2019; 60(12):1743–9.

174. Novy Z, Stepankova J, Hola M, et al. Preclinical evaluation of radiolabeled peptides for PET imaging of glioblastoma multiforme. Molecules 2019; 24(13).

175. Kenny L. The use of novel PET tracers to image breast cancer biologic processes such as proliferation, DNA damage and repair, and angiogenesis. J Nucl Med 2016;57(Suppl 1):89s–95s.

176. O'Sullivan CC, Lindenberg M, Bryla C, et al. ANG1005 for breast cancer brain metastases: correlation between (18)F-FLT-PET after first cycle and MRI in response assessment. Breast Cancer Res Treat 2016;160(1):51–9.

177. Kairemo K, Santos EB, Macapinlac HA, et al. Early response assessment to targeted therapy using 3'-deoxy-3'[(18)F]-fluorothymidine ((18)F-FLT) PET/CT in lung cancer. Diagnostics (Basel) 2020;10(1).

178. Campbell BA, Hofman MS, Prince HM. A novel application of [18F]Fluorothymidine-PET ([18F]FLT-PET) in clinical practice to quantify regional bone marrow function in a patient with treatment-induced cytopenias and to guide "marrow-sparing" radiotherapy. Clin Nucl Med 2019;44(11):e624–6.

179. Kumar A, Ballal S, Yadav MP, et al. 177Lu-/68Ga-PSMA theranostics in recurrent glioblastoma multiforme: proof of concept. Clin Nucl Med 2020; 45(12):e512–3.

180. Arslan E, Ergül N, Karagöz Y, et al. Recurrent brain metastasis of triple negative breast cancer with high uptake in 68Ga-PSMA-11 PET/CT. Clin Nucl Med 2020.

181. Korsen J, Kalidindi T, Khitrov S, et al. Delta-like ligand 3 (DLL3) is a novel target for molecular imaging of neuroendocrine prostate cancer. J Nucl Med 2020;61(supplement 1):133.

182. Puca L, Gavyert K, Sailer V, et al. Delta-like protein 3 expression and therapeutic targeting in neuroendocrine prostate cancer. Sci Transl Med 2019; 11(484).

183. Donabedian PL, Kossatz S, Engelbach JA, et al. Discriminating radiation injury from recurrent tumor with [(18)F]PARPi and amino acid PET in mouse models. EJNMMI Res 2018;8(1):59.

184. Reilly SW, Puentes LN, Schmitz A, et al. Synthesis and evaluation of an AZD2461 [(18)F]PET probe in non-human primates reveals the PARP-1 inhibitor to be non-blood-brain barrier penetrant. Bioorg Chem 2019;83:242–9.

185. Edmonds CE, Makvandi M, Lieberman BP, et al. [(18)F]FluorThanatrace uptake as a marker of PARP1 expression and activity in breast cancer. Am J Nucl Med Mol Imaging 2016;6(1):94–101.

186. Miedema IH, Zwezerijnen GJ, Dongen GAv, et al. Abstract 1136: tumor uptake and biodistribution of [89]Zirconium-labeled ipilimumab in patients with metastatic melanoma during ipilimumab treatment. Cancer Res 2019;79(13 Supplement):1136.

187. Bensch F, van der Veen EL, Lub-de Hooge MN, et al. 89)Zr-atezolizumab imaging as a non-invasive approach to assess clinical response to PD-L1 blockade in cancer. Nat Med 2018;24(12): 1852–8.

188. Li M, Ehlerding EB, Jiang D, et al. In vivo characterization of PD-L1 expression in breast cancer by immuno-PET with (89)Zr-labeled avelumab. Am J Transl Res 2020;12(5):1862–72.

189. Jagoda EM, Vasalatiy O, Basuli F, et al. Immuno-PET imaging of the programmed cell death-1 ligand (PD-L1) using a zirconium-89 labeled therapeutic antibody, avelumab. Mol Imaging 2019;18. 1536012119829986.

190. Daumar P, Wanger-Baumann CA, Pillarsetty N, et al. Efficient (18)F-labeling of large 37-amino-acid pHLIP peptide analogues and their biological evaluation. Bioconjug Chem 2012;23(8):1557–66.

191. Bittner MI, Wiedenmann N, Bucher S, et al. Analysis of relation between hypoxia PET imaging and tissue-based biomarkers during head and neck radiochemotherapy. Acta Oncol 2016;55(11): 1299–304.

192. Cheng J, Zhang J, He S, et al. Characterization of heterogeneity of hypoxia with 18FMISO PET/CT, BOLD fMRI and immunohistochemistry in human breast tumor xenograft: initial study. Q J Nucl Med Mol Imaging 2020.

193. Sachpekidis C, Thieke C, Askoxylakis V, et al. Combined use of (18)F-FDG and (18)F-FMISO in unresectable non-small cell lung cancer patients planned for radiotherapy: a dynamic PET/CT study. Am J Nucl Med Mol Imaging 2015;5(2):127–42.

194. Segard T, Robins PD, Yusoff IF, et al. Detection of hypoxia with 18F-fluoromisonidazole (18F-FMISO) PET/CT in suspected or proven pancreatic cancer. Clin Nucl Med 2013;38(1):1–6.

195. Pell VR, Baark F, Mota F, et al. PET imaging of cardiac hypoxia: hitting hypoxia where it hurts. Curr Cardiovasc Imaging Rep 2018;11(3):7.

196. Imaizumi A, Obata T, Kershaw J, et al. Imaging of hypoxic tumor: correlation between diffusion-weighted MR imaging and (18)F-fluoroazomycin arabinoside positron emission tomography in head and neck carcinoma. Magn Reson Med Sci 2020;19(3):276–81.

197. Hamann I, Krys D, Glubrecht D, et al. Expression and function of hexose transporters GLUT1, GLUT2, and GLUT5 in breast cancer-effects of hypoxia. FASEB J 2018;32(9):5104–18.

198. Metran-Nascente C, Yeung I, Vines DC, et al. Measurement of tumor hypoxia in patients with advanced pancreatic cancer based on 18F-fluoroazomyin arabinoside uptake. J Nucl Med 2016;57(3):361–6.

199. Ventura M, Bernards N, De Souza R, et al. Longitudinal PET imaging to monitor treatment efficacy by liposomal irinotecan in orthotopic patient-derived pancreatic tumor models of high and low hypoxia. Mol Imaging Biol 2020;22(3):653–64.

200. Chang E, Liu H, Unterschemmann K, et al. 18F-FAZA PET imaging response tracks the reoxygenation of tumors in mice upon treatment with the mitochondrial complex I inhibitor BAY 87-2243. Clin Cancer Res 2015;21(2):335–46.

201. Havelund BM, Holdgaard PC, Rafaelsen SR, et al. Tumour hypoxia imaging with 18F-fluoroazomyci-narabinofuranoside PET/CT in patients with locally advanced rectal cancer. Nucl Med Commun 2013;34(2):155–61.

202. Capitanio U, Pepe G, Incerti E, et al. The role of 18F-FAZA PET/CT in detecting lymph node metastases in renal cell carcinoma patients: a prospective pilot trial. Eur J Nucl Med Mol Imaging 2020.

203. Pérès EA, Toutain J, Paty LP, et al. 64Cu-ATSM/(64)Cu-Cl(2) and their relationship to hypoxia in glioblastoma: a preclinical study. EJNMMI Res 2019;9(1):114.

204. Pasquali M, Martini P, Shahi A, et al. Copper-64 based radiopharmaceuticals for brain tumors and hypoxia imaging. Q J Nucl Med Mol Imaging 2020.

205. Vāvere AL, Lewis JS. Examining the relationship between Cu-ATSM hypoxia selectivity and fatty acid synthase expression in human prostate cancer cell lines. Nucl Med Biol 2008;35(3):273–9.

206. Baark F, Shaughnessy F, Pell VR, et al. Tissue acidosis does not mediate the hypoxia selectivity of [(64)Cu][Cu(ATSM)] in the isolated perfused rat heart. Sci Rep 2019;9(1):499.

207. Leung K. l-[methyl-(11)C]Methionine. In: Molecular imaging and contrast agent database (MICAD). Bethesda (MD): National Center for Biotechnology Information (US); 2004.

208. Hasebe M, Yoshikawa K, Nishii R, et al. Usefulness of (11)C-methionine-PET for predicting the efficacy of carbon ion radiation therapy for head and neck mucosal malignant melanoma. Int J Oral Maxillofac Surg 2017;46(10):1220–8.

209. Zhao J, Chen Z, Cai L, et al. Quantitative volumetric analysis of primary glioblastoma multiforme on MRI and 11C-methionine PET: initial study on five patients. Neurol Neurochir Pol 2019;53(3):199–204.

210. Zaragori T, Castello A, Guedj E, et al. Photopenic defects in gliomas with amino-acid PET and relative prognostic value: a multicentric 11C-methionine and 18F-FDOPA PET experience. Clin Nucl Med 2020.

211. Shiiba M, Ishihara K, Kimura G, et al. Evaluation of primary prostate cancer using 11C-methionine-PET/CT and 18F-FDG-PET/CT. Ann Nucl Med 2012;26(2):138–45.

212. Lapa C, Garcia-Velloso MJ, Lückerath K, et al. (11)C-Methionine-PET in multiple myeloma: a combined study from two different institutions. Theranostics 2017;7(11):2956–64.

213. Drake LR, Hillmer AT, Cai Z. Approaches to PET imaging of glioblastoma. Molecules 2020;25(3).

214. Ceccon G, Lohmann P, Werner JM, et al. Early treatment response assessment using (18)F-FET PET compared to contrast-enhanced MRI in glioma patients following adjuvant temozolomide chemotherapy. J Nucl Med 2020.

215. Kumar M, Salem K, Jeffery JJ, et al. Longitudinal molecular imaging of progesterone receptor reveals early differential response to endocrine therapy in breast cancer with an activating ESR1 mutation. J Nucl Med 2020.

216. Grabher BJ. Breast cancer: evaluating tumor estrogen receptor status with molecular imaging to increase response to therapy and improve patient outcomes. J Nucl Med Technol 2020;48(3):191–201.

217. Sipos D, Tóth Z, Lukács G, et al. [F-DOPA PET/MR based target definiton in the 3D based radiotherapy treatment of glioblastoma multiforme patients. First Hungarian experiences]. Ideggyogy Sz 2019;72(5–6):209–15.

218. Kuten J, Linevitz A, Lerman H, et al. [18F] FDOPA PET may confirm the clinical diagnosis of Parkinson's disease by imaging the nigro-striatal pathway and the sympathetic cardiac innervation: proof-of-concept study. J Integr Neurosci 2020;19(3):489–94.

219. Avram M, Brandl F, Cabello J, et al. Reduced striatal dopamine synthesis capacity in patients with schizophrenia during remission of positive symptoms. Brain 2019;142(6):1813–26.

220. Gong K, Han PK, Johnson KA, et al. Attenuation correction using deep Learning and integrated UTE/multi-echo Dixon sequence: evaluation in amyloid and tau PET imaging. Eur J Nucl Med Mol Imaging 2020.

221. Shirvan J, Clement N, Ye R, et al. Neuropathologic correlates of amyloid and dopamine transporter imaging in Lewy body disease. Neurology 2019;93(5):e476–84.

222. Schultz AP, Kloet RW, Sohrabi HR, et al. Amyloid imaging of Dutch-type hereditary cerebral amyloid angiopathy carriers. Ann Neurol 2019;86(4):616–25.

223. Kero T, Sörensen J, Antoni G, et al. Quantification of (11)C-PIB kinetics in cardiac amyloidosis. J Nucl Cardiol 2020;27(3):774–84.

224. Teipel SJ, Temp AGM, Levin F, et al. Association of PET-based stages of amyloid deposition with neuropathological markers of Aβ pathology. Ann Clin Transl Neurol 2020.

225. Palermo G, Tommasini L, Aghakhanyan G, et al. Clinical correlates of cerebral amyloid deposition in Parkinson's disease dementia: evidence from a PET study. J Alzheimers Dis 2019;70(2):597–609.

226. Leuzy A, Heurling K, De Santi S, et al. Validation of a spatial normalization method using a principal component derived adaptive template for [(18)F] florbetaben PET. Am J Nucl Med Mol Imaging 2020;10(4):161–7.

227. Na S, Jeong H, Park JS, et al. The impact of amyloid-beta positivity with 18F-Florbetaben PET on neuropsychological aspects in Parkinson's disease dementia. Metabolites 2020;10(10).

228. Cho SH, Choe YS, Kim YJ, et al. Concordance in detecting amyloid positivity between (18)F-florbetaben and (18)F-flutemetamol amyloid PET using quantitative and qualitative assessments. Sci Rep 2020;10(1):19576.

229. Hellberg S, Silvola JMU, Liljenbäck H, et al. Amyloid-targeting PET Tracer [(18)F]Flutemetamol accumulates in atherosclerotic plaques. Molecules 2019;24(6).

230. Grimmer T, Shi K, Diehl-Schmid J, et al. (18)F-FIBT may expand PET for β-amyloid imaging in neurodegenerative diseases. Mol Psychiatry 2020;25(10):2608–19.

231. Yousefi BH, von Reutern B, Scherübl D, et al. FIBT versus florbetaben and PiB: a preclinical comparison study with amyloid-PET in transgenic mice. EJNMMI Res 2015;5:20.

232. Bensaïdane MR, Beauregard JM, Poulin S, et al. Clinical utility of amyloid PET imaging in the differential diagnosis of atypical dementias and its impact on caregivers. J Alzheimers Dis 2016; 52(4):1251–62.

233. Rowe CC, Jones G, Doré V, et al. Standardized expression of 18F-NAV4694 and 11C-PiB β-amyloid PET results with the centiloid scale. J Nucl Med 2016;57(8):1233–7.

234. Lerdsirisuk P, Harada R, Hayakawa Y, et al. Synthesis and evaluation of 2-pyrrolopyridinylquinoline derivatives as selective tau PET tracers for the diagnosis of Alzheimer's disease. Nucl Med Biol 2020;93:11–8.

235. Schönecker S, Brendel M, Palleis C, et al. PET imaging of astrogliosis and tau facilitates diagnosis of Parkinsonian syndromes. Front Aging Neurosci 2019;11:249.

236. Malpetti M, Kievit RA, Passamonti L, et al. Microglial activation and tau burden predict cognitive decline in Alzheimer's disease. Brain 2020;143(5): 1588–602.

237. Nedelska Z, Josephs KA, Graff-Radford J, et al. (18) F-AV-1451 uptake differs between dementia with lewy bodies and posterior cortical atrophy. Mov Disord 2019;34(3):344–52.

238. Takenoshita N, Fukasawa R, Ogawa Y, et al. Amyloid and tau positron emission tomography in suggested diabetesrelated dementia. Curr Alzheimer Res 2018;15(11):1062–9.

239. Perez-Soriano A, Arena JE, Dinelle K, et al. PBB3 imaging in Parkinsonian disorders: evidence for binding to tau and other proteins. Mov Disord 2017;32(7):1016–24.

240. Salinas C, Lohith TG, Purohit A, et al. Test-retest characteristic of [(18)F]MK-6240 quantitative outcomes in cognitively normal adults and subjects with Alzheimer's disease. J Cereb Blood Flow Metab 2020;40(11):2179–87.

241. Kuwabara H, Comley RA, Borroni E, et al. Evaluation of 18F-RO-948 (18F-RO6958948) for quantitative assessment of tau accumulation in the human brain with positron emission tomography. J Nucl Med 2018.

242. Honer M, Gobbi L, Knust H, et al. Preclinical evaluation of (18)F-RO6958948, (11)C-RO6931643, and (11)C-RO6924963 as novel PET radiotracers for imaging tau aggregates in Alzheimer disease. J Nucl Med 2018;59(4):675–81.

243. Hong CM, Ryu HS, Ahn BC. Early perfusion and dopamine transporter imaging using (18)F-FP-CIT PET/CT in patients with parkinsonism. Am J Nucl Med Mol Imaging 2018;8(6):360–72.

244. Suh M, Im JH, Choi H, et al. Unsupervised clustering of dopamine transporter PET imaging discovers heterogeneity of parkinsonism. Hum Brain Mapp 2020;41(16):4744–52.

245. Yang Y, Cheon M, Kwak YT. 18F-FP-CIT positron emission tomography for correlating motor and cognitive symptoms of Parkinson's disease. Dement Neurocogn Disord 2017;16(3):57–63.

246. Brumberg J, Kerstens V, Cselényi Z, et al. Simplified quantification of [18F]FE-PE2I PET in Parkinson's disease: discriminative power, test–retest reliability and longitudinal validity during early peak and late pseudo-equilibrium. J Cereb Blood Flow Metab 2021;41(6):1291–300.

247. Schmitz TW, Mur M, Aghourian M, et al. Longitudinal Alzheimer's degeneration reflects the spatial topography of cholinergic basal forebrain projections. Cell Rep 2018;24(1):38–46.

248. Cyr M, Parent MJ, Mechawar N, et al. PET imaging with [¹F]fluoroethoxybenzovesamicol ([¹F]FEOBV) following selective lesion of cholinergic pedunculopontine tegmental neurons in rat. Nucl Med Biol 2014;41(1):96–101.

249. Bevan-Jones WR, Cope TE, Jones PS, et al. Neuroinflammation and protein aggregation co-localize across the frontotemporal dementia spectrum. Brain 2020;143(3):1010–26.

250. Herholz K. Cognitive dysfunction and emotional-behavioural changes in MS: the potential of positron emission tomography. J Neurol Sci 2006; 245(1–2):9–13.

251. Kumata K, Zhang Y, Fujinaga M, et al. [(18)F] DAA1106: automated radiosynthesis using spirocyclic iodonium ylide and preclinical evaluation for positron emission tomography imaging of translocator protein (18 kDa). Bioorg Med Chem 2018; 26(17):4817–22.

252. Yasuno F, Kosaka J, Ota M, et al. Increased binding of peripheral benzodiazepine receptor in mild cognitive impairment-dementia converters measured by positron emission tomography with [¹¹C]DAA1106. Psychiatry Res 2012;203(1):67–74.

253. Fan Z, Dani M, Femminella GD, et al. Parametric mapping using spectral analysis for (11)C-PBR28 PET reveals neuroinflammation in mild cognitive impairment subjects. Eur J Nucl Med Mol Imaging 2018;45(8):1432–41.

254. Varnäs K, Cselényi Z, Jucaite A, et al. PET imaging of [(11)C]PBR28 in Parkinson's disease patients does not indicate increased binding to TSPO despite reduced dopamine transporter binding. Eur J Nucl Med Mol Imaging 2019; 46(2):367–75.

255. Herranz E, Louapre C, Treaba CA, et al. Profiles of cortical inflammation in multiple sclerosis by (11)C-PBR28 MR-PET and 7 Tesla imaging. Mult Scler 2020;26(12):1497–509.

256. Tran TT, Gallezot JD, Jilaveanu LB, et al. [(11)C] Methionine and [(11)C]PBR28 as PET imaging tracers to differentiate metastatic tumor recurrence or radiation necrosis. Mol Imaging 2020;19. 1536012120968669.

257. Mabrouk R, Strafella AP, Knezevic D, et al. Feasibility study of TSPO quantification with [18F]FEPPA using population-based input function. PLoS One 2017;12(5):e0177785.

258. Yilmaz R, Strafella AP, Bernard A, et al. Serum inflammatory profile for the discrimination of clinical subtypes in Parkinson's disease. Front Neurol 2018;9:1123.

259. Leung K. N-Acetyl-N-(2-[(18)F]fluoroethoxybenzyl)-2-phenoxy-5-pyridinamine. In: Molecular imaging and contrast agent database (MICAD). Bethesda (MD): National Center for Biotechnology Information (US); 2004.

260. Vasdev N, Green DE, Vines DC, et al. Positron-emission tomography imaging of the TSPO with [(18)F]FEPPA in a preclinical breast cancer model. Cancer Biother Radiopharm 2013;28(3):254–9.

261. James ML, Belichenko NP, Nguyen TV, et al. PET imaging of translocator protein (18 kDa) in a mouse model of Alzheimer's disease using N-(2,5-dimethoxybenzyl)-2-18F-fluoro-N-(2-phenoxyphenyl) acetamide. J Nucl Med 2015;56(2):311–6.

262. Singhal T, Rissanen E, Ficke J, et al. Widespread glial activation in primary progressive multiple sclerosis revealed by 18F-PBR06 PET: a clinically feasible, individualized approach. Clin Nucl Med 2020.

263. Singhal T, O'Connor K, Dubey S, et al. 18F-PBR06 versus 11C-PBR28 PET for assessing white matter translocator protein binding in multiple sclerosis. Clin Nucl Med 2018;43(9):e289–95.

264. Zhang H, Tan H, Mao W-J, et al. 18F-PBR06 PET/CT imaging of inflammation and differentiation of lung cancer in mice. Nucl Sci Tech 2019;30(5):83.

265. Edison P, Donat CK, Sastre M. In vivo imaging of glial activation in Alzheimer's disease. Front Neurol 2018;9:625.

266. Dupont AC, Largeau B, Santiago Ribeiro MJ, et al. Translocator protein-18 kDa (TSPO) positron emission tomography (PET) imaging and its clinical impact in neurodegenerative diseases. Int J Mol Sci 2017;18(4).

267. Datta G, Colasanti A, Kalk N, et al. (11)C-PBR28 and (18)F-PBR111 detect white matter inflammatory heterogeneity in multiple sclerosis. J Nucl Med 2017;58(9):1477–82.

268. Ottoy J, De Picker L, Verhaeghe J, et al. (18)F-PBR111 PET imaging in healthy controls and schizophrenia: test-retest reproducibility and quantification of neuroinflammation. J Nucl Med 2018; 59(8):1267–74.

269. Hu W, Pan D, Wang Y, et al. PET imaging for dynamically monitoring neuroinflammation in APP/PS1 mouse model using [(18)F]DPA714. Front Neurosci 2020;14:810.

270. Van Weehaeghe D, Babu S, De Vocht J, et al. Moving toward multicenter therapeutic trials in amyotrophic lateral sclerosis: feasibility of data pooling using different translocator protein PET radioligands. J Nucl Med 2020;61(11):1621–7.

271. Bahri MA, Plenevaux A, Aerts J, et al. Measuring brain synaptic vesicle protein 2A with positron emission tomography and [18F]UCB-H. Alzheimers Dement (N Y) 2017;3(4):481–6.

272. Serrano ME, Becker G, Bahri MA, et al. Evaluating the in vivo specificity of [(18)F]UCB-H for the SV2A protein, compared with SV2B and SV2C in rats using microPET. Molecules 2019;24(9).

273. Estrada S, Lubberink M, Thibblin A, et al. [(11)C] UCB-A, a novel PET tracer for synaptic vesicle protein 2A. Nucl Med Biol 2016;43(6):325–32.

274. Rokka J, Schlein E, Eriksson J. Improved synthesis of SV2A targeting radiotracer [11C]UCB-J. EJNMMI Radiopharm Chem 2019;4(1):30.

275. Cai Z, Li S, Zhang W, et al. Synthesis and preclinical evaluation of an 18F-labeled synaptic vesicle glycoprotein 2A PET imaging probe: [18F]SynVesT-2. ACS Chem Neurosci 2020;11(4):592–603.

276. Naganawa M, Li S, Nabulsi NB, et al. First-in-human evaluation of (18)F-SynVesT-1, a novel radioligand for PET imaging of synaptic vesicle protein 2A. J Nucl Med 2020.

277. Papadakis GZ, Kochiadakis G, Lazopoulos G, et al. Targeting vulnerable atherosclerotic plaque via PET-tracers aiming at cell-surface overexpression of somatostatin receptors. Biomed Rep 2020;13(3):9.

278. Vachatimanont S, Kunawudhi A, Promteangtrong C, et al. Benefits of [(68)Ga]-DOTATATE PET-CT comparable to [(18)F]-FDG in patient with suspected cardiac sarcoidosis. J Nucl Cardiol 2020.

279. Lee H, Eads JR, Pryma DA. 68) Ga-DOTATATE positron emission tomography-computed tomography quantification predicts response to somatostatin analog therapy in gastroenteropancreatic neuroendocrine tumors. Oncologist 2020.

280. Guirguis MS, Adrada BE, Surasi DS, et al. 68Ga-DOTATATE uptake in primary breast cancer. Clin Nucl Med 2020.

Moving?

Make sure your subscription moves with you!

To notify us of your new address, find your **Clinics Account Number** (located on your mailing label above your name), and contact customer service at:

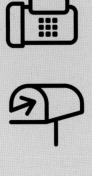

Email: journalscustomerservice-usa@elsevier.com

800-654-2452 (subscribers in the U.S. & Canada)
314-447-8871 (subscribers outside of the U.S. & Canada)

Fax number: 314-447-8029

Elsevier Health Sciences Division
Subscription Customer Service
3251 Riverport Lane
Maryland Heights, MO 63043

*To ensure uninterrupted delivery of your subscription, please notify us at least 4 weeks in advance of move.

ELSEVIER